Community Care

INITIAL TRAINING AND BEYOND

Edited by

David Skidmore MSc PhD RN DipPE CertEd

Head of Department, Department of Health Care Studies, Manchester Metropolitan University, UK

ARNOLD

A member of the Hodder Headline Group
LONDON • SYDNEY • AUCKLAND

First published in Great Britain in 1997 by
Arnold, a member of the Hodder Headline Group
338 Euston Road, London NW1 3BH

British Library Cataloguing in Publication Data
A catalogue record for this book is available from the British Library

Library of Congress Cataloging-in-Publication Data
A catalog record of this book is available from the Library of Congress

ISBN 0 340 61390 4

Composition in 10/12 Palatino by Anneset, Weston-super-Mare, Somerset
Printed and bound in Great Britain by J. W. Arrowsmith Ltd, Bristol

For Brenda: a true community spirit

Contents

List of contributors   ix
Acknowledgements   xi
Introduction   1

PART ONE   **FOOD FOR THOUGHT**   **9**

Chapter 1   Holding the community up for inspection   11
      Joel Richman

Chapter 2   Views of the world   33
      Jim Lord

Chapter 3   What is home?   43
      Eileen Fairhurst

Chapter 4   Promoting health   58
      Sandy Whitelaw

Chapter 5   Models of care   75
      Lynn Sbaih

PART TWO   **MAIN INGREDIENTS**   **105**

Chapter 6   Paediatric care   107
      Bernadette Carter

Chapter 7   Adult care   133
      Eileen Groves

Chapter 8   Elder care   143
      Susan Moore

PART THREE   **ADD A TOUCH OF ENVIRONMENT**   **157**

Chapter 9   The school   159
      Jennie Humphries

Chapter 10   Primary health care   175
      Joyce Green and Bobbie Saltman

Chapter 11   The work place   188
                James Garvey

Chapter 12   Health visiting   208
                Joanna Bateman

PART FOUR   AND THAT SPECIAL FLAVOUR . . .   235

Chapter 13   Learning disability   237
                Peggy Cooke

Chapter 14   Mental health   258
                Len Bowers

Chapter 15   Substance abuse   267
                I. Smith, T. Carnworth, N. Prinjha, and M. Smith

PART FIVE   BAKE FOR SEVERAL HOURS   283

Chapter 16   Asking the questions   285
                Christopher Wibberley

Chapter 17   Closing comments   296
                David Skidmore

Index   303

List of contributors

Joanna Bateman MSc, BNurs, PGCE, RGN, RHV, NDN Cert
Senior Lecturer, Department of Health Care Studies, Manchester
Metropolitan University, Manchester, UK

Len Bowers RMN, RGN, BSc (Hons), MA (Econ), PhD
Reader in Mental Health Nursing, City University, London, UK. At the time
of writing: Lecturer in Mental Health, Manchester Metropolitan University,
UK

T Carnworth BA, MA, MB, BCh, MRC Psych, MRCGP
Consultant Psychiatrist, Trafford Health Care NHS Trust, UK

Peggy Cooke RNMH, BA, MA, Cert Ed, RNJ
Principal Lecturer Department of Health Care Studies, Manchester
Metropolitan University, Manchester, UK

Bernadette Carter PhD, PGCE, BSc, RSCN, SRN
Senior Lecturer in Health Care Studies, Department of Health Care Studies,
Manchester Metropolitan University, Manchester, UK

Eileen Fairhurst BA (Econ), PhD
Senior Lecturer, Department of Health Care Studies, Manchester
Metropolitan University, Manchester, UK

James Garvey BA, MEd, RMN, Occ H, Cert Ed
Senior Lecturer, International Coordinator, Department of Health Care
Studies, Manchester Metropolitan University, Manchester, UK

Joyce Green RGN, RM, RHV, QN, RNT, DNT, BA, MA
Part-time Lecturer, Department of Health Care Studies, Manchester
Metropolitan University, Manchester, UK

Eileen Groves RGN, DN, CPT, DNT, RNT, MA, Cert Ed
Senior Lecturer in Health Care Studies, Department of Health Care Studies,
Manchester Metropolitan University, Manchester, UK

Jennifer C. Humphries MA, BSc, RN, RM, RHV
Senior Lecturer, Department of Health Care Studies, Manchester
Metropolitan University, Manchester, UK

James W. Lord BA (Econ), MSc, PhD
Principal Lecturer, Research Degrees Coordinator, Department of Health Care Studies, Manchester Metropolitan University, Manchester, UK

Susan Moore RGN, MSc, DANS
Senior Lecturer in Nursing, Course Leader BSc (Hons) Community Health, Department of Health Care Studies, Manchester Metropolitan University, Manchester, UK

N Prinja BSc (Hons)
Senior Health Promotion Officer, Trafford Substance Misuse Services, UK

Joel Richman BA (Hon), MA (Econ), PhD
Professor Emeritus in Medical Sociology, Department of Health Care Studies, Manchester Metropolitan University, Manchester, UK

Bobbie M. Saltman BSc, RGN
Practice Nurse, Part-time Lecturer, Facilitator, Marie Curie Cancer Care Practice Nurse Education, UK

Lynn Sbaih MPhil, BSc (Hons), RGN, RMN
Senior Lecturer, Department of Health Care Studies, Manchester Metropolitan University, Manchester, UK

I Smith BSc (Hons)
Drugs Prevention Manager, Trafford Substance Misuse Services, UK

M Smith BA, RMN, RGN, Cert MHS
Clinical Manager, Trafford Substance Misuse Services, UK

Sandy Whitelaw BSc (Hons), PGCE, MSc
Lecturer in Health Promotion, School of Epidemiology and Health Science, University of Manchester, Manchester, UK

Christopher Wibberley BA, PGCE, MSc, PhD
Principal Lecturer (Research Development), Deputy Head, Department of Health Care Studies, Manchester Metropolitan University, Manchester, UK

Acknowledgements

Much gratitude to the individual authors for tolerating my often fictitious deadlines. I am indebted to the late Dr David George for introducing me to primary health care and the late Dr Ted Codogan for stimulating critical thought. I would finally acknowedge Peter Cooke (a man after my own liver) for shaping my appreciation of humour.

Introduction

Community care is with us. Regardless of the debates as to whether community exists or not, the closer the twenty-first century comes the greater the need for alternative methods of care delivery. In the end economy wins out; demographic change has made the provision of a welfare state too costly. Naturally, economy is not an easy bedfellow with quality of care and, at the end of the day, the most practitioners may be able to offer will be superficial intervention. It is for this reason that this text is offered by way of a cookbook. Preparing a meal is largely founded on hope and expectation. The instructions, for preparation, are pretty standard and yet 10 people following the same instructions may produce 10 different tastes. There is that personal touch, that touch which creates the very best chefs. This can not be learned from common text. The chef experiences his or her art and has to have a 'feel' for it to be a success. Delivering care is similar, be it through parenthood, friendship, sexual love or intervention; there must be commitment to the activity. We can never make another love us, nor can we enforce another to care. It is possible to buy mechanical care – that is, practitioners who go through the motions for some type of reward – and this often works within the hospital environment.

People enter hospital with a collection of expectations. They anticipate certain outcomes when engaged in each encounter. By and large hospital patients are quite happy to be treated like cars and do not mind their carers acting like mechanics. There is a certain reassurance in knowing that the problem can be fixed in a relatively mundane way (Skidmore, 1979). This, of course, brings into question all that rhetoric about empowerment. Not everyone wants to be empowered . . . but if we, as practitioners, succeed in empowering clients then we pass on the responsibility for care.

> Ah! . . . it was so much easier in the old days; a place for everything and everything in its place. People knew their location then: if a man got sick, he went to a doctor and he'd be diagnosed, and maybe sent to hospital. Those hospitals, well they might have been a bit scary, but you just knew that you'd get sorted out; . . . and you could slip back into childhood once admitted, and people would tell you how to behave, that is what you had to do to get right again. Then there were the nurses . . . they were so lovely; and everyone pulled together to get you discharged. It was so good that television programmes were made about it, even Carry On films. One can only parody real life, after all.

I mean, where are the community equivalents? District Nurse didn't last long and that lovely Nerys Hughes was in it; and where was Carry On in the District Nurse? Well it just wouldn't reflect real life would it?

The point is that most people in the west, particularly the UK, have been cultured into expecting care as something that is given, not something that is negotiated. There is reassurance in the belief that one's condition can be handed over, like a package, to an expert and be effectively dealt with. To some extent that reassurance is diluted with community care; it may even imply that there is no hope of relief or that a condition is unworthy of attention. Practitioners should take note that many hospitals had religious or charitable origins. Over time, like churches, these places have not come to be associated with evil deeds. Witness the horror, both media wide and publically, at violence in the A and E department . . . *that's the sort of behaviour one expects in a hostelry!* We have lost sight of the fact that hospitals are part of the community. In simple terms, a community is merely a place where people live and work. In an ideal world different environments would not stimulate different behaviours . . . in reality they do and professionals have to deal with this.

The major problem being: people are different, back to cooking again. Okay, so we all have the same basic ingredients, but because we are cooked in an infinite number of ways we end up with different flavours. Schutz (1962) suggests that we are born individuals, but the moment we socialize we become people . . . that is socially desirable types. The influence of the environment can never be dismissed. Each person will experience a different socialization process which will affect the psychological development. In turn, the type of personality persons have will dictate how much power they feel that they have to control their lives. In short, some people will want to be empowered, others will wish to be controlled. How a person initially develops (i.e. how they feel about themselves) will be retained until they shed this mortal coil. My own feelings tell me I am still a young man, empirically I am not . . . logic informs me that I am ageing, but inside I feel young. I am not unique . . . very many other old people do not see themselves as old. Unfortunately, those other people with whom we socialize have definite expectations of what we are, who we are and how we should behave. Just another example of the many problems that the practitioner takes to every encounter.

This text makes some attempt to direct the practitioner, in much the same way as a cookbook. It is, for no other reason than pure artistry, constructed in five parts. *Part One* explores some of the theory that has developed from studies of community care and caring in general. To maintain the culinary leitmotif, these are the theories of cooking. Joel Richman's first chapter may well have been titled: 'What is cooking all about?' since he scrutinizes the very notion of community. This is further developed by Jim Lord's examination of how academic views of the world have developed and exist. From this starting point we become more specific: What is home? asks Eileen

Fairhurst, in an attempt to specify policy and personal decisions about community life. Sandy Whitelaw then examines the potential for promoting health in this context before we are exposed to models of care by Lynn Sbaih. This section is offered as the underlying theory of community cookery: that knowledge which every practitioner should be aware of before attempting to intervene.

In *Part Two* I have taken the liberty of offering a basic, survival menu. Three meals are offered: the child, the adult and the elderly. This was not an easy categorization; my own view is that the elderly (and yes I do have an interest) is an extension of the child. However, the elderly section of most populations is now so marginalized that I felt the need to offer special recognition. This section offers the boiled eggs and sandwiches of community care . . . in other words, the basics. *Part Three* attempts to explore these basics in specific environments and involves quite a lot of overlap. The analogy is the egg, it can be boiled, scrambled, fried and poached, depending upon the environment in which it is placed, or, indeed, that which is available.

Part Three invites you to stretch your skills and concoct some special flavours. These are not definitive, concentrating on only four areas.

However, a small taste of these flavours should entice the practitioner to delve deeper and experiment with his/her own recipes. Some guidance is offered in *Part Four* when direction is offered regarding the safe ingredients to try. This is offered because, like eating, community care is here to stay and all of us have an invested interest in trying to get it right.

Part Five examines the way forward with Christopher Wibberley offering suggestions about the right questions to ask. There is, of course, the inevitable conclusion from the editor. The last chapter is a feeble attempt to draw all these themes together and offer apologies for any omissions. The joy of being editor allows one to lay the blame at everyone else's feet.

The different author styles have been retained in the hope that some culinary variation will whet the reader's appetite. In the style of the cooking leitmotif a person may well enjoy rice pudding, but swallowing rice pudding everyday of his/her life invites interest in sponge and custard now and again. Similarly, the various rhetorical paragraphs about what community is have been retained. The aim of this text is to stimulate thought and this can only be achieved by exposure to various points of view. The text makes no claim regarding the definitive meaning of community.

Mention was made, above, of empowerment. It is the view of these authors that this has become one of the standard buzz words of community care. Many practitioners incorporate the word into their intervention vocabulary to the extent that we are in danger of losing understanding of what the word means. The notion that the client desires to be empowered is dangerous since it has become euphemistic with taking control. True empowerment means having the knowledge to make meaningful choices. Such a choice may involve the client in taking the back seat and allowing the practitioner to direct care and treatment. When a person is ill and worried about the future, s/he might appreciate the actions of the masked therapist who rides in and solves the problem. Others may desire direct involvement and appreciate the therapist facilitating health. People are different but they only have one life; it is their right to decide how they choose to live it. Client-centred intervention must take note of this, regardless of the various fashionable styles and therapeutic rhetoric.

Something else, dear reader, that you need to bring with you when visiting this text: there is a difference between morals and ethics, again buzz words when applied to intervention. Nietzsche (1977) argues that these are created in order to realize the ideals of society's most powerful men (and women). I would argue that there is a fundamental difference, in that morals are personally defined and ethics devised to reinforce the common good. Morals, which may be based on an ethical code, are personally constructed so that the individual can carry out everyday activities and feel comfortable with self; ethics are devised to protect the interests of society. It is the latter that Nietzsche (1977) may have had in mind. It is now ethical, for instance, to discharge the chronically mentally ill into the community without adequate resources. It is ethical to allow a rapist to practice nursing. Those people who define the rules (i.e. the government or the United Kingdom Central Council (UKCC)) define the ethics. To the individual, both activities may be immoral. The latter example is deliberately emotive. I am, of course, referring to the case of the nurse who raped a lady in her seventies 'because' he was drunk (on duty yet) and was allowed back on to the register in 1995. Darbyshire (1995) argues that this is indicative of the UKCC's inability to recognize the moral base of nursing. I would totally agree. The function of the register was to protect the public from 'nurses' who could do them harm; it was the final client advocate, the big one. Those who could not get on to the register could not practice, those who brought the profession into disrepute were struck off and prevented from further practice. The 1995 action, by the UKCC, suggests that the professional body is now more motivated by self-interest than by professional standards. Alternatively, it may be that the few on the council who represent the many are far more liberal and forgiving than the rest of us; since the UKCC refuses to explain its reasoning one can only speculate.

Although one might feel this abhorrent, how different is this from enforcing a practitioner's personal point of view on the client? For example . . . I believe in empowerment, therefore you should be empowered. This is the nub of Nietzsche's (1977) argument, that those who control policy dictate the ethics. There can be no argument with this, since ethics are devised for the common good. The 10 commandments are, perhaps, the most famous example of a code of ethics designed to protect the majority. They 'held' the children of Israel together. Nietzsche would no doubt argue that they enforced order by stopping man doing what he basically enjoyed. I can meet him half way on this. Consider adultery; two people find pleasure in each other which is fine until their partners find out. This leads to hurt, perhaps fighting and breaks down the basic unit of society . . . the family;

which, arguably is the building block of society. If one can prevent adultery and safeguard the family then the society is safe.

Morals, on the other hand, are far more subtle. Certainly attitudes towards adultery have changed over the years. Over the years, in my academic career as a social anthropologist, I have lost count of the number of people, male and female, who insist that adultery is okay as long as nobody finds out or if it is just a one off. Indeed, the tabloid press are, now, only interested in adultery if there is some public figure who can be disgraced with it. During the 1950s even the common man made headlines: *Caught wife in bed with best friend!* Now you have to be a successful actor or a Tory MP to earn copy. Technically, there are no grey areas between right and wrong but we have to understand ethical and moral shift against a backdrop of changing society. Within tight-knit communities with little or no geographic mobility it is relatively easy to adopt the community ethics as a moral code. Primarily, it is difficult to develop a private life and hide activities that we know others will frown upon. Society is much more private now and the consequence is that people have far more opportunity to live their own life. Their activities may clash with our own moral code, but who is to say that we are right?

There is an issue here because morals are personal and should not be inflicted upon clients. The fact that a nurse has a moral objection to abortion should not impede the client's right to obtain quality care. However, where the ethical stance places clients at risk – that is, a known paedophile involved in child care – then the practitioner has to be aware of his/her responsibility to be an advocate. This brings us back to empowerment. The ethical stance of the practitioner is to advocate the client's rights. Professional morals may well impose upon the client's rights. However, the practitioner has an obligation to make known the client's morals whenever the client lacks the voice. This is all the more important when care is offered in the community.

The practitioner carries the mantle of the institution with her/him. This can cause the client to become mute; roles are symbolic and their image conveys far more meaning than that which is seen. Uniforms convey much more meaning than the people wearing them. Carlyle (1908) argues that symbols offer: '. . . concealment and yet revelation . . .'; that is, a uniform can hide the man/woman and yet reveal the power. When the practitioner enters a client's home s/he is likely to dress the client in a uniform, by way of a previously revealed diagnosis or letter of referral. This is another aspect that mitigates against advocacy. Bergsen (1918) suggests that true perception (i.e. seeing things for the first time without ascribing meaning) is only possible in theory as long as we have knowledge of the past. Buber (1976) goes further and suggests that we can only ever gain a perception of another's experience – we can never experience their experience. These issues are crucial for intervention. In the best interests of the client the practitioner must take care that s/he is not misinterpreting or overinterpreting the client's experience. Whilst this has implications for client care in hospital it is far more important within the community context.

Clients take a totally different attitude with them when going into hospital (Skidmore, 1979) and, by and large, are prepared to be passive.

Institutional care can only survive in an ethical context, that is a service for the common good. Community care involves an individual approach . . . a service for the person's good, hence recognition of the moral stance. In other words, one has to respect the person: that is what they want, believe and feel is best for them. Often it will be incongruent with the practitioner's beliefs; but do you really want to be a controller . . . or a facilitator? If your desire is to control, then stop reading now, throw this text in the bin and dedicate your life to watching Claude van Damme movies. You have no future as a community practitioner.

To be a true community practitioner can be a humbling experience. One may be called upon to compromise one's morals or take issue against the profession's ethical stance. In short, the community practitioner has to have confidence in his/her ability to respect the individual. It is easy, and often rewarding, to hide behind the professional mantle, much more difficult to treat the client as a potential equal. Naturally, there are times when the practitioner has to take command. If a client lapses into diabetic coma there is little point in trying to counsel him/her out of it or enter into dialogue regarding whether or not they want to recover. These areas are when professional judgement comes to the fore. This is perhaps a very simple example since medical knowledge allows somewhat mechanical action to enable recovery. There are far more complex issues. Consider the use of synthetic insulin; many diabetics complain that it does not give them the warning signs that they had with animal insulin. Professional knowledge, at the time of writing, argues that synthetic is a better long-term issue, even if the client is more at ease with his/her old regime. There is no choice in that particular argument which, simplistically, states: if you do not follow my advice then you'll have severe problems in later life and may not even have a later life.

Similarly, discharging the long-term mentally ill into the community carries with it the implication that these people are responsible enough to look after themselves and cause no harm to others. Why then are we constructing supervision registers? The simple answer is that these people have brought it on themselves by various acts of violence. Such a response ignores the fact that many of these people have been forced into social isolation by being discharged. The label, mental illness, dresses a person in a very bold uniform. Often, the only way to gain any interaction with one's community is to utilize those behaviours that attracted a lot of attention in the hospital. This is negative empowerment, using deviant behaviour to gain power. The professional should have asked: is it ethical and moral to discharge these people when we have spent a large part of their lives denuding them of social skills? This is a classic area where the professional failed in advocacy. The ethical stance was that it would lead to a better quality of life for the client. How did we arrive at this conclusion? Did a group of professionals think themselves into the 'inmates' position '*I would much prefer to be outside than in this place*'? Of course, based on your experience . . . but you have not had *their* experience. The consequences of the Care in the Community Act are now apparent and the professional response is to paper over the cracks. New courses are devised to equip community psychiatric nurses (CPNs) with psychosocial intervention skills. Very useful, but we now find that a proportion of the population is now ignored because of that intervention which is currently in vogue. Community care should be about facilitating everyone's health. Unfortunately, with regard to psychiatry, it is in danger of developing into community policing.

I hope you have realized that much of this introduction has been devised to stimulate thought before you dip into the chapters below. My colleagues have a wealth of experience in both the academic and practitioner fields but, like sitting at the feet of the guru, if you accept these words as truths, then you are lost. Education is about facilitating learning, not concerned with providing cast iron truths. That is why new theories continue to evolve; if we all thought the same way as our teachers we would have a dull and intellectually stagnant life. Similarly, if practitioners were produced by a mould there would be no innovative practice. With regard to the community, the practitioner has to rely on more than acquired knowledge. These chapters, then, are offered purely to build on your valuable knowledge. I hope you find areas where you disagree with the narrative because that will illustrate your professional confidence.

We have tried to cover the whole area of community care and the various specialist practices that have evolved. It is hoped that this will give a flavour of community practice; the would-be gourmet can find various texts that focus with more depth in a particular arena. However, we wish to emphasize that community care is a complex issue that stretches beyond mere specialism. We offer a glimpse of some of the practitioners that may intrude on a person's life. That same glimpse should inform just how important nurses are. In the context of the community they are required to take their art and skills into the homes of others and adapt them to meet various needs. At the same time they are required to be at the frontline of client advocacy, undergo periodic updating, get on with a personal life and justify why they should receive a meaningful salary. Funny old world! However, if you've read this far it is unlikely that I can talk you out of your career. I hope this text helps you in your professional journey, that it helps you to pass go and meaningfully touch the lives of your clients.

David Skidmore
Manchester, 1995

References:

Bergsen, H. 1918: *The philosophy of change*. London: T.C. & E.C. Jack.
Buber, M. 1976: *I and thou*. Edinburgh: T. & T. Clark.
Carlyle, T. 1908: *Sartor resartus*. London: J.M. Dent.

Darbyshire, P. 1995: Letters. *Nursing Times* **91** (31) 23.
Nietszche, F. 1977: *A Nietszche reader* trans. R.J Hollingdale. Harmondsworth, Middlesex: Penguin.
Schutz, A. 1962: *The problems of social reality: Collected papers.* The Hague: Martinus Nijhoff.
Skidmore, D. 1979: *The hidden machine.* Bournemouth: Verus.

PART ONE

Food for thought

1 Holding the community up for inspection

Joel Richman

Joel Richman illustrates the difficulty of defining community in his opening paragraphs. Drawing on sociological, political and philosophical themes he explores various meanings of community, truly holding the concept up for inspection, whilst, at the same time, directing the reader to study some of the mainstays of sociological and philosophical discussion. For fellow sociologists this chapter could be described as a roller coaster ride through the theory that terminates with an alarming arrival into cyberspace . . . the new community? With the popularity of virtual reality, the keyboard and visual display unit (VDU) may finally replace interpersonal communication in the human sense. This is a fitting first chapter and should prove a useful reference source for that which is to follow.

'Community' is a universal 'unit of meaning'. All societies have a notion of community, often recognized in different ways. Although community is increasingly linked to a variety of descriptors – whether they be care, work, school, therapy, radio, nurse, policing, ethnicity and so on – it is very difficult to pin down and offer a satisfactory definition. The voluminous literature about community has noted that it has been 'lost', 'rediscovered', 'dissolved', 'eclipsed', 'reconstituted', etc., but despite definitional inadequacies the deployment of the term has not been hindered. Cohen (1985: 11) offers a plausible explanation for this apparent paradox.

> Community is one of those words – like 'culture', 'myth', ritual' and 'symbol' – bandied around in ordinary, everyday speech, apparently readily intelligible to speaker and listeners which, when imported into the discourse of social science, however, causes immense difficulty. Over the years it has proved to be highly resistant to satisfactory definitions in anthropology and sociology, perhaps for the similar reason that all definitions *contain or imply theories* and the theory of community has been very contentious (my emphasis).

It is possible to treat community as a 'thing' possessing identifying traits capable of measurement, ignoring social process, as in positivism; offering definitions independent of members' versions of reality invested in community. It is also possible to construct an ideal-type model of community, as used by Max Weber (1968), as a methodological tool for comparative purposes. An ideal-type (which does not mean 'perfect') is a logical construct of the key components of the institution under analysis. Weber composed ideal-types of bureaucracy, besides community. The components of his medieval European model were: demographic density (which would affect interpersonal relationships), types of kinship (especially the degree of ascription, as in clans), types of markets (whether based on autonomous law making) and taxing policies. Weber was concerned in how a medieval city was differentiated from the *polis*, agrarian-based communities common in ancient Rome and Greece. The ancient Greeks, for example, restricted vigorously the size of their city communities, to conserve their value consensus and democracy. All key decisions were taken by free citizens throwing pebbles (*psephos*) on the 'yes' or 'no' pile in the public square. 'Psephology', the science of voting behaviour today, is derived from the same word. Some who advocate the promotion of community today do so on the same grounds as the ancient Greeks – local democracy for empowering people. When communities reached a given size, swarming occurred – the young, primarily, left to form a new community. Aristotle argued that each citizen should know others by sight; that is, have primary groups. Plato put the figure of 5000 on the ideal polis.

Community is high on the agenda as an antidote for most of our 'social problems', whether they be 'mindless' vandalism, increasing welfare costs of 'single parents' or 'unjust' institutionalization of long-stay psychiatric patients, etc. Community's chameleon-like form attracts a multiplicity of competing and conflicting ideologies. Those making strong claims for community rarely do so on a priori evidence, often as articles of faith. Advocates rarely offer a realistic definition of what they propose. Its taken-for-grantedness is notorious. For example, a key conference organized by the Institute of Health Services Management (and supported by the Department of Health), Commissioning for Community Care (1992), produced a plethora of papers by Dr Mawhinney, the then Minister of Health, and by numerous directors of social services but at no time considering it necessary to offer a basic definition of 'community'. Randomly, the Sainsbury Centre for Mental Health report, Making Community Mental Health Teams Work (Onyett et al., 1995), although loaded with data on professionals' troubles, especially 'burn out' and lack of resources, did not regard it necessary to define or question the concept of community. Ironically nineteenth century Conservatives, who lamented the loss of community, today sing its praises, with others. Prime Minister Disraeli in his novel *Sybil* wrote:

> There is no community in England, there is aggregation but aggregation under circumstances that make it rather dissociating than

a uniting principle. In great cities men are brought together by the desire of gain and are careless of their neighbours . . . modern society acknowledges no neighbours. (Disraeli, 1981: 64–5)

Individualism and self-gain, a tenet of Thatcherism is not new, as Disraeli noted. Despite current claims made for community care for the decanted psychiatric patient it can mean a one-room bed-sit. For others it can mean transinstitutionalization; prisons hold 5000 psychiatrically ill out of an inmate population of 50 000. Issues of community were also heavily criticized last century. Maudsley's presidential address of 1871 to the Royal Medical Psychological Association raised the question of 'asylum-made lunatics'. The Lunacy Commissioners reported in 1855 of the reluctance of many of the 'poor classes' to care for their relatives (even when 'harmless incurables'), when released into community care.

The 1950s and 1960s were the great age of community studies, especially in the USA. Arensberg and Kimball (1965: IX) could proclaim: 'We believe the community to be a master institution or master social system; *a key to society* . . . the main link, perhaps a major determinant, in the connection between culture and society' (my emphasis). Elaborating its 'integrative' properties (1965: 3–4)

> Communities do not exist *in vacuo*. Each one occupies its own physical setting and is spatially surrounded by other communities more or less similar in organization, culture as a function. Institutional arrangements provide the framework within which various members of these separate communities relate to each other in transitory or in permanent *co-operative* activities. Within each community one finds the economic, political, religious, social even familiar activities which create *cohesion* among its members and which also extend to or include those of other communities. Taken as a whole, these linkages between communities make up the network called 'society'. (our emphasis)

Following Cohen's advice to decode the implied theory embedded in community definitions, it is apparent that the above is predicated on a consensus theory. Its functionalist stance considers community as the essential building blocks of society, 'lego-fashion', with no problematics about power, legitimacy of rights, class and gender inequalities, etc. Strangely, there is no attempt to enumerate community, a simple matter if the latter is as precise as Arensberg and Kimball declare.

Warren (1956), taking a different tack, was interested in community under change, with its increasing differentiation. Usefully, he conceptualized community along two axes. The *horizontal* axis focused upon spatial locality for analysing how members interacted; coming together for special activities like neighbourhood or residential associations, voluntary or welfare events. The *vertical* axis focused on participation in activities of regional and national import; today this could mean joining animal rights movements. Warren prophetically argued that the horizontal axis would diminish while the vertical one would gain, thereby reducing the locality dimension of community; amplifying community as part of a wider set of interests. Differential changes along the two axes could generate interpersonal conflict, for example animal rights issues promoted by some within a farming community.

Community contains sets of concepts in flux, much depending on the 'dominant definer's' agenda for given audiences or receivers. Community can be a:

- *Moral category*. Those who argue that individualism, fostered by the Reaganism and Thatcherism, had transformed society into an incoherent mass of atomistic individuals, all doing their own thing, regardless, are now promoting 'community' as a moral 'restorative'. A moral category, as described, is also a *'prescriptive category'*. This is one of the planks of New Labour for retrieving 'lost' values hinged to family life, for example.

- *Analytical category*. Putting community under the research microscope, often using rich ethnographic data for analysing, for example, essentially sociological issues. The Lynd (1929) study of Middletown (a pseudonym for Muncie, Indiana) explored the inhabitants' experience of industrialization. Warner's studies of Yankee City (Warner and Lunt, 1941; Warner and Low, 1947) (a pseudonym for Newbury Port, New England), similarly explored the changing employer/employee relations in a shoe factory, the economic locus of the community, after a local, paternal management was replaced by outside, capitalist cosmopolitans. The latter impacted on everyday traditional, interpersonal ties in a one-time 'natural community'. The latter term was used by Loomis and Beegle (1950) designating a long-established community.

- *Organizing category*. This assumes community is underpinned by a central principle which, when exposed, enables the researcher, especially, to make sense of what appear to be 'discordant' activities. Members of the community may have no such 'problems' in explaining these everyday activities – to them their community is a *normative category* expressed in rites and sentiments. For example, Redfield's (1941) study of the peasants of Yucatan, Mexico, discovered that activities such as clearing the bush for an arable patch (*milpa*) was not only an agricultural activity but also a sacred one. The *milpero* (peasant) took only the bush he needed; in return the gods expressed their good faith by preventing his axe from slipping, harmfully. All nature contains specific, spiritual forms, which must be placated or danger occurs, like illness. The X-tabai spirit, which adopts a woman's form, abides in the silk cotton tree. This is capable of tempting men to their death. Thus, *milpa* activities are also contractual with deities and spirits. The same holds for other activities, such as kinship reciprocity. Elders must be shown respect or the moral order is fractured. Some planned communities are explicitly hinged to an organizing principle, religious or political. The Hutterites founded their isolated communities to practise their own biblical beliefs.

After this eclectic overview, sensitizing to its many ramifications, practical and theoretical, community is now nexused into four major themes, often with overlapping interests. These act as a backcloth to later specialized chapters.

1 To locate community within nineteenth-century European thought. Many of today's debates do not always acknowledge this heritage. Tonnies (1955), often referred to, but rarely read like Marx, will be the mainspring.

2 To examine the spatial dimensions of community, from which members' perceptions are shaped. The relationships between public and private spheres have been essential properties of community.

3 To examine the current claims of the 'back to the community' movement – communitarism – overlapping a large segment of competing political interests of 'left' and 'right'.

4 To speculate on the future, with community in tow; essentially how post-industrialization and postmodernism, arguably departures from the present, offer new ways of understanding and recipes for action.

Tonnies, others and community directions

Tonnies' text *Gemeinschaft und Gesellshaft*, known as *Community and Association*, spelt out the transformation of medieval community, subsuming town, village and estate, by modern capitalistic society. Published in 1887, when Tonnies was only 32, its theses had been germinating for several years. Tonnies was one of the few sociologists who came from a peasant background – albeit comfortable. He had personally witnessed the shattering impact of commercialism (his brother was an international trader) on German rural communities. Tonnies' book went through eight editions, the last appearing one year before his death, 1936. Like the young and old Marx, there are differences of ideas over time. It is noteworthy that his representation of community and association are really ideal-types, a vehicle for his version of sociology, hence immune from empirical criticism. Tonnies' originality was also challenged; his before industrialization, and after dichotomy of change resonated in the work of many of his contemporaries.

Marx and Maine were acknowledged; the latter, an English lawyer argued that society had shifted from one based on status to contract. Sorokin (1955) is more seething: 'Hegel's Family–Society and Civic–Society are almost the twins of Gemeinschaft and Gesellshaft'; and Aristotle's distinction between true and false friendship also mirrors Tonnies' dichotomy. However, merit is in how he *synthesized* the range of vibrant ideas concerning issues of social order. Tonnies, unlike his peers, was not pessimistic about the future moving towards association society.

Community was projected as an intimate cosiness, based on mutual support and stability; its three pillars were blood (kinship), place (neighbourhood) and mind (friendship). Everyone knew and accepted 'natural authority'. The mother–child relationship was based on 'pure instinct', secured within the family unit. Paternal authority was also 'natural' as the Pope is identified as papa or father. The house was pivotal; under the protecting roof members sat at the same table, reinforcing kinship ties – the foundation of 'all natural authority'. Family members enjoyed its common goods. The house, argued Tonnies, evolved from a household cult; the hearth transmitting sacredness, the unifying centre of the extended family. Handicrafts and arts taught within the family had sacramental significance, reinforcing its moral foundation. Ways of thinking were based on 'natural will; inherited by all. Memory was an important quality of this type of will, springing from the "organic" essence of community members. Memory was responsible for preserving communities'; history; generating common symbols and language styles enhancing community identity and dignity in the wider moral order of things.

Tonnies' portrayal of 'schmaltze' gemeinschaft has been lauded by others. The Yiddish writer Isaac Bashevis Singer (reproduced in Minar and Greer, 1969: 44–46) regrets the passing of the traditionalism of the Polish, Jewish community Goray:

> Once upon a time everything had proceeded in an orderly fashion. Masters had labored alongside their apprentices, and merchants had traded; fathers-in-law had provided board and lodging, and sons-in-law had studied the holy teaching; boys had gone off to school, and school mistresses had visited the girls at home ... On Thursdays and Fridays the needy went from house to house carrying beggar's bags, collecting food for the sabbath; on the sabbath itself the good women made white bread and meat, fish and fruit for the needy. If a poor man had a daughter over fifteen years old who was still unwed, the community contrived to arrange a trousseau, and give her in marriage to an orphan youth or an elderly widow. The money that the groom received at the wedding sufficed to support them for months.

Conflicts were contained within talmudic (religious) values. At high festivals fights broke out – but over the honour of carrying the scrolls around the synagogue. The community would round on those who transgressed on religious occasions, cursing them in God's name.

Tonnies' association society was the opposite of community. It was underwritten by 'rational will' (*Kurwille*); metaphorically, 'machine built' for specific ends: whereas 'natural will' was organically derived. Each had different emerging consequences. Association was an aggregate of individuals with their own agendas, making calculations about power and money. The TV is now the hearth of the home, each member sharing her own private world, while munching individual TV meals. Kinship and fellowship were inadequate to temper individual excesses; legal contracts were the major bonding for social order. Tonnies agreed with the English philosopher Hobbes (see his book, *Leviathan*) that the relentless seeking of domination over others would only cease at death. Unlike natural will, rational will did not produce 'good will'. The 'egotist' mind is linked to hostility and indifference. Rational will, argues Tonnies, drives man to control nature, regardless. Also, the emphasis on coercion destroys others' freedom. Paraphrasing Adam Smith's marketeering *The Wealth of the Nations*, advocating the virtues of the market, Tonnies sums association's individualism by declaring that everybody, in some respects, becomes a merchant; money becomes the 'absolute' commodity, that is bought and sold transactionally. Timetables set by production overspill into social relationships: 'technology rules OK' would be an apt slogan, with scientific knowledge out of the control and understanding of the majority.

SOME CONTEMPORARY ISSUES

First, Tonnies' analysis of community and association are gendered. Women (and children) by temperament and intellectualism best harmonize with community values, because 'woman is the natural human being and man the artificial one' (p. 178); the home their fitting domain. Some feminists would accept the intimacy between women and nature, claiming that they are the true heirs to the secret knowledge of the muses. Technologically driven men have fractured this intimacy Today, 85 per cent of six million community carers are women, not because of some instinctive impulse. Tonnies could maintain, however, that rationale will design it that way. He also did not regard women's nature as fixed. Entering factory production and the money market, women would develop rational will, becoming calculating and individualistic, although this was alien to their natural will.

The principles of association can be projected into current health issues: the individualism and fragmentation of the biological medical model; the increasing disquiet over genetic engineering and copyrighting of genes; the commodification of health with decisions underpinned more by financial/market constraints. Rational will can be translated, too, into the paper world of care plans, neatly subdivided into calculative stages; contrasting with gemeinschaft spontaneity.

Tonnies did offer warnings about a community's potential to degrade, modifying its glow. Strangers and household servants could be victimized. Tonnies posited that the spirit of community could still be injected into modern industrial society, 'pseudo-gemeinschaft'. One way was by social engineering new community forms; another by education to include social skills – the 'caring' professions claim this attribute. Summarizing, it must not be forgotten that when Tonnies was analysing community he was really describing a society's stage of historical development, not offering the complexities of microsociological analyses.

However, some, like Marx, regarded community as totally negative within his revolutionary scheme. Capitalism (association) was beyond reform. Only its overthrow by the class struggle of urban workers (proletariat) could remove stunting alienation. The parochialism of community (he had in mind French peasants) was an impediment to the formation of class consciousness.

Peasants were mere 'potatoes' tied in a sack, he eluded, mundanely thinking about their patch for sowing and harvesting.

How Marx would regard the fact that the successful, twentieth-century revolutions in the third world have been peasant based (not necessarily led) is difficult to say. Revolutionary socialists today have realized the urban community's potential, arguing that community action over housing or discrimination can be a political catalyst for developing class consciousness. Others differ, arguing that successful community action can be detrimental to others in a climate of restricted resources. The government's encouraging of bids for funding (e.g. inner city community programmes), with its winners and losers, can be interpreted as a ploy to prevent working class cohesion.

Simmel's *Metropolis and Mental Life* (1903) shared much of Tonnies' thesis. Modern urbanities were different. Bombarded with intense, sensory stimuli they had to fragment their lives into separate spheres for survival. The sense of wholeness had gone. Relationships were treated as arithmetical exercises; many had no sense of community, becoming outsiders. Simmel, however, emphasized more the significance of money as the accounting principle of relationships.

Durkheim's *Division of Labour* (1956) shadowed gemeinschaft and gesellshaft with his typology of mechanical and organic solidarity. He believed that the industrial division of labour, potentially conflict ridden and anomic, could be stabilized by clustering around work to constitute occupational communities for support – a modern equivalent of medieval guilds. Occupational communities would be a mediating buffer between the state and individual, preserving civic rights and supporting the family. The professions were the main inheritors of this Durkheimian bequest, the state granting extra rights of clinical autonomy to doctors, for example, in return for their community's peer control over its own members. This professional arrangement has been described as creating a 'community within a community'. Illich (1976), paraphrasing Lenin, criticized it as a 'state within a state'; a monopoly disabling patients by medicalizing everyday life and mystifying medical knowledge. The privileges of professional communities have been attacked – new managerialism demanding stricter accounting of doctors' activities. Durkheim also proposed that the teaching of moral education (including social skills) would cement a value consensus. Psychiatrists, mushrooming counsellors and therapists with claims to be 'people experts' resemble a new spiritual vanguard; clients' self-awareness being gemeinschaft revelation.

'Loss' of community has spurred, naively, some management ideologies. The Human Relations School of Management, owing its inspiration to Mayo (1949) believed conflicts were caused by community's disappearance. Democracy by itself could not save industrial society. Technical skills had outpaced social ones; gemeinschaft had fused the two. Mayo believed that 'man's greatest desire (instinct ?) was to be grouped'. His solution was to make the work place the hub of the community. Salvation was possible if managers were entrusted to create workgroups with 'natural' leaders trained in social skills, to guide workers towards correct goals (managerially defined). Mayo, however, regarded trade union groups as inferior. Mayo never justified, morally, why work and not leisure, for example, should be the hub of the community. Nor did he consider the impact of redundancies when worker integration was breached: communities cannot escape the consequences of globalization. Few communities can sustain self-sufficiency. The new health trusts, interestingly, are concentrating training on leadership skills and group formation in order to get the new, market culture 'right' for employees mainly trained in a non-accountancy ethos.

Some firms, especially in the nineteenth century, did tie workers more closely into new model communities. Robert Owen's New Lanark factories had their own housing, schools and churches, etc. The Owenite movement also spread to America. Paternalistic, company communities created by Quakers at Bournville, for example, had an obverse side to their humanism. Dissent from their philosophy was not tolerated – that is, they were also coercive. Treatment regimes, especially for psychiatric disorders and substance abuse, have been sponsored in therapeutic communities, some heavily imprinted by charismatic founders. Charisma, although a traditional hinge, is unstable: therapeutic communities undergo turmoil on the death of charismatic founders, succession crises occur when charisma has to be routinized for legitimacy.

Summarizing this eclectic trip around community, with Tonnies as a major guide: community has coagulated many interests, often of different intellectual hue and purpose; each has logged it into its own agenda thereby sustaining its psychic potency as a meta-symbol. The political left and right, social atomists and collectivists, humanists and fundamentalists, romanticists harking back to an idyllic past that never was and pragmatists seeking respite from a runaway economic world – all find sustenance under the rubric of community.

NETWORKS AND COMMUNITY

Social networks have been used to make less opaque concepts of community. Networks are the mapping out of linkages between people and institutions. Networks can be classified by their pattern: being open and expansive to admit others or being dense, clustering tightly around a few members. Networks are also transmitters of services, goods and ideas, thereby being classified by the processes or activation of interaction. Some are totalistic, as in closed, religious communities. Others' networks can be used for a range of specific purposes; for example, the house-bound aged may use a child only for running errands.

Boissevain (1974) classified networks into zones and degrees of personal intimacy. First is the personal zone of immediate family, with 'regular' contacts; second is the intimate zone of friends; third is the effective zone of friends and relatives seen infrequently, but which can be activated by, for example, health crises; fourth, is the zone including non-related but strategically important peoples, like doctors and community psychiatric nurses

(CPNs); fifth is the nominal zone, including those of hearsay, only fleetingly
– representatives of agencies or the local MP, for example.

Another classification used by others has been into:

* Categorical set – network of a given category, e.g. kin.
* Action set – network for a given purpose e.g. church going, or football attendance.
* Role set – people in a specific role arrangement with those around you, e.g. patients on a ward relating to doctors, nurses, visitors and fellow patients.
* Field set – common interest or pressure groups, e.g. political networks, sustaining continuous lobbying.

The Barclay Report (1982) subscribed to a romantic version of community, implicitly gemeinschaft. Social workers were accredited with the knowledge of being able to discover, tap into and orchestrate caring networks of relatives and friends, informal resources and community interests, operating within geographical proximity. The Audit Commission's *Homeward Bound* (1992) clarifying roles in the management of cross-professional units and agencies for community care produced two proto models of networks (Fig. 1.1). Interestingly, the client/consumer was not explicity located.

Network analysis was acclaimed by sociologists post 1950s, after its utility had been tested by anthropologists in tribal societies. Prior to the 'discovery' of traditional, working class communities by Young and Wilmott, networks became a convenient methodological tool. Bott (1957), for example, demonstrated that if husband and wife had separate networks of friends within the community then this correlated with separate conjugal roles within the household. Open community networks have been correlated with more immediate medical referral and diagnosis. Closed networks usually mean lingering longer in lay networks (family and friends), not wishing to refuse immediates' advice and offend. The stigma of mental illness affecting marriages can be concealed in some Asian communities; however, when finally seen by psychiatrists, mental illness (e.g. schizophrenia) can be more severe.

Pattison and Hurd (1984) matched different psychiatric disorders with variations in networks. Using the Pattison Psychosocial Inventory of Emotional Intensity, reciprocity and instrumentality, etc., they showed that the neurotic-type network is smaller than the normal one (average of 25–30 persons), with about 15 persons and few relatives. This network supplied negative emotional responses, conducive of isolation and asymmetry in relationships – with little corrective feedback stress tends to spiral. The psychotic-type network is smaller still, 10–12 people are cloistered in an emotionally charged closed system, generating continuous anxiety and conflicting communications.

Criticisms of networks are well known. In Pattision and Hurd's version do psychotics become psychotic then drift to psychotic networks? Or the converse? If the former, then the prepsychotic network, not analysed, becomes more significant. There is always the question of the 'invisible' network, not

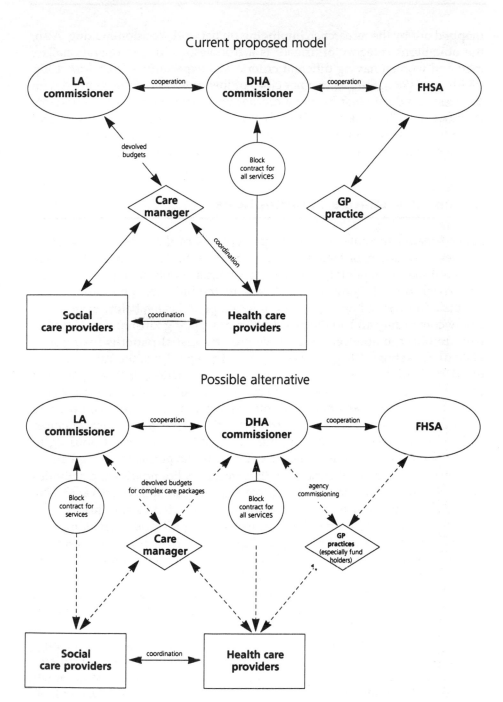

Figure 1.1 Integrated commissioning through care management. LA, local authority; DHA, district health authority; FHSA, family health service authority. Audit commision (1992). Crown copyright is reproduced with permission of the controller of HMSO.

mapped out by the researcher, impinging on network decision-making. Also, the ubiquitous category of 'friend' is a troublesome one to operationalize, men and women having different criteria and expectations from friendship (Skidmore, 1986). Studies in inner cities of low economic status women with depression indicate that having a mother and women friends as confidants is alleviating. The expectation, too, that network analysis would bridge community, with its use of micro- and middle-range sociological analyses with macro-society theories, has largely remained unaccomplished.

Community, space and perceptions

Space broadly mediates members' perceptions of their community, often developing markers of sacred and secular. Sioux Indians venerate the Black Hills of Dakota containing their ancestral spirits, emphasizing their culture. The Welsh proudly sing of a 'welcome in the hillsides' and 'land of our fathers'. The Tiw in Nigeria used to migrate periodically; before structuring a new community all had the possibilities of rejigging kinship ties. New ties were publicly announced in land reciprocity, spatial patterns fusing new kinship obligations. Chagnon's (1992) rich ethnography of the Yanomamo of the Brazilian rainforest, now on the point of extinction, shows again how spatial arrangements of shelters, the subdivision of the *shabono* (communal house) and seating arrangements on the ground, etc., are a community lexicography. Community size is also a reflection of outside political alliances with other villages; the host community must build sufficient housing to accommodate all its visiting allies, together with its permanent members.

Even in our 'urban wilderness', with community boundaries and activities often invisible, latent perceptions of community can still be activated. The National Health Service (NHS) programme of hospital closure has crystallized and mobilized community sentiments, often historical. The long running saga of the closure of Withington Hospital (S. Manchester) has aroused dormant mythology and fact of its historical role in the community. Mothers having babies there 40 years ago praise its community service. The save the tree movement is not just 'bloody mindedness' against motorway 'progress'; long-living trees are valuable remnants, linking perceptions of the community's past and present.

The history of community has been one of shifting perception, coinciding with change in how space has been understood. As Sennett (1991) brilliantly reminds us the eye for Plato, as it was for Saint Augustine, was an organ of conscience; a window on the soul. The Greek for 'theory' is *theoria*, to look at: reflexivity is shaped by experience of that around us. The ancient Greek community was visibly on display in public space. Healing ceremonies for the sick, in temples or on breezy hillsides, were open to all. Community agreement was easily marshalled to sanction inefficient doctors, who were expelled.

Modernity accelerated the trend from public space to private. Medieval community relied on appearential ordering, maintaining social ranking of costume, language and mannerisms for social control. Commoners in Elizabethan England were forbidden to wear clothes from gold or silver cloth, velvet and furs. Spatial ordering with linked activities is now dominant. Variations in policing styles are responsive to their perceptions of appropriate behaviour in appropriate places. Middle class communities are policed differently from inner city ones. The *Scarman Report* (1981) criticized the use of young, inexperienced policemen (outsiders) in aggressively using stop and search (suss law) tactics on young blacks congregating in public places assumed to be 'up to no good'. Community policing has modified police perceptions, by moving more to an insider's view of place.

The decline in the street as a people-centred, public place has transformed semiotic representations. The street inspired Renaissance artists, and biblical events were transposed to European streets. The street and theatre were fused in medieval mystery plays and carnivals, with full community participation, recharging community symbols. For Rudofsky (1969) the shift from the vibrative public sphere is demonstrated by the nadir of Menotti's *Telephone*, a drama with one static set, no action and one actor hooked into an electronic network, the new communicative community. The reconstitution of the family behind closed doors, the rise of the cult of privacy, has drastically reduced opportunities for dispersing tension publicly in prescribed ways. The rise in mental illness has been attributed by the 'radical psychiatrists', such as Laing and Cooper, to the 'pressure cook family'. The retreat from the streets is epitomized by community perceptions of 'dangerousness', especially the elderly who are least likely to be attacked.

Despite the decline in social significance of streets their ecological dominance is heavily reflected in community images. Lynch's (1972) investigation into the images or cognitive maps possessed by community members (his original study was of Boston, USA) were expressed by 'paths', primarily streets but also including canals and railroads. Respondents could reproduce a map image of the community more easily when a regular street mosaic existed.

Streets are important community dimensions for maintaining cultural identity. Street names have proved most loyal to Scottish nationalism. Streets signal community continuity and change and are the first to be refurbished with community transformation. The Ukrainian city of Lvov has recently changed over half its street titles: 'Peace Street' to 'Stephen Bandera Street' – the Ukrainian nationalist with German support who opposed the Red Army, 1944. Lvov is attempting to shed its former USSR associations. Local communities have lobbied their council for a change of street name, if the latter became 'notorious' and casts a shadow over the whole community. Skidmore (1994) has aptly posed the dilemma for practitioners cultured in a 'tourist environment' of the institution, routinized and screened by bureaucratic defences, who now have to leave the citadel and home visit. She then becomes a 'daytripper', carrying the former, institutional perception. As an outsider, communities become immediately taxonomized into 'good' and 'bad' areas, or 'dangerous' and 'safe'; not remaining long enough to learn the social intrinsics. Her vandalized car being sufficient 'proof' of a bad area, despite many cars stolen from 'secure' car parks, etc.

Kostoff (1993) has distinguished five cultural designs of cities: planned as grids; transforming into organic patterns; the symbolic and diagrammatic layout; the Baroque plan; and the urban skyline. The Baroque, supplanting the organic medieval communities, relied on long axial streets. The grid, straight streets meeting at right angles, is the oldest design, used by Babylonians believing they symbolized the apex of community and spirituality. But streets change their sentiments. The same formation indicates impersonality and the rational business ethic. US streets are generally unreflective of topographical, botanical or mythological interests, unlike the European traditions. The grid iron pattern, with large squares for orchestrated, public displays of community feeling toward communist rulers, was also the pattern of the former Eastern Bloc. The conformist grid iron pattern reached exaggerated proportions in San Francisco, where rigid insistence on right-angled intersections and straight-line roads, even on steep hills, caused inharmonious and needlessly steep thoroughfares, used frequently in films with car chases. However, they did not inhibit the formation of communities by gender, ethnicity and class – in the 1960s its hippie community was famous, as is the gay one today.

Summarizing, all communities acknowledge their ecological foundations; the significance given to it in shaping perceptions has been a two-way process. Despite the devaluing of the public sphere, nevertheless it remains the only place where the community can be on show, *en masse*, at critical times as when demonstrating against a 'community threat' of hospital closure. Streets are still impregnated with community values; their projection as community images and neighbourhood compass is more than symbolic. Children's street games (now declining rapidly) are major conveyors of historical remembrances. Roberts (1978) noted that Salford children during his childhood played 'bobbers and kibs', a game illustrated on ancient Greek vases. Communities are not time vacuums.

Communitarianisms, back to community

At crises, 'community' is often elevated to emblematic status, as salvation. Saint Augustine's *The City of God* was one such response to the turmoil following the destruction of Rome (AD 410). His vision of the eternal city blended inner and outer truths. The Reformation spawned a multiplicity of communities espousing versions of the new faith. The nineteenth century, the age of European revolutions, produced a host of 'artificial gemeinschaft'. The French sociologist and socialist, Saint Simon, hoped to create small communities with intimate face to face rapport between workers and owners, overriding class hostility. The 'age of reconstruction', just after World War II, was saturated with blueprints for planned communities, whether they be towns with mixed residential patterns, to initiate egalitarianisms. Some put their faith in the 'new science' of sociometric analysis, claiming to group-match individuals. Moreno's *Who Shall Survive* asserts his technique transformed an American penal agency for women from disruption to communal bliss. The hippies of the 1960s, seeking alternative realities, formed 'wigwam' communities. With high rates of failure, children inevitably dispersed with mothers, as Tonnies would have predicted. New Age travellers, with hot lines to nature, are their successors; medieval pilgrims traversed by church spires, today's often rely on benefit offices.

The kibbutz was a shining beacon for some, founded on a reversal of ghetto values of Talmudic scholarship and commerce dominated by men with women tied to kitchen and children. (Tonnies would have acclaimed the ghetto as a good example of gemeinschaft.) Kibbutz democracy was based upon equality of rights for all, expressed via a communal council; private property was abolished and communal working and dining installed. The family was radically changed; many did not marry and men and women paired off (in Hebrew 'zug'). Children were reared communally, forming age groups; sleeping in their own quarters. Parents were big playmates to their children in the absence of patriarchalism. The expectation that the Oedipus complex would disappear was, however, false.

Post-1949, the egalitarian ideals diminished. A managerial elite emerged with the kibbutz moving from self-sufficiency to market economy, also becoming an employer of labour. Gender typing surfaced; women found themselves in the communal kitchens and laundries. Ideological conflicts, appeared between the young, socialized into the kibbutz ideals, and the elders who wanted more personal comforts. Aspects of the nuclear family developed – women, particularly, demanding that their children slept at home, motherhood compensating for loss of economic prestige. The kibbutz is a good example of how difficult it is for ideologically, planned communities to remain faithful to their ideals when open to dominant, external factors.

The rest of this section is owed to Amitai Etzioni, the influential founder of communitarians and its germane ideas expressed in his *The Spirit of Community*, subtitled aptly *The Reinvention of American Society* (Etzioni, 1993). The challenging ideas (also disseminated in the movement's journal, *The Responsive Community*) appeal to President Clinton, who has called for a new covenant between individual and community. Tony Blair and Gordon Brown, architects of 'New Labour', have appropriated the rhetoric (especially on the need for communities to be revitalized, with more responsibilities to control deviancy). The British right has also latched on to communitarisms; welfare funding to be reined in with the appeal of voluntarism and self-help to maintain services are attractive. Social security spending 1995–96 totals £80 billion, one-third of all government spending.

A personal note, Etzioni, born when Hitler came to power in 1929, was taken to Palestine by his parents. He was a student of Martin Buber, at the Hebrew University, inspired by his ethical writings, especially *I and Thou*, a testament of the necessity for co-operation. Buber's *Between Man and Man* was a distillation of 'self formed clans' (community), including, for example, the Kibbutz, Amish, Shaker and Hutterite, etc., and also influenced Etzioni. Etzioni's personal revelation is signified by a change of name. Born Werner Falk, Amitai is the Hebrew for 'truth' and Etzioni is derived from 'Zion'. His academic career took off in America 1957, first studying philosophy then gravitating to a chair in Sociology at George Washington University. *The Spirit of Community* is climactic; Etzioni's earlier texts include: *An Immodest Agenda: Rebuilding America Before the Twenty-First Century* (1983); *Capital Corruption* (1984); *The Moral Dimensions: Towards a New Economics* (1988); and *A Responsive Society* (1991).

Etzioni's aim is a 'new moral order, social, public order – without Puritanism or oppression' (p. 1), encoded into eight articles of faith (written mimicking the style of the American constitution), for example *'We hold* that the family – without which no society has ever survived, let alone flourished – can be saved without – forcing women to stay at home or otherwise violating their rights' . . . *'We hold* that people can again live in communities without turning into vigilantes or becoming hostile to one another' (p. 1).

The 'moral decay' of society is historically located. The 1950s had certainty of major values, albeit prejudicial to women, minorities and lower classes. The 1960s produced moral confusions, with many into self experimentation and therapeutic reliance, and competing demands of minority rights. The 1980s was the decade of greed, with the promise of golden manacles. The 1990s is the reaping of past influences – the 'parenting deficit', with 'marriage for many as a disposable relationship' (p. 29), undercuts morality. The British scene is only a lesser variation of the USA. Between 1971 and 1991 British single parents with families rose from 1:13 to 1:5; in North Manchester 3:5. For people marrying under 30 years old the divorce rate has quadrupled in 30 years. Divorces for second and third marriages are also increasing, not only harming the young, but also adolescents. Most American child-care centres are inadequate, with staff lacking skills and earnings in the lowest tenth of wage earners. Crime and dishonesty is rampant at all levels. Neighbourhoods have been taken over by drug dealing. For many, the barricaded home is a refuge. The finale is that a quarter of Americans say that if the money was right they would desert their families; seven per cent would likewise kill for money!

The advancment of citizens' rights has far outpaced corresponding responsibilities. People want more rights of privacy and less government, but 'confusingly' also want more government services. America is a litigious society with more lawyers per head than other countries. A common car sticker reads 'let your son become a doctor and employ five lawyers'. Death row inmates suing the government for its denying the rights of future offspring's to be born is an Etzioni illuminative. The 'me society' is shackled to a Faustian end.

Tried solutions have failed. The command economy of communism has been disastrous. Centralized planning failed to meet consumers' needs and give political freedom, producing another serfdom. The other extreme, free market, also produces injustices, the unemployed and poor being regarded as 'natural casualties'. Crime is an alternative economy, money equals success. Communitarianism is also a response to the anxious middle classes, now with fractured careers, restricted incomes and doses of unemployment, impacted by the global economy. Communitarism promises a new stability.

The communitarian essence is 'Communities speak to us in moral voices. They lay claim to their members' (p. 31). The charge that many interests can lay claim to 'moral interest' coercively imposing their will (e.g. fundamentalists, like the creationists who had Darwinism banned from schools) has been raised. Etzioni denies he is the standard bearer of the new Puritans. No *komitehs* (Iranian religious police) will roam the streets. Individuals, however, can be shamed into fulfilling their civic responsibilities. A press column recording neglect of duties will be the modern village stocks. Etzioni does not favour a return to small town communities. Cities have what Gans (1962) called 'urban villagers, replicated worldwide'. There are also ample community catalysts: information technology is accelerating home-working. Gans broadens community to include non-geographic ones. Professional groupings are spending more working time together. Residents of high-rise buildings can be made more community orientated by more in-house services to hang around in. Etzioni favours national service for the young, as community dedicators. New Labour's 'plan' for 'citizen's service' echoes this. Altruism is not dead. Seattle, for example, has 400 000 citizens certificated in resuscitation; 40 per cent of heart attack victims have their resuscitation started by volunteers, prior to the arrival of the ambulance, with a better chance of survival. Communities are to lock into and maintain the supracommunity – society. Idealistically, Etzioni says wealthier communities should recognize the duty to help poorer ones, in his coalition scheme. The major pillars of communitarianism are the family and school. Both parents should revalue children acknowledging their moral responsibility; the community should make a similar commitment. Parents should make a 'precommitment' not to divorce within a given period and not without counselling. (A cooling off period with counselling is proposed within the recent English reform on divorce.) Some states in the USA have Family Preservation Programmes. New York has one caseworker to every two 'welfare families' covered by the scheme, teaching 'parenting', etc. Whether all work organizations will allow flexitime and leave of absence for family crisis, as IBM and Dunlop, is problematic. Two-parent families are not only better for children, without denigrating one-parent ones, says Etzioni, but they are also cost effective: marrieds remain healthier. Adoption and orphanages offer 'unwanted' children more opportunities.

Schools should focus on self discipline, character formation and service to others. Again the question arises of : 'whose morals?' Schools should create 'new experiences'; and counsellors should guide students away from working in fast- food outlets, whose work permits no initiative. What if that is the only employment available ?

Some comment is needed on communitarianisms. In some respects it is at the stage of a secular religion and moral crusade. It is impossible now to say how it will work out in practice. The key ideas have a strong Durkheimian flavour (the latter is not indexed). Durkheim promoted moral education and occupational community as a palliative to anomie. Moral rearmament can be equated with recharging the collective conscience, which was 'above' individual, unrestrained freedom. Like Durkheim, little is discussed about the entrenched power of the state with its powerful elites, or class inequalities with enlarging 'underclass', or the influence of footloose corporations geared to bottom-line accounting. Feminists suspect a subtle plot to drive women back to the home, which Etzioni refutes. Communitarian experiments are in progress. Definition of community poses the same problem Durkheim had in his defining religion. He was forced back on a relativistic position, despite the positivist mission for sociology of discovering the universal – that which people regard as sacred. Etzioni is similarly 'open ended', deliberately, arguing for individual membership of a host of communities with differing criteria, depending on the occasion.

The future of community: postindustrialism and postmodernism

Predicting the future is the graveyard of 'experts', especially economists' short-term forecasts, globalization rendering it impossible to 'hold the world still' for futurology. The predictive optimism of the 1960s, when the western economy promised unlimited prosperity, was gone. The once-firm benchmark of nursing demand predicating P2K has, for example, shattered: between 1989 and 1994 the number of nurses fell 7.7 per cent and is reducing. However, every age has always produced its vision(s) of the future. This section attempts to locate community within the 'grand ideas' of some futurologists. One thing is common, 'community' is mainly 'invisible' within their schemes.

The term 'postindustrial' society is accredited to Daniel Bell's (1973) book of the same title. The approaching 'new society' has many other labels: 'service society', 'late capitalist', 'postcapitalist', 'knowledge society' 'after industrial society' and 'information society'. Technological determinism is a common denominator. 'Modernism' relies on the promise of science to improve upon the laws of nature by reshaping society for the 'common good'. Scientific incrementalism steers the 'march of progress', clearly signposted, runs the argument. Postmodernism posits a radical departure from that certainty.

Kerr et al. (1960) precipitated later debates with their 'logic of industrialism', relentlessly driving all societies – albeit some were at different stages – to converge to one, underscored by the same technological forces. Class conflict would be dead, only minor bureaucratic quibbles of detail would exist. The nuclear family would be universal. Differential communities, apparently, have no overt place. Kerr *et al.* suppose a mass, uniform society, perhaps as one mass community freed from the toils of work, permitting bohemianism within its leisure surplus. There is the 'end of ideology'.

Bell offers more detail of the future. Society will have three spheres: social structure, the polity and cultural, each having its own 'axial principles'. The implications of change in social structure are not necessarily connected with the other spheres. Bell discusses the rise of the new knowledge class (scientists, engineers and economists), to replace industrialists, but again 'community' is not central. Details of their occupational community, moral responsibilities and spatiality are vague. Kerr, Bell *et al.*, like Marx, are more concerned with logical principles. Marx wrote only about 4000 words on the socialist heaven on earth, despite voluminously denouncing capitalism. Man, once freed from alienation, would resort to his true self in harmony with nature: the state would wither away because there would be no need for external constraint. What glimmers are available are that of nineteenth century, country gentlemen where all would hunt in the morning, fish in the afternoon and enjoy conviviality in the evening. Ironically, having once denounced rural communities Marx's vision now exalts them!

Illich (1985) is anti technological progress; future trends will increase its evils. The technological model underpins all institutions: learning is programmed and technological errors threaten the ecology. The professions having adopted the 'engineering model', deskill and pacify clients. His attack on health professions is particularly stringent. They have mystified the world, monopolized medical explanation and practice, reduced civil liberties and generated iatrogenesis; simultaneously addicting us to medicine. The professions cannot be reformed. Illich's postindustrial society involves the abolition of professional credentialism, a reversal of industrialization and decentralization of technology into local control. Communities would be major social units based on an ethic of frugality; leaving Illich open to the charge of religiosity, having trained as a Jesuit. Communities would capture former political and professional decision making. 'Experts' would now be validated by community networks of users, like the ancient Greeks did. Illich's active mechanism for reversing industrialization and emphasizing community development is vague. His diagnosis of the evils of undustrialization is in tandem with Marx, but his 'commune' solution based on self-help and mutuality comforts both the New Right, and Left, yet he called for a Copernican revolution in value and perceptions!

The first to theorize seriously about the impact of new media technologies was McLuhan (1973), arguing that the new electronic age was experiencing the 'Gutenberg configuration'. Just as printing technology revolutionized sensory directions and knowledge development the new media is more revolutionary. All now live in a 'global village', with the abolition of time and space. Simultaneous events, from anywhere, are now in the front room; the 'medium as the message'. From TV we assimilate and 'pass judgement' on Eboli plague or admire death transformed into an electronic show in the Gulf War. It is difficult to challenge the image package, or escape its subliminal impact. Although members of a global community are all not equal; but are increasingly in a symbolic relationship with the other.

McLuhan anticipated the global highway of information, although half the world still lacks access to a phone network. The internet, if permitting open access, allows individuals to generate membership of a multiplicity of new electronic communities, often overlapping in interests; transient or permanent; single or many purposed. The focus of home will be the 'electronic hearth'. Etzioni's vision of interlocking communities, as a moral force, now has the means. 'Interface', once meaning primary or interpersonal relations, takes on sets of different perceptions and meanings, once the world community becomes digitized.

'Postmodernism', once tagged to radical breaks from current fashion in art, architecture and aesthetics is now debated in society terms. Some argue that there is a postmodern society, *per se*: a complete break with linear, historical development of culture and ideas; others argue for postmodernist features within existing society. Details of this controversy are not a concern here. Suffice to say 'core truths' no longer hold; natural science's privileged status has been critically challenged, it can no longer conform to its own orderly, methodological tenets. Reason and justice have lost their anchorage. Magic and science fuse. The postmodern maelstrom of form, value and will further grasp 'community'. Place and space as essential characteristics of society and community are dissipating. For example, hospitals as places of medical diagnoses and treatment can be reduced further in significance with the new electronic communications. Pacemakers are checked by telephone; operations in London are satellited to impoverished doctors in the African bush; UK Cancer Support internets worldwide to fellow sufferers.

Conclusion

Community is not a unitary concept for all to consensually behold. Community is totemic for diverse interests. Those espousing community care feel no necessity to intellectualize its theoretical problematics, but will it to order, according to preconceived policy formulations. The latter themselves often contain unexplications about 'need', 'care', 'empowerment' and 'professional judgement' and so on. Some of community's axial principles have been discussed, showing how nineteenth century debates, especially, are continuously recycled. A version of Tonnies was offered, elaborating his insights, 'errors' and significance for current issues. The new, community guru, Etzioni, was detailed noting how his 'communty panacea' for the social ills of our time permits opposing, political philosophies that find convenient pegs for their clothes. Peter Drucker (1993: 157), for example, argues that 'The community that is needed in post-capitalist society – especially needed by knowledge workers – has to be based on commitment and compassion rather than being imposed by proximity and isolation'.

A crude offering was made of postindustrial and postmodern society, the latter containing confusing and contradictory strands, to locate community in the 'future'. The implications of membership of cyber-communities are still open debates. Exciting contradictions of freedom and coercion embedded in community have still to be played out. Community represents the potential for humanism through caring and sharing with the tension of coercion via compulsory psychiatric supervision orders and other penal orders. Whether we become cyber slaves amplifying what Foucault called 'surveillance and control' following us everywhere, is a strong possibility. For certain space, place and interpersonal relationships will take on new meanings as perceptions of community are reshaped. In Bordieu's (1993) framework of multidimensional space and networks communities become 'social capital'.

References

Arensberg, C.M. and Kimball, S.T. 1965: *Culture and community*. New York: Harcourt, Brace & World, Inc.

Audit Commission 1992: *Homeward bound: a new course for community health*. London: HMSO, p. 35.

Barclay Report 1982 *Social workers: their roles and tasks*. National Institute for Social Work.

Bell, D. 1973: *The coming of post industrial society: a venture in social forecasting*. New York: Basic Books.

Bott, E. 1957: *Family and social network*. London: Tavistock.

Boissevain, J. 1974: *Friends of friends, networks, manipulators and coalitions*. Oxford: Blackwell.

Bourdieu, P. 1993: *Sociology in question*. London: Sage.

Buber, M. 1961: *Between Man and Man*. Boston: Beacon Press.

Buber, M. 1970: *I and thou*. Edinburgh: T & T Clarke.

Chagnon, N.A. 1992: *Yanomamo: the last days of Eden*. San Diego: Harcourt Brace Jovanovich.

Cohen, A.P. 1985: *The symbolic construction of community*. London: Tavistock.

Conference Organized by the Institution of Health Services Management (10th July, 1992) *Commissioning for Community Care*.

Disraeli, B. 1981: *Sybil or The Two Nations*. Oxford University Press (first published 1845).

Drucker, P.F. 1993: *Post capitalist society*. Oxford: Butterworth, Heinemann.

Durkheim, E. 1956: *Division of labour*. London: Free Press.

Etzioni, A. 1983: *An immodest agenda: rebuilding America before the twenty-first century*. New York: Simon & Schuster.

Etzioni, A. 1984: *Capital corruption*. New York: Simon & Schuster.

Etzioni, A. 1988: *Moral dimensions: towards a new economics*. New York: Simon & Schuster.

Etzioni, A. 1991: *A responsive society*. New York: Simon & Schuster.

Etzioni, A. 1993: *The spirit of community: the reinvention of American society*. New York: Simon & Schuster.

Gans, H.J. 1962: *The urban villagers: group and class in the life of Italian Americans*. New York: Free Press.

Hobbes, T. 1957: *Leviathan*, ed. Oakshott, M. Oxford: Oxford University Press.

Illich, I. 1976: *Limits to medicine, medical nemesis: the expropriation of health*. London: Marion Boyars.

Illich, I. 1985: *Tools for conviviality*. London: Marion Boyars.

Kerr, C., Dunop, T., Harbison, F. and Myers, C.A. 1960: *Industrialism and industrial man*. Cambridge, MA: Harvard University Press.

Kostoff, S. 1993: *The city shaped, urban patterns and meanings through history*. London: Bullfinch Press.

Loomis, C. and Beegle, J.A. 1950: *Rural social systems*. Englewood Cliffs, NJ: Prentice Hall.

Lynd R.S. and Lynd H.M. 1929: *Middletown in transition*. New York: Harcourt, Brace & World.

Lynch, K. 1972: *What time is this place?* Cambridge, MA: MIT Press.

Mayo, E. 1949: *Social problems of an industrial civilization*. London: Routledge & Kegan Paul.

McLuhan, M. 1973: *Understanding media* London: Verso.

Minar, D.W. and Greer, S. 1969: *The concept of community*. London: Butterworth.

Moreno, J.L. 1934: *Who shall survive?* Washington DC: Nervous and Mental Diseases Publishing.

Onyett, S., Pillinger, T. and Muijen, M. 1995: *Making community mental health teams work*. London: Sainsbury Centre for Mental Health.

Pattitison, E.M. and Hurd, G.S. 1984: *The social network paradigm*. In O'Connor, W.A. and Lubin, B. (eds), *Ecological approaches to community and clinical psychology*. New York: Wiley.

Redfield, F. 1941: *The folk culture of Yucatan*. Chicago: University of Chicago Press.

Report of an Inquiry by the Rt Hon. The Lord Scarman 1981: *The Brixton disorders*. London: HMSO Cmnd 8427.

Roberts, R. 1978: *A ragged schooling*. London: Fontana.

Rudofsky, B. 1969: *Streets for people: a primer for Americans*. New York: Doubleday.

Sennett, R. 1991: *The conscience of the eye: the design and social life of cities*. New York: Knopf.

Simmel, G. 1903: reproduced in Wolf, K. (ed.) (1950) *The sociology of George Simmel*. Glencoe, IL: Free Press.

Skidmore, D. 1994: *The ideology of community care*. London: Chapman & Hall.

Skidmore, D. 1986: *The sociology of friendship*. University of Keele, PhD thesis.

Smith, A. 1976: *The wealth of the nations*. Oxford: Oxford University Press.

Sorokin, P. 1955: Foreward. In Tonnies, F. (ed.), *Community and association*. London: Routledge & Kegan Paul.

Tonnies F. 1955: *Community and association*. London: Routledge & Kegan Paul. (Translated and supplemented by Charles P. Loomis)

Warren, R.L. 1956: Towards a reformulation of community theory. *Human Organization* 15(2), 174–182.

Warner, W.L. and Lunt, P. 1941: *The social life of a modern community*. New Haven: Yale University Press.

Warner, W.L. and Low, J. 1947: *The social system of the modern factory*. New Haven: Yale University Press.

Weber, M. 1968: *Economy and society*. Berkeley, CA: University of California Press.

Young, M. and Wilmott, P. 1959: *Family and kinship in East London*. London: Routledge & Kegan Paul.

2 Views of the world

Jim Lord

Jim Lord tackles these difficult issues by way of everyday metaphors; do not be surprised if you suddenly find yourself reading about garage doors and central heating one minute, only to leap to war the next. Positivism is a somewhat abstruse area and I urge you to stay with this chapter since it underpins all that follows. Positivism is that school of thought which suggests that there is a natural order to things and it only has to be found and measured. The implication for life is that, because there are fixed laws and knowledge, humans are basically the same and all 'difficulties' can be dealt with in like manner. This is an oversimplification and Jim explores the notion in greater depth before examining other viewpoints.

The term *positivism* originated in the works of the French philosopher Auguste Comte in the early nineteenth century.[1] Comte was not alone in his deep admiration of the achievements of the, still young, natural sciences in discovering and elucidating the laws of nature in their various fields of enquiry. Acquaintance with those laws had already enabled interventions in natural processes either to promote desirable outcomes or to prevent undesirable ones. The future seemed to hold boundless prospects for further empowerment of this kind. His 'positivist philosophy' embraced *both* a vision of what it was that gave the disparate activities involved their status and unity as *scientific* enterprises *and* a programme for the systematic development and expansion of such scientific enquiry – even into areas, such as the social, where the subject matter had, thus far, seemed only dubiously amenable to such treatment.

At the heart of all this was the argument that the sciences were to be identified as such solely in their use of a common method of investigation – this was the unity of the scientific method. Any subject could then, in principle, be studied scientifically. The test of a study's scientificity lay in its meeting a set of methodologically defined specifications or standards. To have done a piece of scientific research was, in this respect, to have followed a set of procedures.

1 See Andreski, S. (Ed.) 1974: *The essential Comte*. London: Croom Helm.

The procedural template involved is clearly of great importance. Yet, on this, Comte himself was relatively sketchy and allusive, though the offerings of contemporary mathematical physicists clearly had a powerful influence. It fell to others[2] to provide the basis for a more detailed account.

The gist of this sees the process as beginning with the systematic observation of the subject matter. In the course of such observation certain recurrent sequences of events may be noted such as to suggest a pattern. This patterning, then, becomes the object of closer scrutiny, ideally revealing a definite correspondence (or set of correspondences) which suggest that whenever events of kind X occur, events of kind Y follow. Here would be grounds for the *hypothesis* that X is the *cause* of Y. However, it remains possible either that the conjunction of Xs and Ys has been merely coincidental or that not all the links in the causal chain have been uncovered. At the simplest, Xs may cause (hidden) Zs which, in turn, cause Ys. And there may be more than one such intervening link in the chain of causality.

The next stage, frequently dubbed 'hypothesis testing', involves the exercise of all available ingenuity to try to eliminate the possibility of 'mere coincidence' or to expose any intervening links in the chain. There are, as yet, unfinished debates about whether either of these objectives can absolutely and finally be achieved.[3] But, with regard to the first, repeated observation over time of the relevant, invariant relationship between X and Y dispels serious doubts about its accidental nature. In so far as science is a communal endeavour, independent testing, which in all cases confirms the findings, provides further grounds for the dissolution of doubt on this score. Much the same can be said on the issue of the existence of intervening causes. Anything less than universally demonstrable, constant conjunction of X and Y must give leave to doubt the existence of a single cause and effect link and lead to attempts at revision of the hypothesis (with further test) until the constancy criterion can be met.

Even now, assuming the hypothesis has passed its test, all that has been attested is that X causes Y. (And this, it has been argued,[4] is provisional upon the subsequent exercise of greater ingenuity revealing that there are, after all, intervening links in the chain of causation.) The move to the establishment of the pertinent laws of nature requires far more. It involves a shift in the level of abstraction away from the concrete particulars of Xs being the cause of Y, to seeing X as but one specific example of a more general phenomenon, which we may call Z, which causes general effects, which we may call W, of which Y is again just one example. Ideally, as far as Comte was concerned, the nature of the relationships between Z and W should be rendered susceptible to precise mathematical formulation and elucidation. This should be such as to allow (ultimately) for complete predictive accuracy of the effects of Zs on Ws.

2 See especially Wright, G.H. Von 1971: *Explanation & understanding* London: Routledge.
3 See Popper, K. 1990: *The logic of scientific discovery* 2nd ed. London: Unwin Hyman.
4 See Popper, K. *op cit.*

Perhaps an example of the major steps in this process will serve to clarify the major issues here. The room in which you are working is periodically beset by a series of clicking and creaking noises, sometimes coming in rapid succession, sometimes in more spaced out form. Discounting the possibility that it is the profoundly disturbed ghost of one Auguste Comte, you decide to investigate the phenomenon scientifically. First, presumably, you would seek systematically to locate the source of the noises. They prove to be coming from the central heating radiator panel and its pipework, specifically from the clips and brackets securing the panel to the wall and where the feed pipes penetrate the floorboards. Closer and now more specific investigation reveals that the noises are being generated by friction-impaired movements between the radiator-mounted clips and the (stationary) wall brackets and between the pipes and the (stationary) floorboards. Yet closer investigation reveals that the movements involved are to do with the fact that the radiator and its pipes increase in size by small but measurable amounts in all directions at certain times, and alternately decrease in size at others. Moreover, this growth and shrinkage coincides with the thermostatic cycles of the heating system; when the thermostat switches the pump on and starts the water circulating in the system the increase in size occurs (and this fairly rapidly), when the thermostat switches the pump off and the water circulation ceases, the decrease in size occurs (though this occurs at a much more modest rate). Hence the differing tempo of the clicks and creaks.

Continued observation of the phenomenon leads you to discount the possibility that the juxtaposition of these phenomena is merely coincidence, and that some kind of causal relationship obtains. Perhaps now is the time for some preliminary hypothesizing as to the nature of the causal link. Two possibilities suggest themselves. The first of these is that it is the circulation of the water in the pipes that is the cause of the size changes (maybe the increased pressure when the pump is on serves to inflate the system; when it is off the system deflates). The second of these might be that it is the temperature of the system which causes these changes (the hot water causes enlargement, system cooling causes shrinkage – this is more promising as it accords more closely with the observations, the heating up of the system is faster than its cooling down though the 'mechanism' through which it might happen is more difficult to speculate about). Of course there could be an interaction between these processes.

You arrange for a test of the first hypothesis by turning the boiler off so allowing the pump to circulate only cold water. Over repeated trials no perceptible difference in size occurs either when the pump is switched on or off. No pattern emerges at all, the hypothesis is abandoned. The second hypothesis fares much better, however. The test reveals a satisfactory level of constancy in the relationship between temperature and size. A thermometer strapped to the system shows a remarkably strong relationship between the two.

You are aware, though, that this primitive test falls well short of the levels of accuracy that might be obtained. So in true scientific spirit (and being totally obsessed – Ed.), you arrange to remove the radiator and its pipework to a place in which these matters can be addressed more minutely – a place where controlled and measured amounts of heating and cooling can be applied and temperature and size changes monitored closely. Having, perhaps, discovered that changes in atmospheric pressure and humidity interfere with the pattern, you arrange that the testing is done in a vacuum to eliminate these distractions. Soon a distinct pattern emerges between increments and decrements of heating and size changes. The copper pipe behaves differently from the steel radiator and this leads to checks against other samples of copper and steel. Copper, it seems, has a consistent reaction to temperature across many samples and trials. So too does steel.

Having set up the apparatus for the relevant tests, why stop at just steel and copper, why not check the phenomenon in relation to other metals too? Given time and patience, you discover that there are quite specific, measurable and predictable reactions to temperature changes and that each metal has its unique pattern consistent across all samples tried and confirmed by each new instance tested. You are on your way to being able to give coefficients of expansion for each metal (stating its peculiar pattern of growth per unit of heat applied). And these, in turn, inform an explanation of the general laws of nature in relation to the expansion and contraction of metals.

Now this example may be terminated here with the enunciation of some of the laws of nature in the relevant area. Of course, the story need not have ended here. A question was raised earlier about the mechanism involved in the process. How does heating cause expansion? This might have led off into an investigation of molecular excitation and subsequently into atomic physics. The point is, however, that such investigations would, in their formal and procedural features, be repeats of the foregoing.

The example was drawn from Comte's beloved physics, but a major strand in positivism is that this scientific method should be deployed outside its traditional preserves such as physics, chemistry, anatomy and physiology, most particularly in relation to a *science of society*.

At the time he was writing, Comte was unable to cite much in the way of contributions to such a social science. To account for this he advanced two explanations. First came the view that, lacking a clear vision of what was involved in working scientifically, those writers who had tackled social matters had been unable, in general, to wean themselves from commonsense preoccupations with goals, motives, intentions and purposes. This involved *teleological* or *finalistic* explanations in which the achievement of some anticipated state-of-affairs is adduced as accounting for current conduct. This implies that present effects have future causes and this reversal of the sequence of cause and effect was to be regarded as a logical nonsense and, therefore, as profoundly unscientific. Second came the argument that nature gives up its secrets only reluctantly. The fact that physicists seemed to have superior penetration of their universe to that enjoyed by the other sciences was not to do with the superior intellectual powers of physicists or to do with more concerted efforts in that domain than in others, but was rather a function of the fact that nature's secrets were more easily uncovered here than elsewhere. There were good grounds for believing that, in the case of his hypothetically assumed general laws of human and social nature, discoveries would be at their most difficult. Social science would be the hardest of them all – it may even require considerable advances in the other sciences before it could attain more than the status of a prospectus.

Such then were the origins of positivism. Of course, the debates have ranged widely since then. Ideas as to what constitutes a science have sophisticated and multiplied.[5] But 'positivism' remains in use to describe the view that the methods of the natural sciences (however construed) should be adopted in the pursuit of social research. Alternative methods must needs be seen as unscientific or, at best, prescientific.[6]

Antipositivism, was the term coined to cover the broad set of (antagonistic) philosophical reactions to positivism which emerged later in the nineteenth century. There was no single proponent or programme. The antipositivists were a diverse group of historians, philosophers and social scientists of German, British and Italian extraction[7] who each contributed differing elements to the overall position. In fact, it could be argued that anything like a fully articulated 'position', such as that outlined below, was close to a century in the making.

The first set of differences with Comtean positivism derived from worries concerning subject matter and the objective(s) which led to its engagement. Taking a historian's question such as, 'Why did Napoleon declare war on the Russians?', it was argued that what was interestingly at issue here were the individual and unique features of that specific decision. The resulting investigation would indeed reveal a chain of putative (hypothetical) causal links leading up to the event in question, but after that the positivist template seemed curiously unhelpful. How might these hypotheses be tested? The idea of a universally demonstrable, constant conjunction presupposes that the phenomenon under scrutiny is *reproducible*. When it was thought that the workings of the central heating system caused the size variations in the radiator, repeated checks could be carried out by turning the system on and off. Once the radiator had been taken off to the laboratory, the issue generalized to the heating of steel and the test more closely defined, anyone, anywhere, at any time could recreate the experiment and corroborate the results.

Even were it possible to turn the clock back (with a cast of millions!) and recreate the original conditions in which Napoleon's decision was taken, it seems unlikely that the sequence of events would follow the same course. This might be, not least, because Napoleon and others involved had learned from the consequences of their actions the first time round. In that sense, it

5 See Bhaskar, R. 1975: *A realist theory of science*. Hassocks: Harvester Press, and Gleick, J. 1988: *Chaos*. London: Heinemann.
6 See Weber, M. 1968: *Economy and society*, (2 vols). New York: Bedminster Press.
7 Droysen, Dilthey, Windelband, Rickert, Croce and Collingwood.

would not be a reproduction of the original sequence at all. Arrangements would have to be made for all the participants to be afflicted with amnesia for precisely the relevant time period and necessarily that they had not aged in any other way.... There is a vast list of such stipulations which would have to be made for just one reproduction of the events and the achievement of any of them seems equally improbable!

Suppose, however, that these difficulties could be surmounted – that the hypothesis could be tested in the approved fashion – a vital question still remains. All that would have been established, at this stage, is the existence of a set of causal relationships. How might progress be made towards the general laws which are specified as the apex of scientific endeavour?

Two observations may be made. First, that the historian's question with which the investigation started does not require it. Second, as the strictures with regard to the reproduction of the event demonstrate, this kind of causal relationship is situationally and temporally quite specific. It is difficult to see this example as just one instance of the generic type 'declarations of war' (or similar). If that were possible, then specified, relevant features of any declaration of war would have done as a test of the hypothesis.

It could be argued that this is simply a case of failure to move to the appropriate level of abstraction. In the central heating case, temperature and size were selected as meeting this requirement. What are the equivalents in the historical case? Perhaps a 'bellicosity index' should have been devised and monitored against a 'declaration threshold score'. The former could be measured, say, by some amalgamation of an individual's blood pressure, heart rate, respiration, and a variety of electrical brain wave readings. Given that declarations of war are unlikely to be the outcome of one person's initiative, it would be necessary to monitor all of those likely to be involved, for example all members of all nation states' ruling groups and their advisors. What might be found from such an exercise is that whenever the mean average bellicosity index between two (or more) national ruling groups rose above a certain score (the threshold) there would be a declaration of war. Further, the ruler with the highest personal index would declare war on the ruler with the next highest and so on. ... Thus, Napoleon declared war on the Russians because these two ruling groups had reached the threshold score and Napoleon's personal index was the highest (statistics quoted).

Were such a study to be undertaken and were it to produce such results, it would undoubtedly qualify as good positivist science. What it would not do is answer the historian's question which was why it was Franco-Russian indices which had risen to this climax at that moment and why, specifically, it was Napoleon for the French whose index had peaked at the crucial point. And these causes are as unique as was the event itself. The general laws would have been bought at the expense of changing the historian's subject matter out of all recognition.

Perhaps then, there are differences in subject matter which make some accessible to scientific investigation and others not. Significantly, it is not necessary to stipulate that steel or copper be afflicted with amnesia or prevented from ageing. Previous experience of expansion seems to have no bearing. And this lies at the heart of the matter: the conundrum can be seen to arise from the fact that the notion of 'cause' as employed in the physical sciences is somehow different from the notion of 'cause' as employed by the historian. The physicist's 'causes' are items like heat, atmospheric pressure and humidity in their 'effects' on the expansion of metals. The historian's 'causes' are items like Napoleon's plans for European domination, calculations of the relative strength of the Russian military, the strategic skill of its generals, and the chances of intimidating success in battle in their 'effects', namely, the decision(s) taken to wage war.

This last type of 'cause' concerns thinking things out or reasoning as a prelude to the 'effect' which is action to (attempt to) realise that which has been thought *in practice*. And this kind of cause–effect linkage may be seen as the archetype of human action. It is, too, a very odd kind of linkage, in which the immaterial world of thoughts is somehow directly involved with the material world of physical action.

To capture the sort of process involved in practical reasoning, reference is made to Aristotle's conception of the *practical syllogism*.[8] This is reconstructed in the following terms: the major premise of the syllogism is a statement of some wanted thing or end in view (in Napoleon's case, say, the definitive removal of potential threats to his empire from the northeast); the minor premise relates some most likely means to secure the wanted thing or to achieve that end (a swift and successful military thrust on the probable adversary's seat of government); the conclusion consists in using those means to obtain the desired end (arranging for the engagement of the opposition's forces at specified locations and in strength deemed to be sufficient).

A number of things may be noted at this point. There is, here, an adequate account of why war was declared. However, there is also a clear sense in which the cause did not produce the originally envisaged effect. The ignominious French retreat from the outskirts of Moscow, defeated partly by the Russian army and partly by the Russian winter, can be understood in terms of defective reasoning: mistakes over the prospects for speedy victory, misjudgements concerning the strength of the opposition, ignorance of the climatic rigours, and so on. All of these are acceptable in the world of logical connections and the always dubious truth value of the premises of a syllogism. They are equally unacceptable within the framework of positivistic causal connection. If, in the controlled environment, the steel failed to expand when heated, this could not be attributed to a mistake on the metal's part. It would be a powerful counter instance leading (especially if confirmed by other observations) to a refutation of the original hypothesis and a major review of the laws of nature based upon it. And yet in the world of human action, causes are, as above, frequently greeted by unintended effects.

8 See Anscombe, G.E.M. 1957: *Intention*. Oxford: Blackwell.

On these grounds, antipositivists have argued for a radical separation between those subjects (like the natural sciences) in which the relationships between the phenomena involved are causal and those (like the human sciences) in which the relationships are logical. The former lead on to the discovery of general laws, the latter do not. On this basis, antipositivists have freed themselves of the prohibition on examining intentions, motives and purposes. These are no substitutes for more rigorous causal explanations, but valid in and of themselves. The injunction is to seek the reasons for, not the causes of, developments where the subject matter so requires.[9]

Importantly, from the point of view of research in the human sciences, the methods by which the existence of causal relationships may be identified and established are very different from those by which logical relationships are elucidated and warranted.

A final example may serve to illustrate what is at issue here. A car being driven along a road mounts the pavement and collides with a pedestrian. How might an account be given of this development? Assuming that this can be attributed to the driver's agency (and not to mechanical failure or the impact of a crash), it is still entirely possible that the explanation is a causal one. A heart attack and the associated muscular pain spasms would be a case in point. But where the driver cannot be shown to have suffered illness, or been blinded by a flash of lightning or whatever (all matters where the operative laws of nature are well established and/or tests available), then the possibility opens up that this was a deliberate act or a failure involved in performing a deliberate act. In the terms above it must be seen as the conclusion of a process of practical reasoning (a practical syllogism) – including the possibility that the outcome was an unintended consequence not entertained in and by the original premises.

It may be shown that, for example, the driver's desired end was to get to work. The means to be employed to that end had been to drive by car along an appointed route to the place of work. The conclusion was to take those means to that end. However, crucially entailed in the minor premise is the assumption of competence to handle the vehicle to the required level. This assumption did not hold and, in losing control, the car mounted the pavement. . . .

Alternatively, it may be shown that, with the syllogism as before, the driver spotted a friend and, going through the syllogism involved in waving, failed momentarily to attend to the original syllogism with the same tragic result.

Finally, it may be shown that there were no mistakes, no failures and no distractions; that the collision was the conclusion of a successful practical syllogism; that the result was fully intentional; that the driver aimed to hit the pedestrian, say, in pursuit of a quarrel.

9 See Winch, P. 1990: *The idea of a social science and its relation to philosophy* (2nd edn). London: Routledge.

This is not, of course, anything like an exhaustive list of the possibilities. It is unlikely that an exhaustive list is possible, given the open-ended nature of reasoning processes. These three examples are put forward rather to examine what might be involved in establishing them. How may it be shown that, as in the first example, it was a case of simple incompetence, the result an accident – an unintended consequence? What evidence would count as adequate in support of this contention?

The driver's account would be given considerable weight here, but it would not necessarily be definitive. Suppose a witness had observed the driver in heated argument with a passenger just prior to the event and that the passenger, when interviewed, confirmed that such was the case. Again, it may emerge that the driver was seen saluting an acquaintance in the instant before the happening. Perhaps the driver was attested by intimates to be involved in a long-running and violent quarrel with the victim and had been threatening physical injury if the opportunity arose. Should any of these accounts be given, it may be appropriate to set the driver's account aside as an attempt to dupe us (to redescribe the actions as resulting from a syllogism other than the actually operative one).

Whether this 'setting aside' is appropriate is clearly to do with the weight of evidence for each of the candidate syllogisms and their consequences. But the weight involved is not such as to yield to being measured by the kilogram, it is rather a question of logical consistency, congruence and connection. The matters at issue are those which would emerge from any thorough forensic investigation or, indeed, from any exhaustive investigation which any member (of the society in question) could, given the time and other resources, carry out. The competencies required to conduct such investigations are formal: they concern knowing what is involved in 'driving', 'waving', 'quarrelling' and 'feeling murderous towards'. What specifically is being driven where, what the argument is about, at whom and why we are waving, between whom and why there is a quarrel; all of these are unique and contextual matters requiring *ad hoc* accounts.

If, then, the antipositivist position is accepted, a number of possibilities open up. The first is to examine topics in their unique and contextual aspects (such as was the concern of the historian above). Another is to elucidate the formal elements involved. So, in a society where vehicles are unknown, giving an understanding of what is involved in 'driving' requires particular care in showing what is presupposed by and entailed in that activity. That is what *ethnographers* do. Thus, the anthropologist Malinowski introduced his readers to the society of the Trobriand Islands.[10] In this process and among many other things, he showed how their much more extensive blue/green colour vocabulary was to be understood in terms of the significance of ocean fishing to their livelihoods and the need to assess complex combinations of sky/sea colour and the way in which these were affected by the presence of different kinds of plankton. Such complex

10 See Malinowski, B. 1978: *Argonauts of the western Pacific*. London: Routledge.

readings were necessary to identify the kinds of fish likely to be present and so the strategy and equipment likely to be required for a good catch. Others[11] have sought to give similar accounts, not of such complete and different cultures, but of subcultures within their own society. So, to understand or to enter as a member the occupational world of British lorry driving, it is necessary to understand, for example, what is involved in and the differences between 'trunking', 'shunting' and 'tramping' – not something to which outsiders are normally privy.

Finally, there are those who regard any kind of (social) order as a contingent achievement-in-context of members. The subject matter for them is the ways in which members contrive this on each occasion of its achievement, the (artful) practices involved, the methods employed – hence, *ethnomethodology*.[12]

These, then, are the basic outlines of the differences between positivism and antipositivism. The arguments have become more sophisticated, and there are differing positions within each of the camps. There have been attempts to argue that the divide can be transcended either through combining the approaches[13] or through denying that the division has any final validity.[14] But so far, none has successfully claimed a large following. There remains a deep difference between those who wish to adapt the methods of the natural sciences as a template for their work in the human sciences, and those who see the human sciences as requiring separate and fundamentally different methods appropriate to their very different subject matter.

11 See Ditton J. 1977: *Part-time crime*. London: Macmillan, and Hollowell P.G. 1968: *The lorry driver*. London: Routledge.
12 See Garfinkel, H. 1967: *Studies in ethnomethodology*, Englewood Cliffs, NJ: Prentice Hall.
13 See Weber, M. *op cit.*
14 See Bhaskar, R. *op cit.*

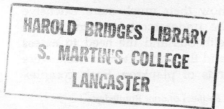

3 What is home?

Eileen Fairhurst

Most of us will have our own views of what home is; some will see it as synonymous with family, others as a place of privacy. It is one of those words that suggests a commonality of understanding and yet carries with it various and diverse meanings. Eileen Fairhurst explores the concept and locates its position with regard to community; she offers useful commentary on the sociological and anthropological views of community and home.

Clarke (1982) in one of the many recent examinations of community care policies posed the question, 'Where is the community which cares?'. His focus on the concept of community fits into a long tradition of sociological concern which stretches from Tonnies (1955) to Skidmore (1994). This kind of conceptual scrutiny is increasingly being directed to the term 'care'. Thomas' (1993) work is a contribution to this current interest. She addresses Graham's (1991) and Ungerson's (1990) conceptualizations of care and argues that care has been taken as given. She aims to introduce a unified concept of care with the intention of developing its theoretical status. Whilst sharing such a concern with developing the theoretical status of those categories from which the notion of community care is constituted, my interest is rather different to most others' (e.g. Glennerster and Falkingham, 1990). A major feature of community care policy is the emphasis on the individual's home as the setting for care as opposed to some kind of institutional setting, conventionally referred to as residential or nursing homes. Whilst academic commentators on community care have often pointed out that the policy assumes there are willing individuals available to care, few have deemed the location in which care takes place as worthy of examination. Community care as a policy, then, is contingent upon there being a home in which care can be located. Despite the category of home being logically prior to the attainment of the policy and being a conceptual pivot upon which community care rests, the former, on the whole , has been viewed unproblematically. The purpose of this chapter is to explicate the concept of home with particular reference to community care for older people. To paraphrase Clarke (1982) 'What is the home in which caring is done?'

Although there has been little examination of the category home in the literature on community care, this is not the case in wider anthropological and sociological writings. Such literature is the spring board for embarking upon a conceptual unravelling of the category home. Having outlined how the house and home have been studied as symbolic systems, the first section of this chapter concludes with a brief examination of how the category of home was treated in the community studies tradition of British sociology and anthropology of the 1950s and 1960s. Given the particular focus on community care and older people, attention is then directed towards how the home has been studied in relation to later life. These two sections provide the context for me to pinpoint a theoretical shortcoming running through this range of literature and, in turn, to propose a way forward which employs the ideas of Schutz. I argue that his conceptualization of the home as a location where spatial and temporal matters meet has great relevance for understanding how older people may experience community care in their own homes. The final section of this chapter identifies some of the implications of community care for the meaning of home to older people.

Domestic architecture and home as symbolic systems

Social anthropologists' interest in domestic architecture and homes reflects Durkheim and Mauss' (1963) pursuit of the classification of social life. They distinguished between symbolic classifications of a moral or religious nature and technological classifications referring to practical schemes of distinction. They argued that these ideas were based on models of society held by different cultures. Douglas (1972) observes this is the foundation of the anthropological critique of a deterministic interpretation of domestic organization. She suggests the latter,

> demands an ecological approach in which the structure of ideas and of society, the mode of gaining a livelihood and the domestic architecture are interpreted as a single interacting whole in which no one element can be said to determine the others. (Douglas, 1972: 514)

Anthropologists have pictured domestic architecture and home as models of society so that the more elaborate their structure in terms of separate rooms, the more complex the society. Donley-Reid (1990) documents how anthropologists' purpose has been to criticize technological and geographical determinism as keys for interpreting domestic organisation and to stress symbolic and social values. Thus, she refers to Fortes' (1949) identification of the 'psychological power' of the Tallensi household and to Cunningham's (1973) point that the floor-plan of the Atoni house conveyed social structure from one generation to another. Tambiah (1969) examined a northeast Thailand village in which age, sex and social intimacy and distance were reflected in social relations sanctioned around the household's east–west line of orientation and on ascending floor levels.

Such concerns, though, are not necessarily the preserve of far flung 'exotic' cultures. Douglas' (1972) reference to the physical layout of houses and social relations along north–south or east–west axes as indicators of genealogical and age distinctions has been noted in the British Isles. Arensberg and Kimball identified the phenomenon of the 'west room' in rural areas of western Ireland. This was that part of the farmhouse to which the 'old couple' moved upon the marriage of their eldest son. Not only did the move to the 'west room' involve a change in the living space of the old couple but also it marked the father's retirement from running the farm and the son's social maturity in assuming control of it. These changes in physical location served as rites of passage for two generations of the family (Arensberg 1959; Arensberg and Kimball, 1965, 1968). Similarly, Goffman's (1966) fieldwork in the Shetland Isles where he observed actions surrounding visitor's approaching relatively isolated crofter's cottages led him to develop the distinction between 'front' and 'back' stage activity as tools for understanding general social action.

The anthropological concern with domestic architecture emphasizes the linkage between homes/houses and social structure. Social psychologists amplify this model in their focus on homes and identity when connections are made between social structure, individuals and their social worlds. Homes are pictured as symbols of the self so that identity is expressed through them: the type of homes in which we live and their contents convey our personalities/our selves (Duncan, 1981). Lloyd Grossman's television programme, 'Through the Keyhole', relies upon such a conceptual framework. In the programme 'celebrities' are steered through a vacant home and are invited to deduce from its perusal and examination of interior decor the owner's identity. The owner's identity is not revealed until the end of the 'guessing game'.

Whilst anthropologists would seek to offer a cross-cultural analysis of the relationship between domestic architecture and social structure, Rapoport (1981) cautions social psychologists against such an endeavour. He notes the ethnocentric overtones of emphasizing the primacy of individual identity, since many non-western cultures do not share this.

Just as Goffman used the home environment to make theoretical points about space and actions in general so did Harris and Lipman (1980). In their examination of space usage in open plan offices and homes for the elderly, they argued that spatial arrangements reflected the hierarchical status distinctions found in those settings. These themes of status and power pertaining to the use of space and the household are evident in Giddens' (1979) theory of structuration. Within such a framework, the house is the domain where symbolic systems arise and are maintained through 'practice', that is, daily household and ritual activities and these, in turn, create social hierarchies and power strategies.

So far the focus has been on the different ways in which house and home have been springboards for making general theoretical points about society and social relations. Argument proceeds, then, from the particular to the general. Now I intend to turn to that literature which reverses this path and examines the house and home in terms of what we learn about general social matters within that particular arena. Specifically, it is that literature on the meaning of home which I now examine. A particular theme running through this is the idea of home as a seat of social relations. Sixsmith (1986) specifies this in terms of modes of experience. She identifies home as providing three modes of experience: personal home, social home and physical home. Willcocks *et al.* (1987) focus on this idea of the personal home and, for them, control is an important feature. They argue that the boundaries of home serve as markers for interaction so that their violation by strangers is not expected. Conventionally, individuals are invited into our homes and the type and nature of interaction may vary according to its location. Matters discussed on the doorstep when paying the milkman's bill are likely to be of little consequence when compared with the personal concerns shared with a confidant in the lounge.

Attempts to explore the meaning of home may rest upon a contrast between the concepts of home and institution (Dant, 1988; Higgins, 1989). For Dant, home is a dwelling place wherein types of personal activity seen as essential to being human are found. Moreover, the materiality of a home and the possessions within it are indicators of continuity of identity but, by contrast, 'an institution threatens to institutionalize the activities of dwelling and thereby threaten the ability to live as human'. (Dant, 1988: 12)

Higgins' (1989) critique of 'community care' policy in terms of its neglect of the meaning of home is of particular relevance to this chapter. She contends that the term 'community care' is a redundant notion as the real distinction is between institution and home. Higgins seeks an unambiguous definition of home and institution but notes the difficulty of this as the former may be a physical location, may have metaphysical and psychological dimensions and involve subjective definitions. She opts for an ideal-type approach of identifying key characteristics distinctive of home or institution. Contrastive categories are offered which include, *inter alia*, the absence or presence of privacy, intimacy, strangers and the exercise of choice and personal freedom in living arrangements. Higgins concludes with a call for the abandonment of the term community care from social policy and for its substitution with the distinction between home and institution. Although this critique of community care is a welcome addition to the literature, it nevertheless falls into the trap of reification which Higgins herself associates with the term community care. Since she sets herself the task of providing an unambiguous definition of home and institution, she cannot do other than picture their existence *sui generis*. Unlike Dant (1988), she allows no place for context.

Saunders and Williams (1988), on the other hand, are concerned with the way home constitutes and reproduces elements of the public and private sphere of social life. They see the concepts of privacy, privatism and privatization as three distinct but related aspects of the home as a private sphere. They suggest that the meaning of home varies in three different ways: first, between household members so that it is here that age and gender relations of society are articulated; second, between different types of households according to social class, household composition, ethnicity and housing tenure; third, according to different regions and/or societies. Overall, their concern is with how 'home is lived by different groups in our society' (Saunders and Williams, 1988: 91).

This focus on the public and private spheres of social life and, particularly, the connections between home and family in contemporary society is the concern of Allan and Crow (1989). They and their contributors formulate home in three broad ways: home as a private place but one which may be as much a 'cage' as a 'castle'; home as a place of security, control and freedom; and home as a place of creativity and expression. In general, then, home is portrayed as a physical location, constructed around the 'family' and where the modern domestic ideal of home and family are synonymous. The home is a black box the unpacking of which is pursued primarily, though not exclusively, via an emphasis upon gender relations in a similar way to that done in relation to the distribution of money (Pahl, 1983; Wilson, 1987) and food (Charles and Kerr, 1990) within the household.

Arguably viewing the home as a black box is a characteristic feature of contemporary British social science and no more so is this apparent than in that genre of the 1950s and 1960s – community studies. Although these have been subject to critical reviews which have noted both the conceptual inadequacy of the term 'community study' (Stacey, 1969) and the methodological limitations of the studies for the claims being made about 'working class life' (Platt, 1971), they are, for my purposes, worthy of comment. It might have been thought that community studies would have played close attention to the home: what it meant to people, what activities took place in the home, what types of social relations were found in the home, etc. An examination of some of this literature reveals this not to be the case at all. Indeed the category is conspicuous by its absence in the indexes of Frankenberg (1966), Kerr (1958) and Young and Willmott (1962). Whilst there is discussion of what happens on the doorstep (Young and Willmott, 1962) and in the street (Kerr, 1958), any focus on action within the home is in terms of the mother–daughter relationship. Young and Willmott (1962) ostensibly acknowledge the importance of the home in Bethnal Green for they note that the ideal is to have a 'home of your own' and that anything else is 'second best'. Yet this acknowledgement is more apparent than real in their analysis. Their examination of the meaning of home and what goes on inside it tends to be rather elliptical. What we learn about these matters is revealed from Young and Willmott's focus on the role of 'mum'. According to them, mothers help daughters find houses in which to live, mothers look after grandchildren while their daughters work and after school until they return home and daughters 'pop in and out' of their mother's home. The point is that from Young and Willmott's approach the home is the black box in which mother–daughter relationships are laid bare. Moreover, from their account the only houses which existed in Bethnal Green were 'mum's homes': all events took place there so that, for example, grandchildren were taken there to be baby sat when daughters went out in the evening rather than 'mum' going to her daughter's home.

The emphases found in the literature on the symbolic meanings of home and the connection of home with community (however unsatisfactorily this is dealt with) have recently been brought together by Douglas (1991). She approaches the meaning of home from a Durkheimian concern with solidarity and pictures it as an 'embryonic community'. She dismisses attempts to define home by its functions. For her, home is a kind of space which has some structure in time. Douglas considers that home is a place in which memories may be institutionalized and that, 'memory institutionalised is capable of anticipating future events' (Douglas, 1991: 294) These temporal and spatial features account for, 'the home's capability to allocate space and time and resources over the long term' (Douglas, 1991: 296). She applies these ideas to the store cupboard and argues that by surveying the types and range of goods found there and their accessibility within it, an inkling can be gained of the types of events likely to take place throughout the coming year. Douglas (1991: 307) with a Durkheimian flourish concludes that the home will survive only as long as 'it attends to the needs of its members'.

The home and later life

Having outlined some of the major features of the literature on the symbolic meanings of home, our interest can become focused on the place of home in the lives of older people. Two major themes can be identified in the literature on home and later life: first, home as an implicated but unexplicated notion in studies of kinship relations between older people and their children; and second, a social policy emphasis on living arrangements, especially in terms of 'special' housing needs of older people.

Currently, politicians and journalists are venting their angst on the alleged 'demise of the family'. Such heart searching is not new for in the 1950s and 1960s, in the wake of Parsons' (1949) influential formulation of the joint conjugal nuclear family as the only structural form functional for an industrialized society, attention was directed towards the decline of the extended family and particularly to the relationship between its older and younger members. These cross-generational relationships were specified in terms of older people being neglected by their children; the extent to which contact existed between the generations. These empirical concerns were prompted by Cumming and Henry's (1961) disengagement thesis which postulated, as a functional prerequisite for the maintenance of society, the inevitable disengagement of older people from society in preparation for their death. Hence, Shanas et al.'s (1968: 3) claim that, at that time, social gerontologists were proccupied with integration versus segretation. 'Are old people integrated into society or are they separated from it?'

Unlike the community studies literature of the 1950s, studies of later life did attend to the notion of home; but the manner of its indexing warrants comment. Townsend's (1957: 279) listings of home in his index refer to 'description', 'attachment' and number of generations domiciled there, for example, one, two or three. Arguably, such insertions serve to implicate/associate home with kinship relations rather than focus on the concept of home *per se*. The only other inclusion of home in the index is in relation to home helps.

Similarly, the index of Tunstall's (1966: 340) study of socially isolated old people reflects a predominant emphasis on home helps and a perceived unmet need for them. A further entry for homes is qualified by the category 'old people's'. Where Tunstall's text does explicitly focus on the home it is in relation to 'home centred activity' and includes matters such as cooking, reading, watching television and listening to the radio.

The category of home, then, was not ignored in empirical research of the 1950s and 1960s on later life but neither was it subject to conceptual unpacking. A reference to what happened in the home, however mechanistically this was undertaken, was integral to an examination of the integration–segregation polarity of older people's relationship with the wider society for there was an assumption of their spending a majority of their time within the home. Moreover, the lack of conceptual scrutiny of the category home in the literature of the period was a direct consequence of the theoretical stranglehold held by structural functionalism on the substantive field of the sociology of aging. As Atkinson's (1974: 5) trenchant critique of the integration–segration debate makes clear, the research reflected two sides of the same coin.

> For in formulating the big theoretical issue in terms of social integration and in arguing as to whether or not old people are integrated into society, both are accepting the importance of the question and by implication are also accepting a societal model characterised by order, consensus and stability and in which people and groups are integrated via mechanisms such as the family. Attention thus was directed not at the problem of whether or not this was the best way of conceptualising social structure, but at the precise *form* that integration took – was the integration of the elderly something special to old people as a group as is suggested by the disengagement theory or were they integrated via the same mechanisms that anyone else in society could be integrated as seemed to be the alternative implied in the counter arguments?

That the concern with living arrangements of older people is firmly rooted in social policy is evident with its focus on 'housing' as opposed to 'home'. By concentrating on the former as opposed to the latter, the home as a built environment is manifested solely through its material constituents rather than a locale in which social relations take place. Hence, despite 'ordinary' housing being the type in which the majority of older people live, social policy literature is characterized by an emphasis on their 'special needs' associated with declining physical capabilities. (Bond (1993) offers a review of this literature but see Fairhurst (1994a) for a different perspective.)

Two notable exceptions to the analytical stranglehold wrought by functionalism and social policy concerns on the study of home and later life are Steinfeld (1981) and Mason (1989). Steinfeld employs a symbolic interactionist framework to argue that decisions made by older Americans to move home are most approriately understood in terms of the relationship between status passage, identity and the meaning of home. A status passage, such as retirement or death of a spouse, of itself cannot account for residential mobility. Rather, it is a matter of whether the symbolism of home maintains or threatens identity; if the former, older people are likely to remain in their home and, if the latter, to move home. Mason (1989) notes that the rather stark contrast made between the public and private domains of domestic and social life are not so straightforward. She shows how the meaning of home is negotiated between married couples in later life. Retirement and ageing are the mechanisms through which home's meaning is negoiated and reconstructed.

Schutz on the home

Although the literature considered in the previous two sections embraces a range of different disciplinary and theoretical perspectives, there is an epistemological unity linking it. Without exception it is all underpinned by a correspondence theory of truth in which it is assumed that that being studied has an existence and reality of its own which is independent of the text. In this way, home is viewed as a resource in the analysis rather than a topic for analysis in its own right. It is this latter approach, relying upon a coherence theory of truth, which I am suggesting will further our understanding of the category home in commmunity care policy. (For some explorations of this approach see Fairhurst, 1993; 1994a, b.)

Schutz's (1964) neglected ideas on the home offer us a way forward. For him, the home is an environment of familiarity and predictability, shared with others and located in time and space. 'Life at home' consists of an organized system of routines, patterned in such a way that traditions and habits surround all kind of activities. Such is the extent of this patterning and shared relevancies that not only tomorrow's events may be accurately forecast but also plans for the future may be laid. This substantive focus of Schutz's reflects his general theoretical concerns with the intersubjective nature of social life. The way in which we interpret the intersubjective world which we inhabit is through typifying social action. Since we possess common-sense knowledge, we are able to identify and categorize our experience in terms of typical aspects of things, events or actions. It is through the operation of these processes that we can have ideas about 'life at home'.

The crux of Schutz's ideas are the way home is a locale in which the interstices between the spatial and the temporal are blended. As he declares (Schutz, 1964: 107):

The home is a starting point as well as a terminus. It is the null-point of the system of co-ordinates which we ascribe to the world in order to find our bearings in it. Geographically 'home' means a certain spot on the surface of the earth. Where I happen to be is my 'abode'; where I intend to stay is my 'residence'; where I come from and whither I want to return is my 'home.' Yet home is not merely the homestead – my house, my room, my garden, my town – but everything.

It is precisely such matters which may be called into question in community care, a policy which by its very purpose entails changing the detail of the spatial location in which one lives. It is the 'everything' identified by Schutz which potentially may become problematical. For Schutz, 'home as everything' embraces, 'a scheme of expression and interpretation' which governs 'not only my own acts but also those of other members of the in group' (Schutz, 1964: 108). Moreover,

> life at home means [having] in common with others a section of space and time . . . and interests based upon an underlying more or less homogeneous system of relevancies. . . . To each of the partners the other's life becomes, thus, part of his own autobiography, an element of his personal history. (Schutz, 1964: 111)

Subsequently the implications of this for older people remaining at home will be considered.

Schutz's focus on the spatial arrangements of the everyday life world continued to link the spatial and the temporal (Schutz and Luckman, 1973). Three distinctions are made between actual, restorable and attainable reach as aspects of our everyday experience. Experience within our actual reach refers to the here and now and rests upon our immediate experience. Physical experience, though, is not the only way to know of our experience. Since we can have a remembered past, our experience can be restored. That we can have a restorable reach implies also we can have an attainable reach. Just as physical presence is not a prerequisite for a remembered past, so is this the case for the future: our actual reach can inform our attainable reach. The future can be brought into our own experience even though it may still be unknown. Unfolding past, current and future experience hinges upon memory. It is precisely those kinds of processes which underpin the assessment and articulation of the notion of home (Fairhurst, 1993).

At this point let me return to my earlier reference to Douglas' (1991) conceptualization of home as 'embryonic community'. Lest it be thought that, since both she and Schutz have recourse to ideas about temporality, space and memories, there is no difference in their analytical approaches it must be made clear that this is not the case at all. Whilst both hold a 'storage' view of memory (Sacks, 1979), Schutz's pivotal notion of intersubjectivity is in direct contrast to the Durkheimian structuralism informing Douglas's work. It is not surprising, then, that she reifies the concept of home in claiming that 'The home's capability to allocate space and time and resources over the long term is a legitimate matter for wonder' (Douglas, 1991: 296).

Some implications of community care for the meaning of home

From the perspective of practitioners, enabling an individual to remain at home rather than be cared for in a nursing or residential setting may require adaptations and/or alterations to be made to the physical fabric of a house. As demonstrated elsewhere (Fairhurst, 1993), such actions intend to minimize risk to which older individuals may be exposed so that home becomes as safe an environment as possible. Whilst a carpet rug to an older person may serve to enhance a room by 'brightening it up' to a remedial therapist it may represent a potential hazard: someone who is 'unsteady on their feet' may trip up over it. Thus the picking up of rugs transforms the home from a dangerous to a safe environment. Home as a safe environment is one which aims to stave off the possibility of accidents. More importantly, though, such a practice conceptually redocuments the home as a normal environment.

Let me elaborate further on this matter of the home as a physical entity, as a location in space. So far my discussion has been primarily in terms of the home as a spatial location. Implicit in this standpoint is the assumption that there is some kind of physical boundary between inside and outside the home. Conventionally, we would identify the walls of the house as indicators of these markers so that we would have little difficulty in deciding what was 'home' and what was 'not home'. Community care, however, may render such a categorization of home as acutely problemmetical in at least two ways: first, home becomes not only a place in which to live but also a place of work and second, home becomes home within home.

Individuals remaining at home may receive care from a variety of sources such as nurses, social workers or volunteers. In coming into an individual's home to deliver care, that home becomes a place of work. The claim that home may be a place of work is not new. Outworking, whereby piece work is undertaken at home, has been a traditional form of employment for working class women unable because of domestic commitments to leave the home to go out to work. Currently the rise of information technology not only facilitates home-working but also extends it from being primarily a female and working class phenomenon to being increasingly male and middle class. Furthermore, a prominent feature of that feminist analysis which makes a distinction between the public and private spheres of social life is the identification of the home as the domain in which the private occurs. In focusing upon the home as part of the private sphere, the former becomes the place in which domestic work gets done and in which labour is reproduced: the home is the seat for the reproduction of the family. Indeed the adoption of this analytical standpoint leads some feminists to prefer the term housing rather than home.

The implications of home as a place of work within the context of community care policy, however, are quite different to those noted above. The point is that the inhabitants of home are not themselves working. On the contrary, they are the objects of someone else's work so that they are the worked on rather than the workers. In this sense, then, home as a place of work is a place of work for others rather than for oneself. Medical care given within the home and the kind of interaction so generated has attracted increasing attention. In general, studies of this kind have shown that work undertaken in a client or patient's home is done in a different way to that done in a conventional medical setting. These studies have also challenged that orthodoxy which subscribes to the dominance of the medical expert in medical lay interaction. Bowers (1992) has teased out some of their main features. Although some research has focused on medical students' work in patients' homes (Sankar, 1986), most has highlighted that of district nurses and health visitors. Sankar demonstrated that the interaction of medical students on home visits to the chronically ill reflected features of a guest–host relationship so that the former had less control over communication. That being both a guest and a 'professional' at one and the same time may pose difficulties for medical work in an individual's home was previously noted in McIntosh's (1981) observational study of district nurses. She suggested that district nurses had to juggle the complementary roles of guest–host and nurse–patient. Whilst McIntosh's study directs us to medical lay interaction within the home, Luker and Chalmers (1990) take us one step further back. Their research on health visiting practice reveals the strategies used to enter the home in order to do health visiting work. Bowers' (1992) own focus is on community psychiatric nurses. Using an ethnomethodological approach he is concerned to explicate how a 'home visit' is accomplished. He demonstrates that typifications of 'being a friend' and 'being a nurse', which draw upon both community psychiatric nurses' (CPNs') and patients' commonsense knowledge of 'nurses' and 'patients', inform 'being in the home' and are the ways in which the CPN exerts control over work.

These studies encourage us to think about the home as a place of medical work and they are united by each focusing on one occupational group so that the home is viewed as a place of work for one specific occupation. Therein lies a limitation for my interest in the practice of community care within the home. A probable feature of community care work is that it entails the recipient having care from more than one source, for example social services, health services or voluntary organizations. Thus, the home now becomes a potential place of work for more than one occupational group. Whilst the literature examined above informs us about the workers' perspectives on the home as a place of work and how they undertake it, we know little of how the recipients themselves accomplish 'being worked upon' in relation to one occupational group, never mind more than one likely to pertain in community care. As yet, we have no empirical evidence on how individuals manage the home as a site of multiple work. Schutz's (1964) point that life at home calls upon the relevancies of all those participating therein is pertinent here: how and in what ways do the autobiographies of the workers and the older person mesh together to transform life at home.

Much of the work undertaken within a home may be of that type which Hughes (1971) conceptualized as 'dirty work'. Hughes' use of this term is not restricted to its hygienic aspects but it also embraces matters of status. Hughes notes that 'dirty work ' often consists of what is ascribed as 'menial tasks' which are deemed as less important than others. These attributes of work are transferred to its doers so that just as the work itself is seen as of less importance than other types of work so are the workers. In general, then, 'dirty work' attracts little status. Now whilst much of the work of district nurses may fit within this classification and, arguably, compared with health visitors who also work within individual's homes, the former have less status, current events are presenting some interesting variations on these matters. Given the perceived financial pressures on health care expenditure and the high proportion of expenditure accounted for by overall labour costs and, within those, particularly for nursing, attempts are being made to reduce labour costs. One such attempt is 'skill-mix' whereby the overall composition of nursing backgrounds is being scrutinized with the consequence that tasks previously undertaken by district nurses or health visitors may be done by individuals with less education and training. Irrespective of whether this process constitutes 'deskilling' or not, there are potential consequences in terms of Hughes' idea of 'dirty work', especially for the recipients of care. For instance, how do they assign status to these workers or are such matters of little salience to them? In addition, given my earlier point that community care is likely to involve members of more than one occupational group, do older people differentially value them and, if so, on what bases are these differential evaluations made?

Since remaining at home may result in fewer rooms being used, home as a physical location may be liable to reduction. In this sense, then, home becomes within one's former home and the walls of rooms, rather than the exterior walls, mark the boundaries between 'home' and 'not home'. At its most extreme this is demonstrated when the living room is also the bedroom. An examination of the social processes underpinning such a scenario allows us to identify some of the, as yet uninvestigated, empirical issues arising from community care.

Living in part of rather than the whole of the house results in the concentration of social life in a specifically bounded physical area. Practically this entails a consideration of which objects both functional, for example, furniture such as seating, tables or beds, and non-functional, for example, photographs, books or ornaments are to be placed in the room. The logic of such a course of action demands that, since less space is to be inhabited, a limited number of objects can be placed in it. This would seem to require that decisions must be made about which objects are to be retained and which to be discarded. (See Fairhurst (1994b) for how older people may call upon their notions of home in such decision making.) The matter is much more complicated in instances of reduced physical space for it is not just a question of fewer objects fitting in less space: at one and the same time space is occupied by both fewer and extra objects. For instance, a zimmer frame may be required as an aid to walking or a commode may be placed in the room. Murray (1993) has highlighted how towels, soap, bowls and scissors may be reserved for the exclusive use of district nurses visiting clients in their own homes. Moreover, such features of everyday life are kept permanantly visible and accessible in the room of the dependent so that they become what she refers to as 'shrines'.

Conventionally in everyday life, accoutrements of washing and toileting are restricted to specific physical locations within the home. The separation of such activities reflects our cultural classifications of dirt and danger. Following Douglas (1974) dirt is 'matter out of place'. Living in one room of one's home, then, calls into question our ideas about 'the right and proper place' to wash and toilet. It may be that individuals map out their 'room as home' in terms of symbolic boundaries between different areas appropriate for particular activities. How individuals identify what constitutes 'matter out of place' and how this may reflect the meaning of home are empirical matters. Their investigation, however, would enable us to flesh out the experience of community care.

Summary

The purpose of this chapter has been to draw attention to the neglected scrutiny of the category home in community care policy. I have shown that, whilst there is a body of sociological and anthropological literature on the topic of home, there is little within the substantive domain of community care. This omission is surprising for the realization of community care policy is predicated upon there being a physical space, conventionally called home rather than 'a (residential) home'. Despite the disciplinary and analytical diversity evident in the literature on home, it is characterized by a common epistemological framework. Its reliance upon a correspondence theory of reality entails pursuing a line of enquiry such that home becomes a resource in analysis. I have argued that a Schutzian framework with its proclamation of an intersubjective social world allows the category home to become a topic for analysis. I have indicated some of the issues arising out of community care policy, the empirical examination of which may advance through following the suggested Schutzian route.

References

Allan, G. and Crow, G. (eds) 1989: *Home and family*. London: Macmillan.
Arensberg, C. 1959: *The Irish countryman*. Gloucester, MA: Peter Smith.

Arensberg, C. and Kimball, S. 1965: *Culture and community.* New York: Harcourt Brace.

Arensberg, C. and Kimball, S. 1968: *Family and community in Ireland,* 2nd edn. Cambridge, MA: Harvard University Press.

Atkinson, J.M. 1974: Social integration as a limiting feature of theoretical approaches to the sociology of aging. Paper presented to the VIIth World Congress of Sociology, Toronto.

Bond, J. 1993: Living arrangements of older people. In Bond, J., Coleman, P. and Peace, S. (eds), *Ageing in society.* London: Sage, 200–25.

Bowers, L. 1992: Ethnomethodology II: a study of the psychiatric nurse in the patient's home. *International Journal of Nursing Studies* **29,** 69–79.

Charles, N. and Kerr, M. 1990: *Women, food and families.* Manchester: Manchester University Press.

Clarke, M. 1982: Where is the community which cares? *British Journal of Social Work* **12,** 45–60.

Cumming, E. and Henry, W. 1961: *Growing old: the process of disengagement.* New York: Basic Books.

Cunningham, C. 1973: Order in the Atoni home. In Needham, R. (ed.), *Right and left: essays in dual symbolic classification.* Chicago: University of Chicago Press. Cited in Donley-Reid (1990).

Dant, T. 1988: 'Home is everything' – the significance of home for social policy. Paper presented to the Annual Conference of the British Society of Gerontology, September, Keele.

Donley-Reid, L. 1990: A structuring structure: the Swahili home. In Kent, S. (ed.), *Domestic architecture and the use of space.* Cambridge: Cambridge University Press, 114–26.

Douglas, M. 1972: Symbolic orders in the use of domestic space. In Ucko, P., Tringham, R. and Dimbleby, G. (eds), *Man, settlement and urbanism.* London: Duckworth, 513–21.

Douglas, M. 1974: *Purity and danger.* Harmondsworth: Pelican.

Douglas, M. 1991: The idea of a home: a kind of space. *Social Research* **58,** 287–307.

Duncan, J. (ed.) 1981: *Housing and identity: cross-cultural perspectives.* London: Croom-Helm.

Durkheim, E. and Mauss, M. 1963: *Primitive classification,* trans. Needham, R. London: Cohen & West.

Fairhurst, E. 1993: Caring for the elderly in the community: home and the documentation and re-documentation of a normal environment. Revised version of a paper presented to the International Conference on Caring for the Elderly in the Community, University of Plymouth, April.

Fairhurst, E. 1994a: Utilising space in sheltered housing or fitting a quart into a pint pot: perspectives of architects and older people. Presented to the Conference on Ideal Homes? Towards a Sociology of Domestic Architecture, University of Teeside, September.

Fairhurst, E. 1994b. Recalling life: analytical issues in the use of 'memories'. Presented to the Annual Conference of the British Society of Gerontology. Royal Holloway College, University of London, September.

Fortes, M. 1949: *The web of kinship among Tallensi.* London: Oxford University Press. Cited in Donley-Reid (1990).

Frankenberg, R. 1966: *Communities in Britain.* Harmondsworth: Pelican.

Giddens, A. 1979: *Central problems in social theory: actor, stricture and contradiction in social analysis.* London: Macmillan.

Glennerster, H. and Falkingham, J. 1990: How much do we care? *Social Policy and Administration* **24,** 93–103.

Goffman, E. 1966: *Asylums.* New York: Doubleday.

Graham, H. 1991: The concept of caring in feminist research: the case of domestic service. *Sociology* **25,** 61–78.

Harris, H. and Lipman, A. 1980: Social symbolism and space usage in daily life. *Sociological Review* **28**(2), 415–28.

Higgins, J. 1989: Defining community care: realities and myths. *Social Policy and Administration* **23**, 3–16.

Hughes, E.C. 1971: *The sociological eye*. Book 2. Chicago: Aldine-Atherton.

Kerr, M. 1958: *The people of Ship Street*. London: Routledge & Kegan Paul.

Luker, K. and Chalmers, K. 1990: Gaining access to clients: the case of health visiting. *Journal of Advanced Nursing* **15**, 74–82. Cited in Bowers (1992).

Mason, J. 1989: Reconstructing the public and the private: the home and marriage in later life. In Allen, G. and Crow, G. (eds), *Home and family*. London: Macmillan, 102–21.

McIntosh, J. 1981: Communicating with patients in their own homes. In Bridge, W. and MacLeod Clark, J. (eds), *Communication in nursing care*. London: Heyden, 77. Cited in Bowers (1992).

Murray, Y. 1993: *An investigation into the roles and relationships of the district nurse with family carers*. Unpublished M.Phil. thesis, Manchester Metropolitan University.

Pahl, J. 1983: The allocation of money and the structuring of inequality in marriage. *Sociological Review* **31**, 273–82.

Platt, J. 1971: *Social research in Bethnal Green*. London: Macmillan.

Parsons, T. 1949: *Essays in sociological theory: pure and applied*. Glencoe, IL: Free Press.

Rapoport, A. 1981: Identity and environment: a cross-cultural perspective. In Duncan, J. (ed.), *Housing and identity: cross-cultural perspectives*. London: Croom-Helm, 6–35.

Sacks, H. 1979. Lecture notes, Vol. I. Unpublished, UCLA.

Sankar, A. 1986: Out of the clinic and into the home: control and patient–physician communication. *Social Science and Medicine* **22**, 973–82. Cited in Bowers (1992).

Saunders, P. and Williams, P. 1988: The constitution of the home: towards a research agenda. *Housing Studies* **3**, 81–93.

Schutz, A. 1964: The homecomer. In *Collected papers II: studies in social theory*. The Hague: Martinus Nijhoff, 106–19.

Schutz, A. and Luckman, T. 1973: *The structure of the life world*. London: Heinemann.

Shanas, E., Townsend, P., Wedderburn, D., Hemming, F., Milhof, P. and Stewhouwer, J. 1968: *Old people in three industrial societies*. London: Routledge & Kegan Paul.

Sixsmith, J. 1986: The meaning of home: an exploratory study of environmental experience. *Journal of Environmental Psychology* **6**, 281–98.

Skidmore, D. 1994: *The ideology of community care*. London: Chapman & Hall.

Stacey, M. 1969: The myth of community studies. *British Journal of Sociology* **20**, 134–47.

Steinfeld, E. 1981: The place of old age: the meaning of housing for older people. In Duncan, J. (ed.), *Housing and identity: cross-cultural perspectives* London: Croom-Helm, 198–246.

Tambiah, S. 1969: Animals are good to think and good to prohibit. *Ethnology* **7–8**, 423–59. Cited in Donley-Reid (1990).

Thomas, C. 1993: De-constructing concepts of care. *Sociology* **27**, 649–70.

Tonnies, F. 1955: *Community and association*. London: Routledge & Kegan Paul.

Townsend, P. 1957: *The family life of old people*. London: Routledge & Kegan Paul.

Tunstall, J. 1966: *Old and alone*. London: Routledge & Kegan Paul.

Ungerson, C. (ed.) 1990: *Gender and caring: work and welfare in Britain and Scandinavia*. London: Harvester Wheatsheaf.

Willcocks, D., Peace, S. and Kellaher, L. 1987: *Private lives and public places*. London: Tavistock.

Wilson, G. 1987: Money: patterns of responsibility and irresponsibility in marriage. In Brannen, J. and Wilson, G. (eds), *Give and take in families*. London: Allen & Unwin, 136–54.

Young, M. and Willmott, P. 1962: *Family and kinship in east London*. Harmondsworth: Pelican.

4 Promoting health

Sandy Whitelaw

Sandy Whitelaw explores the ideologies of health promotion within a community setting. Health promotion is an important tool for the community practitioner and offers much in the way health can be facilitated. In recent years it has attracted bad press because we still have the same health problems and the blame is laid at the feet of health educators. Education and promotion are not the same thing, as Sandy illustrates. He examines the notion of 'community' before going into an exploration of the ideologies that underpin health promotion.

Introduction: the origins of 'community' health

The addition of a 'community' perspective to a range of health and social services has clearly been an important factor in recent health policy development (DoH, 1987, 1989, 1992). The desire to add a 'community' ingredient to existing service provision in, for example, education, town planning, social services, policing and, most importantly in this context, the health sector can easily be recognized. As we shall see, this movement contains differing motivations, covering a range of perspectives.

In specific terms, the health sector has seen two types of development:

- the re-alignment of what were previously institutionally based formal agencies to take on board a 'community' label (for example, health visiting, district nursing, community psychiatric nursing, community drug services);
- and the encouragement of 'informal' initiatives with an emphasis on encouraging grassroots 'neighbourhood' activity.

Whilst both hope to be able to promote health, we should be aware of the complexity of this desire and be clear that the *means* by which the task is seen to be achieved varies greatly.

In summary, we should be wary of seeing 'community health promotion' as a single practice. Rather, our perceptions of the nature of 'communities', our view of health and its determinants (as suggested by the Health Field Model) as well as our beliefs on the role and scope of health promotion will contribute to the existence of a wide range of activities. It is at these levels that the links that exist between perceptions of 'community' and 'health promotion' will initially be considered, with an emphasis on the founding 'roots' of community development. The chapter considers the practical consequences of these broad influences.

Views of 'community'

Just as the values of practitioners can dictate the emphasis they place on particular aspects of the Health Field Model, so it is the case that definitions of what is considered to be a 'community' are individually constructed. Richman (1987) for example, notes:

> ... the term 'community' is one of indefinite elasticity. For those promoting reforming or peddling panaceas for our social, economic and political dilemmas, community has instant appeal. Its chameleon-like form has been blended with a multitude of competing ideologies. Although most of its recent purveyors take care not to offer detailed descriptions of what a community actually is, their policies are predicated on the understanding that it does actually exist (or can be stimulated into existence) and that it is endowed with beneficial qualities. (Richman, 1987: 185)

If we start with a general consideration of what we understand a community to be, a range of images can be identified; spanning the notion of a warm and home-like collection of individuals with a common identity or purpose through to a more pessimistic view of ambiguity and even a fundamental denial of existence.

The first is a positive and optimistic image, reflecting a hope that such a thing as community actually exists. The image is then given the qualities of a 'traditional' family within which mutual support between individuals leads to a better collective end-point. The ideal of a collective fabric holding communities together and being used actively to improve the health of that grouping is therefore pursued. This perspective has evolved against a perceived drift in social trends towards competitive and uncaring individ-ualism as a result of excessive 'modern' political, social, economic and spiritual pressures. This has led to the condemnation of such trends and calls for the restoration of a more 'old fashioned' collective lifestyle.

For many, the need for such a social arrangement has rested on the acceptance of inherent inequalities in opportunity between individuals and groups along with a belief that individual potential is limited by a range of social and political barriers. As such, it is hoped that these differences can be minimized via collective responsibility and action. As we shall see later, community activity of this sort has an explicit desire to address social and political structures that are felt to be 'unfair' and thus detrimental to individual health.

Still operating within an acceptance of the concept of community, a second type of work can be identified; one which though embracing the ideal of collective and mutual support, seeks to direct this force inwardly, encouraging communities to cope with – though not necessarily change – hostile circumstances through self-help and mutual support. Here, rather than community initiatives being seen as a means of redressing injustices within an environment by struggle, the emphasis would be placed on the expectation that communities should revert back to traditional self-help ethics rather than what is felt to be an unreasonable reliance on formal service provision.

Whilst appearing to be located in a 'collective' framework, it should be noted that this perspective exists within a highly ambiguous context and starts to point towards a different view of the structures and roles of communities. In many ways, it can be seen as an extension of an 'anti welfare' sentiment, seeking to encourage independence and motivation with reliance on only the smallest of collective units – the family.

This notion introduces perspectives which favour the right of individual expression in opposition to what is considered to be the constraint to freedom contained within the obligations of collective responsibility. They have arguably enjoyed a political renaissance over the past decade (see Shand, 1990) and Rentoul (1989) points out that:

> Critics call it selfishness, defenders call it self reliance. More neutrally it is called individualism, and everybody seems to think there is more of it. (Retoul, 1989: 2)

Clearly, such views cast doubt over whether there can ever be such a thing as a community and perhaps more importantly, if there is, whether this is a useful tool to carry out health-promoting activities.

There is little doubt that the above values exert a powerful influence on the ways in which health-promoting activities in the broadest sense are delivered. How these broad perspectives of community are practically applied and expressed is dependent upon both professional and public perceptions and motivations as well as the general political climate. We can now consider in more detail the features of these three factors.

The role of professionals in community health promotion

At least at a superficial level – and despite their arguably individualistic orientation – professional health practitioners would appear to have rallied around the concept of community. The extent to which this has happened and the substance that lies behind the term 'community practice' will be questioned later. At this point, it is enough to say that health and social professionals, such as nurses, social workers, probation officers and general practitioners have (at least in a rhetorical sense) attempted to use the concept of the collective community in pursuance of their objectives.

The source of this desire is perhaps predominantly and simply the advantage of the perceived effectiveness of community work; that is, objectives that relate to individuals are more efficiently achieved within a community context. Willmott (1988) notes that many community initiatives originate from a formal central source and have, as their main thrust, a desire to provide centrally driven services in a more efficient manner, preferably drawing on informal support to fill in service gaps. Such arrangements would merely use the community as a vehicle for the more efficient execution of existing strategies. For example, a community-based approach to immunization, would be concerned that centralized services lead to low uptake and would, therefore, see the advantage of going out to the community only in terms of improved uptake rates.

More profoundly, some professionals and policy makers have viewed the medium as a profitable setting for altering the nature of the relationship that exists between professionals, communities and state and as such have stimulated the development of new and innovative approaches to providing health services and improving health (Richardson, 1983; McEwen et al., 1983; Kerans et al., 1988; Dominelli, 1990). All see it as a means of overcoming what is considered to be major failings in existing political structures and subsequent health service provision. This desire is summarized by Baum (1988):

> the approach advocated by the World Health Organisation and endorsed by governments throughout the world suggests a shift away from a primary stress on curative health care and illness prevention, to a stress on the importance on health promotion that provides people with opportunities to exercise control over their health. Central elements of this new public health policy are well integrated primary health care services with a strong preventative element *and an emphasis on the importance of community participation in health care decision making.* (my italics) (Baum, 1988: 259)

For most, the perceived advantage has been the overcoming of the dominance of the formal medical sector (Watt, 1987). There is also, for many, an associated issue of altering what is perceived to be the inappropriate and iniquitous relationships which exist between them and the people they serve. This issue introduces the importance of our expectations of the nature and role of 'community' groupings themselves.

Public involvement in community activities

Earlier discussion suggested the possibility of a range of differing definitions of communities. Such arrangements imply differing types of public/ professional interaction in the process of promoting health, ranging from the dominance of professional and state perspectives to a more participative and questioning role stressing an active and potentially confrontational relationship.

The former suggests an arrangement with professional and political groupings having responsibility implicitly invested in them by a passive and acquiescent public to serve them as they see best. Such an arrangement is allied to the notion of increasingly centralized and distant authority groupings (Willmott, 1988) and the corresponding failure of individuals and groups to contribute actively or significantly to the political process. This arrangement can be viewed in two ways: as being either a satisfactory one, which in practical terms allows societies to be governed in a sensible and efficient way as would be suggested by 'functional' and consensual social models; or one which, in democratic terms, is unsatisfactory, and which results in respectively, a disenfranchised, disinterested public population and a powerful distant ruling 'elite' (George and Wilding, 1989).

This notion of public disenchantment with political structures (Navarro, 1978) and thus a desire to be more actively and critically involved in decision making is central to this latter theme. As a result of increased centralization and 'undemocratic' relations, some would argue that we are seeing an opposing 'counter' force centred on what Navarro (1978) calls a 're-discovery of human rights'. More specifically there exists a perception of a growing tendency for the public to question authority in all its manifestations (Richardson, 1983). Such views suggest the emergence of a more 'conflict'-based relationship between public and professional with the former attempting to be more actively involved in decision making.

The broader political context

Clearly, the conduct of both professional and community groups does not operate within a political vacuum, but rather reflects the climate of particular administrations and eras. Certainly, the past two decades have seen significant shifts in socio-political values that have in turn had a bearing upon the role of communities, professional groupings and the whole concept of welfare provision.

In the broadest of political terms, many would point to the general unresponsiveness of government to large sectors of the population. Sustained by substantial electoral majorities derived from an unrepresentative electoral system, the potential for administrations to largely ignore grassroots community views has been high. In this context, democratic community orientated 'fightback' has become, for many groupings, the only means of redressing this fundamental political imbalance.

It would, however, be improper to characterize all of the political climate as hostile towards community structures. Indeed, much of the developments within health policy over the past 10 years have explicitly sought, in a range of respects, greater community involvement. The reasons for such enthusiasm are, however, clearly varied and reflect a range of different motives. Most positively, there exists a recognition of the worth of enlisting the support and co-operation of community groups in the identification of health priorities and development of services. These trends can be associated largely with the increased emphasis placed on the 'primacy of the consumer' within the public sector (Allsop, 1989).

However, more ambiguous and, arguably, questionable forces are also at play. First, there is a notion that 'primary'-orientated community services can be more cost-effective in a time of economic hardship; similarly, community services can better meet the ever-increasing demands being placed on services by demographic changes and demand. This also conforms to suggestions that the inclination to decentralize and devolve responsibility to communities can be politically prudent in recession. Most significantly, the favouring of community policy solutions has also been linked to the ideological preference of self-care within the community as opposed to formal State services (Loney, 1987; Lee and Raban, 1988; Harrison *et al.*, 1990).

These intentions conceal a host of hidden influences on the preference of community health promotion and as such, lead to a range of approaches under a common heading. It is argued that such themes are reflected in a range of practices. In this respect, Beattie (1986) notes that community practice:

> ... encompasses a wide range of very distinct and disparate ways of working; and the relationships of power and control in these different modes need the most careful critical analysis ... I think it is helpful to regard community work as consisting of a repertoire of alternative approaches, where each alternative represents a major root (or 'route') in the historical development of state welfare interventions. (Beattie, 1986: 13)

What this suggests is that, as a result of the values and motives of professional and public groupings, community participation can be reflected in a number of ways. It is to the central issue of 'participation' that we will now turn.

The concept of 'participation' and community health promotion

Perhaps, as has already been suggested, the most crucial element of the range of such practice is the perceived nature of the relationship that exists between the formal health sector and the recipient community and, as such, the way determinants of health are subsequently defined. These considerations introduce the concept of participation and it is with this concept in mind that the range of health promotion strategies that can be identified within a community setting can be considered. Within such a context, the potential to emphasize particular aspects of the Health Field Model will be considered.

The notion of client participation for health is clearly not new, though for many reasons, the concept, in the face of a reluctance on the part of health services to permit client involvement, appears to be in the ascendency (Maxwell, 1989). Some of the forces that shape this movement are common with those outlined above in relation to community approaches. That is, the realization that health cannot be guaranteed by health professionals alone and that in some cases professionally dominated decision making can in fact be counterproductive to health and perhaps most importantly the ethic of consumerism which sees health service users as customers. Of most importance to our discussion, participation is considered by some as an inherently collective phenomenon; allowing communities to act co-operatively upon forces that shape their health, but which are beyond the scope of any single individual. A number of writers (Arnstein, 1969; Adams, 1989; Bracht and Tsouros, 1990) have considered participation in relation to a range of potential activities or relationships in a series of 'models of participation'.

In summary, the models present participation as a wide-ranging concept, taking in a continuum of activities which range from a position of non-participation and community passivity/professional dominance through to a relationship which shows high citizen control and power over the formal decision-making agencies. Between these end-points a range of central types is identified, relating to the tokenistic models of placating communities and consultation. We can now consider the range of types of health promotion which are located within the context of participation.

Specific approaches to community health promotion

'TYPE 1': COLLECTIVE AND CRITICAL ACTION

Drawing on a perspective of 'active' communities, an 'ideal' model of health promotion practice has developed which essentially draws upon the twin themes identified earlier of the perception of the existence of a collective community structure and iniquitous forces on health that are largely beyond the control of many individuals. Furthermore, elements of political disenchantment with the failure of formal, centralized and bureaucratic welfare agencies to improve the circumstances of those at greatest disadvantage can be detected.

In this sense, the adoption by health promoters of a community-orientated mode or what many have termed, 'community development' (Smithies and Adams, 1990) can be regarded as the genre attempting genuinely to tackle source determinants – mainly socio-economic and environmental – of individual health status. For example, groups may address localized environmental threats to their well being, such as polluting factories, unsafe roads or poor recreational facilities. Also, they may be concerned with responding to socio-economic disadvantages, for example unemployment.

More specifically, French (1990) identifies this type of practice as 'community empowerment' and sees it as a process by which health educators try to enable people to increase control over their lives and health.

Similarly, and under a classification of 'community action', Beattie states that this practice:

> ... takes a stand and mobilises against in-built bias within existing authority structures and agency policies. It is essentially a style of 'protest', of 'fight back', in a long tradition of social action movements, seeking to redress grievances, to correct injustices, and to reclaim resources where they are unequally distributed. (Beattie, 1986: 15)

As such, some would argue that, due to its explicit orientation towards social change, such an approach is openly 'political' and potentially confrontational (Tones, 1991).

In its purest form, this type of health promotion activity is, thus, based on a perception of society as essentially one of inherent inequality and is as such aligned towards attempts to alter radically the perceived cause of these differences – based essentially on socio-economic circumstances. Of the perception of the basic nature of society, Caplan and Holland (1990) note:

> Theories concerned with radical change view society in terms of structural and other social conflicts such as that between capital and labour, the fight against racism and other forms of discrimination. It is these contradictions and tensions reflected in various modes of domination of some classes and groups which lead to various forms of social, economic, political and cultural deprivation of other classes and groups. (Caplan and Holland, 1990: 11)

Of responses to these circumstances, they conclude:

> Radical change is thus concerned with the dynamics of change best described in such terms as emancipation realised through the potential of deprived classes and groups to transform the social, economic-political and cultural conditions which sustain their deprivation. (Caplan and Holland, 1990: 11)

These perspectives can be viewed in the context of participation. Any aspiration to redress such fundamental imbalances strikes at the heart of traditional relationships between powerful and active professionals and respectively powerless and passive public groups. Additionally, it takes our understanding of health on to new grounds – essentially away from individualized and physical dimensions on to collective and socio-economic/environmental grounds.

In efforts to redress the imbalances that exist between community and professional views, any participation of these groups would go beyond placatory relationships. Despite a tendency for health services to be reluctant to involve community groups in substantial decision-making process along with the powerful centralizing tendencies within politics as a whole, many writers talk of a 'rediscovery', particularly at local levels, of democratic principles within the health service. Based on the seminal guidance given by the World Health Organization (WHO) 1978 Alma Ata declaration, a broad consensus has developed on the need for participatory mechanisms within health provision. This accord is, however, loosely constructed and as Haro (1987) recognizes, the understanding given to the concept by differing agents may be at odds with each other:

> ... there are many alternative ways of organising participation which, at least in theory, satisfy the minimum requirements ... (though) the objectives often contain more verbosity than fact. (Haro, 1987: 62)

What is clear, here, is that the key feature of the principle of participation concerns the extent of the responsibility devolved to the individuals and groups as well as the degree to which their decisions can actually be facilitated, accommodated and translated into tangible action. Croft and Beresford (1988) make the crucial distinction between whether it is a matter of feeding into the organization's own decision-making process or having some real power to change it.

Therefore, the crucial factor in participation would appear to be the extent to which community decisions will be re-enforced by statutory and professional groups. In this respect proposals made by communities in a participative context should strengthen community authority and legitimize the competence of 'popular' activities. In other words, community decisions should be decisive rather than advisory.

In practical terms and specifically in relation to the role of health professionals, such work has been orientated around two broad and potentially interactive approaches. The first adopts a predominantly 'top down' focus, the health promoter attempting to directly and unilaterally act upon the structures and processes that fundamentally shape health and which have traditionally been exclusive in the sense that they are predominantly the domain of a narrow grouping of influential individuals. The active nature of such an approach is highlighted by Kennedy (1982) when he expresses a desire that health promotion should:

> look beyond individual orientated health education towards the creation of teams which will promote health on behalf of the individual. (Kennedy, 1982: 15)

Perhaps the most important feature of such work is its desire to exert positive influence directly upon decision makers whilst at the same time keeping in touch with the broad wishes of communities. The work would, for example, attempt to improve accountability and communication between organizations and departments or 'democratize' decision-making procedures, making them more open and accountable to public interest.

The second would align itself towards a more 'bottom up' approach, working actively alongside individuals and communities in a context of partnership. Boot (1986) describes such a strain of work as involving processes by which local people are able to identify their own problems and needs and by various democratic processes obtain solutions to these problems and needs.

This type of work is centred on the notion of fostering skills within disadvantaged communities which will enhance their potential to have an affect upon the forces which shape their health. It operates largely within a context that believes that (nominally) democratic political processes are divisive in that they effectively exclude certain sectors from active participation. As suggested earlier, such groupings could be constructed along the lines of, for example, class, race or gender and as such community action has tended to be orientated around, for example, geographical housing estates, ethnic groupings or women's groups.

The common role of the health promoter in both circumstances can perhaps be most succinctly classified as 'advocate'. Baric (1988) conceptualizes this work in the following way:

> ... the main ingredients ... are the contribution of necessary expert knowledge and understanding of complex systems and sophisticated mechanisms, as well as ensuring a competent and effective community participation in the complex decision making process. (Baric, 1988: 53–54)

Davies (1985: 68) envisages a more fervent role in saying that advocacy can 'take up cudgels' on behalf of an entire community.

Irrespective of the specific details of the role, it is clear that professional advocacy within the context of a close relationship with communities can be effective. For example, Croft and Beresford (1988) recognize that some of the best and most valued health promotion work has been in the field of professional advocacy including the work of, for example, MIND and Age Concern.

Inevitably, there has been criticism of both styles. Any 'top down' orientation is open to the allegation that one dogma is merely being replaced by another and that distanced professionals can never truly act on behalf of the real interests of communities. Similarly, within the 'bottom up' empowerment models, critique has arisen in two respects. First, the contention has been that much of the work towards empowerment has been directed towards individual betterment rather than the intended collective base of the whole community. As such, critics would suggest that the rationale for the work deviates from the acceptance of the social determinants of health. Second, some would argue that the fostering of individual or even group empowerment separately from any attempt to structurally alter profound influences on health determinants is ultimately futile, leading at best to merely the ability for individuals and groups to cope within existing circumstances or at worst disillusionment and a re-enforced sense of powerlessness. Tones (1991) optimistically tries to overcome this by calling for a comprehensive approach to empowerment strategies involving both inwardly orientated work centring on individuals and groups alongside more far reaching processes of 'critical consciousness raising'. This theme will be returned to later.

In summary, a notion of a 'pure' form of community-orientated health promotion activity has been developed. Most importantly, such work can be seen to be fundamentally different to conventional practice. As opposed to more orthodox models of health promotion which have largely focused on individualized, behaviourial and biomedical dimensions within the context of professional superiority and expected conformity from clients, community models offer a means of working which is essentially critical of these methods. Therefore, some forms of community health promotion have been characterized by a recognition that individuals are exposed to profound external and largely uncontrollable influences on their health. Consequently, activities are orientated towards these forces and tackled in a predominantly collective fashion.

'TYPE 2': COMMUNITY HEALTH PROMOTION AS TRADITIONAL PRACTICE

The certainty and stability of such community structures and the associated form of 'idealized' collective and critical health promotion practice has, as is suggested above, been rigorously questioned. Referring back to the earlier theme, which suggested that there are fundamental difficulties in defining communities, which in turn potentially undermine the whole rationale for collective health promotion action, one can more specifically identify a range of perspectives that are critical of community health promotion models.

Primarily, critics would doubt the very existence of entities definable as communities. Seedhouse (1986) fundamentally questions the objective existence of community units, whilst Baric (1990) sees such structures as at best merely loosely formed 'free associations' of individuals with vague similarities.

More importantly, objections to the actual nature of community-orientated work have been forwarded. Rather than such practice possessing the ideal features of collective and participative action against health inequalities, it has been argued that the work does not in fact deviate significantly from the more traditional forms of practice that emphasize active professionals and passive communities.

Principally, as opposed to community practice adopting alternative non-medical orientations, there has been a tendency for practice to conform to established norms. For example, Baum (1988) states:

> ... current knowledge of community health services shows that, despite policy statements to the contrary, much community health activity falls within a traditional medical model that emphasises curative intervention. (Baum, 1988: 259)

Therefore, as opposed to practice favouring the promotion of values that attempt to redress inequalities and work for those communities most disadvantaged, they have had the potential merely to re-enforce existing power structures and influential groupings.

The ability to fulfil this can partly be located in the way communities are 'created'. It has been argued that the very construction of communities around which health promotion activity is focused is potentially divisive. Seedhouse (1986) contends:

> ... communities do not exist in any objective sense but are constructed. And they are constructed by people with certain sets of beliefs and values which are not universal. (Seedhouse, 1987: 15)

Since those who construct these communities and select some to receive attention (at the expense of others) are professionals, it is their values that will normally prevail. Within such a scenario there exists the potential, for those with power, to co-operate selectively with existing communities who are perceived to be sufficiently worthy or vocal to seek attention. Of most significance within such a relationship is the dangerous possibility of a mutually advantageous 'corporate' relationship developing which both fulfils the image of a caring community-orientated professional grouping and devolves power to selected preferred communities. Critics of such a relationship would point to its essentially conservative orientation, constructing actions as a means of maintaining existing order and stifling attempts to challenge it.

Rather than community approaches being seen as 'neutral' attempts to redress inequalities in health which exist between groupings, it is, therefore, argued that such work inevitably involves value judgements which are likely to be professionally derived and ultimately discriminatory against other communities not deemed favourable within the context of these values.

We can go farther than a critique of the existence of the concept itself; we can bring into question the very values and practices that constitute community health promotion models. The ability of influential professionals to set community health promotion agendas which are not necessarily of most benefit is recognized by Tumwine (1989) who, with reference to community health workers, contends that:

> ... our perception of the causes of health problems is influenced by our class interests, and interests are often at variance with those of the diverse sections in the community. At times our interests may even be antagonistic and hostile towards the poor and other disadvantaged members of the community. (Tumwine, 1989: 157)

Within this scenario, the fundamental values of seeing health as a consequence of social causes addressed most effectively by way of collective publicly orientated practice are compromised. There are many reasons for such a departure. McQueen (1989) locates the potential for duplicity between intentions and outcomes within a broad political tendency for 'global' collective ideologies to be stylistically and superficially favoured whilst 'micro' individualism remains dominant at a local level. He suggests:

... the rhetoric of health promotion and public health is social, but the actions, the behavioral base, are at an individual level. How else can one explain a public health rhetoric which argues that social conditions affect health outcomes and then, in turn, argues that the appropriate solution is to eat better, exercise more, drink less and give up smoking? (McQueen, 1989: 342)

Breihl (1978) takes this notion further by suggesting that community-orientated health services not only maintain an ambiguous position but actively perpetuate particular conservative norms. In other words, within what appears to be an open and progressive arrangement, community health projects manage to generate a discreet form of power that is both subtle and repressive.

In this political context, it is clearly expedient for the state to adopt a perspective which sees health status as a consequence of a multitude of individual choices and actions rather than a product of wider social forces and deficiencies. Such a tendency towards the individualizing and internalizing of health behaviour is similar to the perspectives of a medically dominated health sector and the professional status of the people who work in it. Most significantly, and with respect to the concept of participation, many would argue that the very basis of pure community-orientated health promotion, with its emphasis on active participation via empowerment, is directly at odds with the ethic of professionalism with its desire to retain independent influence and autonomy. Jones (1985, 1991) recognizes this gap that separates the ambitious aims of community practice and the restrictive and insular nature of political and professional life, suggesting that their perspectives are essentially at odds with each other. She points out:

... in the main, the audience for declared strategies and policies are the health professionals, health educators and civil servants in the health ministry – not the most likely groups of people to be actively involved in putting health on the agenda, reducing their own power, demystifying their own knowledge or validating lay experiences of health needs, in other words acting against their own interests ... the principles (of community development) if acted upon would mean fundamentally reforming health care services. (Jones, 1985: 4)

As a result of these pressures, the 'ideal' (suggested earlier) of sensitive empowerment-based approaches involving full and active participation are discarded in favour of more conventional approaches. The ability for community-based approaches to reflect a range of activities has already been recognized. In the context of a distorted notion of such work, a type of work can be identified that, though oriented superficially to the physical idea of a community setting, possesses none of the philosophical substance we would expect of 'genuine' community models. The principal features of such work are its desire to extend the role of the state and professional values into 'deficient' communities within a context of what Beattie (1986) calls 'moral entrepreneurism'. Most importantly, the nature of the relationship between workers and client groups is one of inequality – the dominant role of the professional remaining paramount.

In relation to the concept of participation, actions on the continuum of activities identified earlier are very much towards the end of 'non-participation', involving at best tokenistic placatory consultation, at worst no interaction at all. Critics of such models would point to their potential to be deceptive. Primarily, the notion that communities are cosmetically involved in decision making has the tendency to placate such groupings. Of such a style, Beattie notes:

> ... it lends itself to a kind of patronage, pacification or 'colonisation', whereby the surplus energy of local communities is raked up to be 'cooled out' on preserving the status quo. (Beattie, 1986: 14)

The purpose of consultation here is not to find ways of responding in any serious way to the wishes of those consulted, but rather to assess likely opponents, thus enabling counter arguments to be prepared well in advance. Additionally, such processes tend to 'exhaust' community groups.

This notion of appeasement is central to another form of health promotion practice which we have discussed earlier. In relation to self-empowerment models, it was suggested that such practice had the potential to act independently of structural changes, restricting itself to an inwardly looking role of self-help and coping. The ability to create such groups is clearly attractive to providers of statutory services in that it both diverts attention away from structural sources of ill health and places responsibility firmly back with individuals, families and communities.

Conclusion

Initially, this chapter, within the context of the Health Field Model, developed the notion that health promotion can be best forwarded within a flexible and multidimensional understanding of health and its determinants. This chapter has subsequently outlined a vision of what are the most salient features of attempts to practice health promotion in a community context. It could appear that, rather than community methods attaining such an encompassing perspective, they have, at least in their ideal form, tended to emphasize specific aspects of the model. Therefore, rather than community health promotion practitioners unquestioningly accepting, for example, the importance of biological predeterminants and individual actions and motives on health, they have sought to critically challenge these perspectives in favour of an understanding that emphasizes socio-economic influences on health. Positions of critical conflict rather than consensus would therefore appear to be the norm. This situation may not, however, be what it appears.

One must remember that many examples of community practice arose in opposition to what was considered dominant though erroneous approaches to health. In other words, community work has commonly been a radical oppositional force, reacting against entrenched modes of practice supported by powerful groupings. It is therefore unsurprising that the minority rhetoric of community practice has appeared to be strident; efforts to redress imbalances in perspectives arguably requires such a 'single-minded' outlook. Beyond these images, very few community-orientated practices manage, or indeed would want to exclusively operate along these one-dimensional lines. A range of factors contribute to such a situation.

First, the value of individual and group preferences is largely maintained within such structures. Therefore, it is unlikely that in the context of working within the demands of a range of expressed needs, that one-dimensional perspectives will be taken.

Second, and perhaps most importantly, such is the strength of 'conservative' perspectives, favouring the elements of the Health Field Model which stress the importance of dimensions other than socio-economic influences, it would be extremely optimistic to expect such views to gain any sort of real dominance. Realistically, viewpoints which support socio-economic explanations of health exist in a context which has been traditionally hostile towards them and as such practitioners with such values have been forced to operate within existing boundaries. For this reason, practice with a nominal community heading and apparently strong views on the importance of socio-economic influences on health is still forced to work within a climate which demands more conservatively orientated work within relatively restricted confines. These tendencies are clearly made worse by the topic and disease orientation of *The Health of the Nation* (DoH, 1992).

Rather than there being a danger of overemphasizing socio-economic approaches to health within a community-orientated model, the danger of exclusivity lies with the possible exclusion of such a dimension. A strain of practice which, although ostensibly community orientated, in reality possesses few of the features which would suggest any attempt to authentically respond to the characteristics and needs of communities has been identified. This type of work is considered to be conservative, in that it conforms to traditional modes of practice, accentuating the importance of individual lifestyle and biomedical conceptions of health within a context of an iniquitous power relationship between professional and client. Because of its inherent hostility towards an acceptance of socio-economic influences on health, it is arguably practice of this type that is the biggest obstacle to achieving community health services which display a true synthesis of the elements of the Health Field Model.

More positively, and despite these difficulties, there would appear to be some optimism for the continued development of community-oriented health promotion. The notion that such practice provides the most ethical and acceptable form of health promotion still prevails (Naidoo and Wills,

1994). For many, the ability to democratically listen to community groups, to act at levels that will in theory have a profound impact on health, and to avoid naive and simple models of practice is extremely beneficial and vital to health promotion in general. Also, in terms of being able to pursue such work, many will argue that the political environment is not so bleak as is sometimes painted. In particular, the concept of healthy settings and its endorsement within *The Health of the Nation* (1992) and various WHO declarations potentially provides a fertile ground for community work.

Irrespective of the practical consequences of these political forces, what this chapter has sought to emphasize is the need for health promoters with a community orientation to be acutely aware of the values and practices they employ in this setting. It has been suggested that community health promotion cannot be seen as merely a technical exercise nor an implicitly 'ideologically sound' exercise. Whenever such work is undertaken, it will be drawing upon profound and powerful ideological roots and it is these that practitioners must be aware of.

References

Adams, L. 1989: Healthy cities, health participation. *Health Education Journal* 48(4), 179–82.

Allsop, J. 1989: Health. In McCarthy, M. (ed.), *The new politics of welfare: an agenda for the 1990s*. Basingstoke: Macmillan.

Arnstein, S. 1969 Eight rungs on a ladder of citizen participation. *AIP Journal* July. 216–24.

Baric, L. 1988: The new public health and the concept of advocacy. *The Journal of the Institute of Health Education* 26(2), 49–55.

Baric, L. 1990: Health promotion and education in a situation of radical change. *The Journal of the Institute of Health Education* 28(4), 105–8.

Baum, F. 1988: Community based research for the promoting of public health. *Health Promotion* 3(3), 259–68.

Beattie, A. 1986: Community development for health: from practice to theory? *Radical Health Promotion* No. 1, 12–19.

Boot, N. 1986: *Community development*. Trent Health Authority Publication.

Bracht, N. and Tsouros, A. 1990: Principles and strategies of effective community participation. *Health Promotion* 5(3), 199–207.

Breihl, J. 1978: Community medicine under Imperialism – a new political police? In Navarro, V. *Class struggle, the state and medicine*. London: Martin Robertson.

Caplan, R. and Holland, R. 1990: Rethinking health education theory. *Health Education Journal* 49(1), 10–13.

Croft, S. and Beresford, P. 1988: The new paternalism. *Social Work Today* 25 Aug, 16–17.

Davies, M. 1985: *The essential social worker: a guide to positive practice*. London: Gower.

DoH 1987: *Promoting better health*. London: HMSO.

DoH 1989: *Caring for people: community care in the next decade and beyond*. Cmd 849. London: HMSO.

DoH 1992: *The health of the nation*. Cmd 1986. London: HMSO.

Dominelli, L. 1990: *Women and community action*. London: Venture Press.

French, J. 1990: Boundaries and horizons, the role of health education within health promotion. *Health Education Journal* **49**(1), 7–10.

George, V. and Wilding, P. 1989: *Ideology and social welfare.* London: Routledge.

Haro, A. 1987: Community development and health. *Health Promotion* **2**, 60–8.

Harrison, S., Hunter, D. and Pollitt, C. 1990: *The dynamics of British health policy.* London: Unwin Hyman.

Jones, J. 1985: On being radical. *Radical Health Promotion* **Summer 1985**, 3–5.

Jones, J. 1991: Community development and health education: concepts and philosophy in Open University Health Education Unit. *Community Development and Health Education,* Vol. 1. Milton Keynes: OU Press.

Kennedy, I. 1982: Medicine and health: great equation or great myth? In *Lifeline Report no 6. Progress in health promotion.* Wessex: Wessex Positive Health Team.

Kerans, P., Drover, G. and Williams, D. 1988: *Welfare and worker participation.* London: Macmillan.

Lee, P. and Raban, C. 1988: *Welfare theory and social policy: reform or revolution?* London: Sage.

Loney, M. (ed.) 1987: *The state or the market: politics and welfare in contemporary Britain.* London: Sage.

Maxwell, R. 1989: *Second thoughts on the White Paper.* London: King Edward's Hospital Fund.

McEwen, J., Martini, C. and Wilkins, N. 1983: *Participation in health.* London: Croom Helm.

McQueen, D. 1989: Thoughts on the ideological origins of health promotion. *Health Promotion* **4**(4). 339–42.

Niadoo, J. and Wills, J. 1994: *Health promotion: foundations for practice.* London: Baillière Tindall.

Navarro, V. (ed.) 1978: *Imperialism, health and medicine.* New York: Baywood.

Rentoul, J. 1989: *Me and mine: the triumph of individualism* London: Blackwell.

Richardson, A. 1983: *Paticipation.* London: Routledge & Keegan Paul.

Richman, J. 1987: *Medicine and health.* London: Longman.

Watt, A. 1986: Community health education: a time for caution? In Romell, S. and Watt A. (eds), *The politics of health education: raising the issues* London RKP.

Seedhouse, D. 1986: *Health: foundations for achievement.* Chichester: Wiley.

Shand, A. 1990: *Free market morality.* London: Routledge.

Smithies, J. and Adams, L. 1990: *Community participation in health promotion.* London: HEA.

Tumwine, J. 1989: Community participation as myth or reality: a personal experience from Zimbabwe. *Health Policy & Planning* **4**(2), 157–61.

Tones, K. 1991: Health promotion, empowerment and the psychology of control. *Journal of the Institute of Health Education* **29**(1), 17–26.

Watt, A. 1986: Community health education: a time for caution? In: Rodmell, S. and Watt, A. (eds), *The politics of health education: raising the issues.* London: Routledge & Kegan Paul.

Watt, A. 1987: Room for movement? The community response to medical dominance. *Radical Community Medicine* **Spring,** 41–5.

Willmott, D. 1988: Community initiatives: patterns and prospects. *PSI research report* **698.**

World Health Organization 1978: *Primary health care report of the international conference on primary health care Alma Ata, USSR.* Health For All Series No. 1. Geneva: WHO.

5 Models of care

Lynn Sbaih

This chapter reviews models of care prior to utilizing Orem's model as an exemplar. The important area of needs assessment is visited and the whole notion of theory is explored. Lynn Sbaih offers some useful objectives concerning models and effectively explores the arena of assessment.

Introduction

This chapter examines the place that various models of care may have within the community. Certain models of care are introduced for consideration by the reader but particular emphasis is placed upon Orem's (1991) model of care. The reasons for this are that Orem has been used in the community (Cookfair, 1991) and, therefore, offers a basis upon which to examine the nature and process of nursing as viewed by one particular model.

From the examination of Orem's (1991) model of care it is anticipated that other models of care can be examined by the reader using the framework of examination put forward within this chapter. The underlying argument that runs through the whole of this chapter is how and when have models of care been developed and how can models, written with reference to the hospital setting, be used in the community setting. The reader should keep this in mind as they move through this chapter.

One of the first issues to be addressed is the environment of the community and the settings in which carers work.

Revisiting the community

Current thinking about community care relates to meeting the needs of individuals within the community (DoH, 1989). Meeting needs means providing a service that encompasses care delivery in the community.
This raises a number of questions including: what is the nature of care delivery in the community? How is nursing organized? How is it communicated? How is it documented? How is continuity of care encouraged? How do all these issues fit into a model of care?
To begin to examine some of the issues raised by these questions, the key

objectives set out in the White Paper, *Caring for People* (DoH 1989) should be reintroduced:

BOX 5.1

Develop the right services to help people live in their own homes wherever this is possible and sensible

Make sure that those who provide services give high priority to giving carers practical support

Make proper assessment of need and good case management the cornerstones of high quality care

Develop a flourishing independent sector alongside good quality public provision

Make sure health and social services are clear about their responsibilities and promote better co-ordination in providing services

Obtain better value for money in providing care (CCSF & RCN, 1993: 2)

With reference to the above, the points relating to assessment of need, good case management and agency co-ordination are the current issues to be addressed by community practitioners. Within this chapter, the issue of assessment is developed and related to frameworks for care. It is anticipated that other issues will emerge from the debate and include involvement of the patient, family, friends and carers in the planning and delivery of various care strategies devised as a result of the exploration of various frameworks for care. To some extent these additional themes are addressed.

Revisiting a definition of the community

To help establish a basis to the chapter it may be useful to be clear about the definition of community in this context and to consider who is included. Is it those who are accommodated in regular housing, or does it include the homeless? Is community about geographical boundaries or the boundaries created by the health centres and general practitioner (GP) surgeries? All of these issues need to be considered if the nurse in the community is to consider the use of theory and models of care and nursing in relation to nursing practice within the community.

The community may be defined as a group of people living in a specific place (Cookfair, 1991). This definition views community within a geographical frame. Community may also be viewed as a 'social system' (Cookfair, 1991: 39). Within the social system practitioners assess the environment, group and individual needs through communication and interaction (RCN, 1992). Both definitions encompass communication with and within groups. The community is a place where the practitioner can manipulate the environment and make decisions. This takes place within the process of assessment, planning, implementation and evaluation (Cookfair, 1991).

BOX 5.2 Nursing within the community

Assessment – planning – implementation – evaluation

OF
the environment
social needs
physical needs
health needs
psychological needs

VIA
communication & interaction

Ways of identifying various needs by way of communication and interpersonal interaction play a part in the way the client and practitioner view health, ill health, needs and problems. All such factors need to be considered within an organization of care framework, within which decisions about various needs and identified problems can be made by the practitioner and patient. The alternative may be considered to be a haphazard approach to care delivery, or guess work. This does not sit well with Table 5.1 *A manifesto for community health nursing for the 1990s* (RCN, 1992), which puts forward a number of community nurse commitments and

Table 5.1 Powerhouse for change. With permission Royal College of Nursing (1992)

A Manifesto for Community Health Nursing for the 1990s
Commitment and Responsibilities

As community health nurses we accept our responsibility to:

1 Use our knowledge and skills to promote the health of the population and of the individual and groups within the population

2 Contribute to the determination of national and local health priorities, the assessment of community health needs, and the planning, commissioning and management of community health services

3 Ensure that our services are accessible, equitable, flexible and responsive to people's needs and wishes. Our services should recognize their right to be informed about their health, their right to choose amongst available options, and to be involved in decisions about their treatment and care

4 Act as advocate for people when they are unable to achieve these rights for themselves

5 Recognize our personal and professional values and health beliefs and also recognize when these differ from those of patients and clients

6 Constantly evaluate our practice, and maintain, monitor and improve standards of nursing services, treatment and care

7 Communicate and collaborate with other health workers to ensure co-ordination and continuity of care

8 Strive to ensure adequate levels of resource provision for community health nursing and use them effectively and efficiently

9 Ensure our own competence by continually updating our knowledge and skills

---

responsibilities. All relate to action based upon clear thinking and an organized, team approach to care delivery incorporating assessment, planning, delivery and evaluation of care. The question to be asked, now, is: does all of this mean using a model of care or nursing? It may mean the adoption of a model of nursing; it may mean the development of another approach. The issue here is that an organized approach to care in the community is required, an approach that is communicated and known to all involved in the process of care and one that encourages partnership between the client and nurse. The starting place for whichever approach is adopted is the process of assessment, action and evaluation, the nursing process. This is considered important as recent initiatives in the community now place considerable emphasis on the assessment of client needs. The beginning of the examination of such issues involves the exploration of theory, for much of what is to be addressed within this chapter may be considered to be grounded in theory.

What is theory?

Hardy (1988) views theory as thinking and inquiring and this is done by most nurses. Nurses have to think about what they do and why they do certain things at some point in their working lives; this may be regarded as theorizing. Theorizing is about thinking and working out how things are organized and employed and this may be done informally or formally. Formal application of thinking and theorizing may be employed within various types of research (McCaugherty, 1992). In nursing, theory tends to be viewed as developing as a result of investigation and organization. The question that may now get asked is what is the value of theory in community nursing practice?

> A common response to inquiries about the value of theory is to point to past and present professional ills in nursing, accounting for them in relation to a paucity of theory and the processes required for its development. (Chinn and Jacobs, 1987)

It may be suggested that, in the past, nursing has had some problem responding to theory development and understanding its use in relation to the delivery, monitoring and development of nursing practice. One of the reasons for this may be a limited appreciation of the need for theory to develop and reflect changes in nursing. Theory, once developed, has to keep up with changes in nursing and nursing practice. This means that a theory has to be constantly evaluated and considered in relation to changes in nursing (Chinn and Jacobs, 1987).

With reference to the community – if community nursing, and the setting in which nursing is delivered, is growing then so should the theory grow. Perhaps one of the issues to be addressed, within the nursing theory/model debate, is that theory should be expected to grow with nursing if the theory is to have meaning to begin with and continue to have meaning who use it to shape their practice. This is an issue to be considered care by nurses in the community as they adopt and develop existing the

A second perceived problem related to the use of theory, is the nature of nursing as a 'doing' occupation (Dingwall *et al.*, 1988) rather than a 'thinking' occupation. Using theory in practice means that nurses have to adapt to different types of information and use knowledge in various other ways which incorporate the use of reflective and analytical skills on a regular basis. Such an approach to practice should then lead to more informed action (Chinn and Jacobs, 1987), rather than a reaction to events within the setting (Walsh and Ford, 1989).

Chinn and Jacobs (1987) suggest that there is much to be gained by using theory. Again the development of thinking is put forward as a means of considering problems, decisions and work from a number of perspectives. Therefore, the use of theory in this context is about thinking about what you know and relating it to what you do and concluding about whether or not this is the right thing or not. To some extent it may be considered that community nurses do this to a certain extent already. However, it is the awareness of the process that Chinn and Jacobs (1987) are perhaps attempting to get across.

Theory has to be considered in detail and, if developed, developed carefully. However, the development of theory is not the end, the constant evaluation and application of theory is just as important. Community nurses cannot accept and make assumptions about theory just because it is a theory. Theory has to be evaluated by community nurses before they can decide on the value or non-value of the theory. This involves knowing about and using frameworks for the evaluation of theory, including various models of nursing.

Nurses do make assumptions about theory and these may relate to theory being believed to improve nursing practice. Alternatively, nurses may view theory as standing in the way of the development of nursing practice (Marriner, 1979). All of this returns us to the need to evaluate theory (Hardy, 1988; Jolley & Allen, 1989). Nurses in the community need to evaluate the

---

BOX 5.3 Evaluating a theory

How does the theory view the patient?

How does the theory view the environment, e.g. the patient's home?

Does the theory address issues of partnership?

Does the theory address issues of collaboration?

Does the theory address issues of accountability?

Does the theory recognize the nature of community nursing?

Is the theory compatible with the philosophy of community care?

... and consider its value in terms of the individual, the ... ...ving and receiving of care. Nurses in the community ... ... the concept of participation in relation to theory ... . The evaluation of theory in this way is important if ... ...munity is to consider the use of theory and to take part ... ... that applies to the provision of nursing within the

Problem solving and the nursing process

Thinking, analysis and evaluation can all be described as part of the process of problem solving. The approach to problem solving adopted by nursing in recent years is often referred to as the nursing process. The nursing process is made up of a number of stages: assessment, planning, goal setting, implementation and evaluation. This appears to be very straightforward, in theory, but the reality of the use of the nursing process appears to be very problematic.

> The nursing process was heralded as a major innovation which was to revolutionise nursing, resulting in a far higher standard of care for patients and more job satisfaction for nurses ... The nursing process is also misunderstood and abused by nurses from one end of the country to the other. (Walsh and Ford, 1989: 141)

On a positive note, Hurst et al. (1991) believe problem solving to be a significant contribution to modern nursing. As a result, nursing has reconsidered its approach to persons and adopted a more individualistic approach. The first stage of the nursing process is assessment.

Assessment in community nursing

The CCSF & RCN (1993) believe that community nurses have an important contribution to make to the assessment of individuals in the community. What community nurses now have to do is to establish their role in the assessment process and place their assessment process within a framework for care – a framework that encompasses collaborative care with other agencies such as social services, partnership with the individual and family and the documentation of care. To address these issues, the current concept of assessment in the community needs to be revisited.

Assessment in the community is currently being addressed. Current examination stems from April 1993 when it was stated that social services would play a lead role in the assessment of persons with social needs (CCSF & RCN, 1993). With reference to this, it is recognized that the community nurse has a role to play in the assessment of patients by way of collaboration with social services. Nurses have a part to play in the assessment of various care needs; what is important is that the right needs are assessed by the right persons. This means that an understanding of collaboration and communication is required by all community nurses involved in the evaluation and development of nursing models/frameworks for care in the community.

Collaborating and communicating in the community assessment process

Problems have arisen in relation to the collaboration of nursing and social services. According to George (1994) as few as 4 per cent of community nurses may have contact with social workers. In addition, the social workers are more likely to be managing the care given whether by nurses or social workers. This is a very interesting comment considering the way that the RCN (1992) and CCSF & RCN (1993) talk about the role of the community nurse and social worker in relation to the assessment of the patient in the community and hospital setting. According to the comment page (Nursing Standard, 1993: 3):

> Many aspects of the new-look community care are currently matters of faith, rather than known facts.

This means that community nurses need to establish their approach to care assessment in the 'new look' community as soon as possible.

Collaborative assessment or lack of collaborative assessment has led to some concern and social workers are finding themselves in a position of attempting to assess health needs (George, 1994). According to Heath (in George, 1994) community nurses need to have a higher profile in the assessment process. This raises the issue of how the assessment is organized and communicated to others, including other nurses both in hospital and the community, other agencies, the patient and family.

> But various groups representing clients or service users have taken a contrary view. Furthermore, there is an additional problem; the community care reforms have occurred against a backdrop of many other related changes. In theory, there could now be several purchasers of health and social care for a patient/client and proposals for both health and local government reorganisation have created uncertainties about who should be doing what joint service planning and with whom. (George, 1994: 18).

This has implications for community nurses attempting to develop frameworks for care in collaboration with other community workers (CCSF & RCN, 1993). Unless joint assessment and planning are considered in detail by all involved parties, including patients and their families, then the development of assessment, planning and evaluation of care by community nurses is doomed from the beginning and community nurses will be in danger of failing to make a mark for themselves; particularly when the nurse is the 'lead carer' for the patient (CCSF & RCN, 1993). The lead carer should be in a position to put forward and devise frameworks for care and decision making by all involved in the care giving and receiving process.

> Although several attempts have been made to assess the impact of community care, the impact on nursing staff has been under explored. (George, 1994: 18)

The question here is why? Why has community care not been investigated by the very people involved in the care giving and receiving? It may be easy to ask such a question but more difficult for the ones involved in the care to be able to step back and consider the changing role of the community nurse in relation to changes in the provision of community care. However, if nurses in the community wish to take a lead role in assessment then they need to consider strategies for the evaluation and development of assessment and the process of nursing within the community in collaboration with other agencies and not remain passive participants in the scheme. Patients also need to be brought into the process and encouraged to give their views about the delivery and receipt of care.

Returning to the 1993 guidelines, the outcome of assessment in the community is viewed as that which identifies the individual's capabilities and how support should be allocated (CCSF & RCN, 1993). Again this refers to the lead role as adopted by social services; however, nurses need to consider what role they have to play in such an assessment. They also need to consider how the assessment process may be developed within a recognized framework for care. Frameworks for the organization of nursing care may then help community nurses to collectively put forward their role in the assessment of such individual needs as mobilization and the ability to care for self. Community nurses need to ask themselves: is the assessment solely part of the social services agenda, or should community nurses be involved from the start? How far can social assessment be separated from the nursing assessment? Again this raises the issues of teamwork and collaborative care as raised earlier.

According to the CCSF & RCN (1993), the assessment of need arrangements 'will build upon existing good practice' (p.6). It is anticipated that nurses will be involved as shown in Box 5.4.

This raises a number of issues that need to be addressed, by community nurses, if assessment of needs in the community is to be established and developed:

- What is good practice and how is it recognized?
- Is it recognized through good documentation and good use of communication using a suitable framework for care?
- Is it dealt with in some other way in the community?

BOX 5.4

Nurse to social services referral following nursing assessment and recognition of social care needs in the individual

Social services to nursing referral for individuals with health needs

Hospital to community nursing and social services referral for persons discharged from hospital for all patients who are discharged from hospital with health and social needs

. . . in some cases, depending on local arrangements, nurses may be the 'lead' assessor. For example, this could happen where health needs are greater than other needs.

(CCSF & RCN, 1993: 7)

Discharge planning: the start of the community assessment process?

With reference to the initial point of contact for assessment in the community, should the assessment of the patient begin when the patient arrives home? If so, how soon after arriving home should the patient be assessed? Or should the community nurse be more actively involved in the discharge planning of the patient before the patient leaves the hospital? That is, the community assessment of the patient begins with the hospital discharge of the patient. Or should the community assessment of the patient begin even earlier? For example, it is no good assessing the home conditions of the patient as they are about to leave hospital, perhaps the assessment of the home conditions should begin earlier.

Community nurses need to consider when assessment begins and may decide that assessment begins prior to discharge of the patient from hospital; that is, the community nurse is involved with the patient in discharge planning. Less than 10 per cent of community nurses are actively involved in discharge planning. Issues such as inappropriate preparation of the patient's home, lack of time to communicate with various agencies and inappropriate recognition of lay carers' problems were all issues of concern and inadequately addressed. This raises a number of issues relating to time and access to patients and their families. However, they are issues to be addressed by community nurses if the assessment process within the community is to be challenged and updated.

Continuity of care from hospital to home raises issues relating to the continuity of frameworks of care from hospital to home. Community nurses need to be speaking to hospital nurses so that the similarities and differences relating to frameworks for care can be acknowledged. This means working and communicating together (CCSF & RCN, 1993). If blended hospital and community frameworks of care are not possible then community nurses need to consider how and why the approach to assessment, care planning and evaluation of care may be similar or different and plan their approach to problem solving accordingly. This also raises the issue of continuation of documentation from hospital to community to hospital. Can this happen? Is it a realistic option for community nurses,? Have community nurses considered this as an option?

> All patients who are discharged from hospital and who have long term needs either for support in their own homes or who need nursing home or residential care, will need to be assessed. They will also need a package of care put together for them. Hospital social workers will coordinate these assessments, but you will also have a key role as part of the multidisciplinary team.
>
> You should be familiar with:
> – arrangements and guidelines for hospital discharge
> – how patients who have long-term care needs will be assessed;
> – who will be responsible for arranging the assessment;
> – any agreed time scales for carrying out an assessment; and
> – how care will be arranged, including nursing home or residential care. (CCSF & RCN, 1993: 8)

All of this suggests that assessment in the community underpins everything that will follow. Therefore, it seems necessary and important that the assessment is done properly. Community nurses need to seek collective definitions of assessment and establish the place of assessment within any developed or adopted framework for care. The ways in which that assessment is addressed within various models of care should be explored as this seems to be a logical starting point for the examination of nursing models which may be viewed as models for care in the community.

Such an examination will raise the issue of collaboration; that is collaboration with hospital multidisciplinary staff as well as collaboration with community agencies. However, what the community nurse should remember in all of this is that the process of assessment, which is the beginning and a fundamental part of the nursing process, underpinning the use of a framework for care which may be a nursing model, is the foundation upon which all these issue are being addressed. The other point to be raised here is that many nursing models have been developed within the hospital setting and need to be examined from this perspective. Ultimately, it should be remembered that community nurses have a right and indeed an obligation to patients, clients and families to address such issues in depth before any decision relating to adoption or avoidance of them is considered.

The impact of assessment on care planning in the community

It has already been established that social services will initiate the development of a care plan for the assessed individual. The development of a plan will be related to the resources available (CCSF & RCN, 1993). Again, community nurses need to consider their role in care planning to meet the health needs of individuals in the community in collaboration with social services. A definition of what constitutes health needs may be useful here and how such identified needs relate to the use of various frameworks for care by community nurses, patients and their carers. Recognition and a consensus on the definition of health needs by the nurse, patient and family should lead to a recognition of partnership in the assessment, care planning, implementation and evaluation of care in the community by nurses in collaboration with social services personnel.

Documenting assessment in the community

Where is all the information that relates to the process of nursing? Is it all in your head? If so how do patients gain access to the process of assessment, planning and evaluation and the basis upon which decision making is undertaken? The nurse may state that they tell them but is this enough to create a basis for a partnership in care? Is partnership in the community based upon one person (the patient) having to wait to be told a number of factors by the other (the nurse) before a decision effecting the person's care can be made by both parties? This aspect of documentation of care in the community by nurses requires some consideration.

All patients are now required to be given a copy of their care plan, whether this be developed by social or nursing services (CCSF & RCN, 1993). This has implications for the way that community nurses document care and share such documentation with the patient, family and carers. For example, one way of documenting care in the community would be to facilitate the patient and carers to document their own care and keep diaries. This may be developed into a contract of care between the nurse and individual and reflect the framework of care used in the way that assessment, implementation and evaluation of care is organized. The nurse could supplement this with other care documentation (UKCC, 1994).

There are advantages to this approach in that the client has a degree of involvement and helps set the agenda for care in that they identify problems and issues of importance to them. They have ownership of the care episode and it is not solely directed by the nurse. Documented issues written down in the time and comfort of the home without the nurse present with time to think about issues may also provide a different slant to the nurses question of 'what do you think/want?'

There are also disadvantages associated with patient-monitored documentation of care. Documentation of care would depend upon the patient's/carer's motivation to document issues and problems and evaluation of care. Also the person would need to be literate, understand and be comfortable with reading and writing in English and be happy to document in the nurse's absence. The person may see this as the nurse opting out of caring for them and getting the patient to do their work. Of course the physical and mental condition of the patient may also make it difficult to pursue this approach to documentation but it is worth a try.

Staying with documentation, the CCSF & RCN (1993) suggest that community nurses should be familiar with local assessment procedures and the use of assessment forms. The use of assessment forms raises a number of issues:

- It is clear that the role of the community nurse is seen as valuable but how does the use of predeveloped assessment forms reflect the organization of the nursing assessment within an identified framework for care?
- Who has agreed the assessment form?
- Have community nurses been involved, if so which community nurses?
- Those that provide the regular care through contact with the patient and carer are the ones who will need to complete the assessment form. Does the form reflect the organization of the nursing assessment?
- If such a form is now in use how does it reflect a framework for care that has been devised by community nurses?
- How does it reflect community nurses' philosophy of care?
- Can one form be used in all areas of the community?
- Is not the development of the form influenced by the environment and client groups served and the sort of issues, problems and needs of various client groups?
- Can a generic form do all of this in a realistic way?

All these questions illustrate documentation-related issues that need to be addressed by community nurses. All have implications for nurses in the community as well as for the patient and family. A framework for care or a problem-solving approach to the process of assessment should be reflected through the documentation. Generic documentation may promote the value or undervalue the assessment of the nurse in terms of the patients' health needs.

Rituals and routines related to the nursing process

In Walsh and Ford's (1989) work, the examination of the ritualization of use of the nursing process takes place in the hospital setting. They explore the task-centred approach and conclude that such an approach reduced people to '. . . a collection of tasks' (Walsh and Ford, 1989: 141). They also view task-centred nursing as reducing the initiative of the individual nurse and patient. Lack of preparation to utilize the nursing process is viewed as one of the main stumbling blocks to the inappropriate introduction and use of the nursing process. However, can this be stated in 1996 or are community nurses now comfortable with nursing theory and its application in practice?

Walsh and Ford (1989) conclude that there continues to be a lack of understanding as to the use and meaning of the nursing process.

> To the average nurse the nursing process means patient allocation and care plans. (p. 143)

Most of the examples in the chapter relate to the hospital setting so it is difficult to establish whether the ritualized practice exists in the community. So where does that leave the community nurse? To begin with nurses in the community need to consider how they approach problem solving in relation to the delivery of nursing care.

Systematic, deliberate thought is related to the process of consideration and reflection (Benner, 1984) and is fast becoming a requirement for all nurses actively involved in the delivery of care in the community (RCN, 1992). Therefore, the need to consider theory in practice is required by way of a thoughtful and organized approach. This means that the nurse has a rational argument upon which to accept the theory that, in turn, has been developed as a result of rational, thoughtful and organized approach to its development. This is in contrast to the use of rituals which are grounded in gossip and unrigorous practices (Walsh and Ford, 1989). Perhaps one of the starting points to address the many issues further is to establish the philosophy of care in the community.

So far this chapter has considered the assessment process in the community and suggested that community nurses explore the process in

---

BOX 5.5 Nursing in the community: a basis or a philosophy of community nursing

What do community nurses do?

What is the role of the nurse within the community?

How do nurses assess, identify problems, plan and evaluate care?

What do patients do?

What is the role of the patient?

How is the patient involved?

How is the carer involved?

How do they all participate?

How does the nurse document care episodes?

How does collaboration with other agencies taken place?

detail and the role that they have to play within it. This now needs to be considered in relation to philosophies and frameworks for care in more detail.

Answering the questions in Box 5.5 in partnership with clients will form the basis for a philosophy of community care. The term *with clients* suggests that any team of nurses set up to examine a philosophy of community nursing will have within it representatives of client groups.

In addition to the questions in Box 5.5, the reader may have other questions they wish to answer. Addressing issues raised as a result of answering the above questions leads to a need to explore other factors such as the historical background to community nursing, the organization of nurses' work in the community by doctors, other agencies, the patient and carer and skill mix.

The values and beliefs which direct community health nursing in all its forms are reflected in the following statements:

- Community health nursing is directed towards the achievement of the goal of health for all. We believe that health is a fundamental human right and that all people have an equal right to health and access to health care.
- We accept the definition of primary health care contained in the World Health Organization declaration at Alma Ata in 1978 and are committed to the strategy for achieving health for all through the development of primary health care, of which community health nursing is an integral part. (RCN, 1992: 1)

The RCN (1992) also believe that:

... community health nursing makes a major contribution to primary health care at all levels and that community health nurses must be involved in policy decisions and the planning, commissioning and management of services as well as the provision of care. (RCN, 1992: 1)

This leads to a need to consider assessment in the wider sense – to consider assessment of the community as a whole – as this may help community nurses set the pace for the development of needs meeting in individuals in the community. Again a recognized framework for care that recognizes the definition of community, the philosophies of nurses and individuals receiving care in the community may encompass assessment of the community as well as the individual. The question that community nurses need to ask is – are models of nursing able to assist community nurses to define the community and assess the community in the wider sense? This is an issue to be considered when analysing the value of various nursing models in the community.

Frameworks for care – the story so far

... people have the right to make informed choices and to be involved in their own health care. Therefore, we are committed to promoting services which are responsive to people's wishes as well as their needs. We believe that people's needs should be the main determinant for deployment of nursing skills and resources. (RCN, 1992: 1)

This brings us back to some issues already addressed within this chapter including partnership in care, information giving, communication and documentation, all of which could be organized within a recognized framework for care, namely a model of nursing. Do nursing models address the issues of partnership and communication? If they do, how is this done? Do nursing models consider partnership and communication in relation to hospital settings? If so, can these be translated into the community and if so, how?

... health education and health promotion are an essential part of the role of every community health nurse. Community health nurses are an important resource to which people should have direct access for education, information and advice as well as treatment and care. (RCN, 1992: 1)

Organization of health education may take place within a recognized framework for care. Community nurses need to examine frameworks for care to establish whether they can adopt frameworks for care to address health promotion issues (see Chapter 4). Also community nurses need to consider how health promotion is viewed within various models for care and whether issues relating to health promotion at the time the model was devised, in the hospital setting, can be translated into the community setting in the 1990s. This relates to the ability of theory to be subject to development and the ability of nurses to develop theory (Chinn and Jacobs, 1987).

... community health nursing contributes to primary health care both independently and in partnership with carers, statutory and non statutory agencies. We are committed to inter-disciplinary approaches to health care based upon team work and partnership. (RCN, 1992: 1)

When examining nursing models and their place in the community, community nurses need to establish how various models for care delivery encourage collaborative care. Or do nursing models tend to see nursing in isolation of other agencies? If nursing is seen in isolation of other agencies, this raises problems for the community nurse, as partnership and collaboration in care are very much part of the current community care agenda (CCSF & RCN, 1993).

... qualified nurses, whatever their field of practice, are accountable for their professional decisions and actions, and every community health nurse must be a safe and competent practitioner, appropriately prepared for whatever work is undertaken. (RCN, 1992: 1)

The exploration of nursing models, therefore, requires community nurses to consider how accountability is viewed and addressed. Is accountability implied or made explicit within nursing models? How do such approaches influence the use of a particular model in the community? To continue this debate further, an introduction to various models of care is required. The most established one will be introduced first.

The medical model

The principles of the biomedicine have been used as a model and knowledge base for Western health care practice for over three hundred years. . . . However, although the medical model may be considered appropriate for dealing with the physical aspects of a person, there are many who feel it is of limited use as a basis for delivering nursing care. (Kendrick and Simpson, 1992: 92)

It has already been established that community care is about reflection, communication, interaction, documentation, participation, collaboration and evaluation. The medical model may be unable to provide a basis for the organization of care based upon these factors.

Nursing models: an introduction

Nursing models represent nursing (Sbaih,1992); therefore, the model of nursing should represent community nursing and the belief, values and ideas held by community nurses and clients within the community. This is reflected in commonly used nursing models; Roper *et al.* (1983) view nursing as activities of daily living and Orem (1991) views nursing in terms of self-care principles. What community nurses have to establish is how close are these views of nursing to that of community nursing. If the model of Orem was to be adopted within a community setting would the nurses and clients view the organization and outcomes of nursing as Orem would? This question needs to be addressed before adoption of the model of nursing can take place.

Nursing models, like many other professional models, are constructed through the use of words. (Sbaih, 1992: 64)

Use of words by the author of the model may make access to the literature about that particular model difficult. Nurses in the community need to consider this aspect of nursing model adoption also, as this may increase the time it takes to examine a model within the nursing team. MacFarlane (1986) believes that all nurses know how nursing should be practised; that is, they carry their own model of nursing in their head. After all, nurses in the community are qualified and have been prepared through various educational initiatives to practice nursing. It may be stated from this that community nurses do indeed have a set of organized ideas, a model, of how nursing should be practised. With reference to philosophies of care and the process of nursing, such ideas need to be made explicit and shared with other community nurses and clients. Emphasis should be placed upon the sharing of ideas for this may be the key to the development of nursing models in the community. The use of a framework for care should provide a common starting place for all nurses and clients and provide a guide for the development of questions by the nurse, client and family to gain information. It should provide a basis for reflection of care giving and receipt, participation, collaboration within the process of assessment, action and evaluation.

This should then provide the basis for the development of an organized team approach to nursing in the community.

Models of wellness

An important aspect of community nursing may be the emphasis on well being and so many of the models of nursing constructed to care for ill health may have limited suitability. However, it is accepted that most models of nursing do consider the individual in good health as well as ill health (Cookfair, 1991).

The self-efficacy model

This considers how individual behaviour contributes to wellness and includes the motivation and skills required to pursue and maintain good health (Desmond and Price, 1988). Within this model, the issues of difficulty, belief in personal skills to achieve health and the application of specific health acquisition skills to other health-related situations are examined. The authors of the model suggest that a contract between the individual and nurse may be one way of increasing health-related skills. To this should be added support: support of the nurse, other community agencies, the family, friends and carers.

Holistic nursing perspective

This is another health-related model of care (Blattner, 1981). This framework concentrates on the relationship of nine parts to each other: communication, human development, self-responsibility, problem solving, caring, stress, lifestyle, teaching–learning and leadership which incorporates change. All nine areas are required if the client is to achieve and maintain wellness. They are connected via a process of interpersonal, which includes the family; intrapersonal, which includes the relationship between the client and nurse; and community, which includes specific organization of individuals into groups.

As stated earlier, the choice of any model of care should be based upon examination of personal and group philosophies within the nursing and client team and should include the following:

- the community
- the setting/the home
- the client/family
- partnership
- community nursing.

An awareness of all the above factors may be closely associated with an understanding or awareness of personal values and beliefs and how these relate to the provision of nursing in the community. This in turn leads to the need to be clear about personal philosophies and the philosophy underpinning nursing in the community. To begin with this should be viewed as personal beliefs and values and then local and national beliefs and values about community nursing should be considered. How do all these relate to each other? Are they compatible? Or not? This can be related to previous discussions about the development of nursing and patient philosophies in the community.

The nursing model of Orem: an introduction

The following is an introduction to the theory of nursing as generated by Orem and which resulted in the development of the Self Care Deficit Theory of Nursing (Orem, 1991). The detail given in relation to the theories of Orem should provide a framework for community nurses to consider other nursing models available and to consider them within their own practice.

CHARACTERISTICS OF NURSES

Nurses need to be aware of strengths and weaknesses and the impact that various judgements have upon themselves, patients and the delivery of patient care. The nurse needs to have an understanding of what nursing means to them and the patient. Both parties need to understand who is to do the 'doing' of care – the patient or the nurse? The relationship should be seen as one of 'helping' (p259). Orem suggests the following as 'desirable nurse characteristics' (p. 261):

- To be knowledgeable about the situation and have specialized knowledge about various social and legal issues relating to the given situation.

- To be aware of culture and its impact on the person and family and how it may influence communication with others perceived to be in and outside the identified culture.
- To be able to communicate effectively using listening and other techniques.
- To view the development of self and others in positive terms and recognize the differences between developmental needs and wants.
- To accept responsibility for the delivery of nursing care to patients in a calm and courteous manner.
- To understand what nursing is and the goals of nursing and appreciate that nursing may be viewed in different ways by patients and their families, and community trusts.
- To appreciate the development of relationships both with colleagues, managers and patients and their families.

This can be related to page 87 of this chapter and the formulization of a nursing philosophy that reflects the thoughts, beliefs and values of the community nurses and client groups served by the community nurses.

OREM'S VIEW OF NURSING

Form: this is expressed through 'helping and taking care of characteristics' (p. 57). It also refers to the ability of nurses to deal with life situations. Involvement in such situations produces 'goal orientated deliberate actions of nurses and their patients' (p. 57). Both form and situations influence the development of theories relating to nursing. This is because form should take on a reflective nature. It should be about developing and discussing the issues found in any one helping or caring situation and being able to develop strategies for future similar situations; that is, it should contribute to theory development by way of its predictability factor.

   Orem asks a number of questions:

- What do nurses intend to do when they nurse?
- What do nurses make when they nurse? (p. 57)

The first question relates to nurses being able to explore what nursing is to them and this then should lead to the production of a philosophy of nursing. This is an important step when considering the delivery of nursing in the community, either through nursing models or by way of other means or frameworks. It is useful to be able to consider the definitions of what you believe you are doing as you may need to discuss these further with various patients and clients. That is, you will not be asked: 'what is your philosophy of nursing?' but may be asked: 'why do you need to do that or why do I have to do this?' Both questions refer to what you and what the patient understand to be the nature of nursing and both refer to what you and what the patient understand to be the reason you are there, all of which relates to your philosophy of nursing and the patient's philosophy of nursing.

OREM'S THEORY OF NURSING

Orem suggests that a theory of nursing is necessary if the nursing is to be structured and able to meet the demands of the patient by way of a sound relationship. It is also about having nursing situations analysed and considered, reflected upon and decisions made from these that may influence similar, future nursing situations. Good theory development therefore involves recognition of situations and the form they take and reflection upon these situations and the evaluation of actions taken as a result of strategies developed in response to the original situations and form taken.

According to Orem (p. 59) one of the reasons that theory development took place in the USA was because of nurses':

> ... questions about their proper work, about time available for nursing, and their relationships to persons seeking and receiving nursing and to members of other health care disciplines.

This is an interesting point when related to community nursing in the UK, as these may be some of the questions currently being asked by community nurses, managers and the managers of community trusts.

Orem found that stable conditions in any working group allow all group members to continue to work in the ways that they always have done but instability and in particular issues surrounding the boundaries of nursing care led to a need to consider the questions as raised above. Again thoughts about UK nursing in the community relate to rapid change which has resulted in role boundaries being discussed and disputed at times. In particular, issues associated with the role of the health care support worker have led to nurses asking questions similar to those raised by Orem.

OBSTACLES TO THE DEVELOPMENT OF NURSING THEORY

Orem recognized that there were many obstacles in the way of theory development. These could come from persons outside nursing not understanding the nature of nursing but also from inside nursing as well.

> Some recognised internal barriers to the advancement and development of nursing included the continuing focus of nurses on tasks and procedures, many of which were outmoded; demands of nurses that exceeded their preparation; the unstructured state of nursing knowledge; the inability of many nurses to formulate goals of care specific to nursing; and the inability of many nurses to communicate adequately about nursing with persons under nursing care and their families and with members of other health care disciplines, administrators, and officials of governments. (p. 60)

OREM'S DEVELOPMENT OF NURSING THEORY

First, Orem considered her own experiences of nu
consideration as to how nursing may meet the various fe
condition, she formulated the following statement in 195.

> The inability of a person to provide continuously for se.
> and quality of required self-care because of the situation
> health. (p. 61)

She continued by stating that:

> Self care was conceptualised as the personal care that human beings
> require each day and that may be modified by health state,
> environmental conditions, the effects of medical care, and other factors.
> (p. 61)

Through these statements Orem was able to answer the question 'what is nursing?'; that is, she had begun to think about and formulize her philosophy of nursing – a philosophy that was to shape the development of a theory of nursing that shaped the process of the delivery of nursing care to patients. That is, Orem had found the beginnings of her nursing model.

This raises a number of issues for nurses working in the community:

- What is your view of nursing?
- What is the client's view of nursing?
- What is the client's family's view of nursing?
- Do any of you recognize or identify with Orem's understanding of nursing?

If the answer to the last question is YES then you may be able to use Orem's model of care as a framework for your care delivery. If the answer is NO then you need to think why this may be so. Is it because you/the patient/ the family have never given these issues much thought, or is it because you view nursing in some other way? If you do view nursing in another way then this may lead you to consider an alternative model of nursing that does reflect your beliefs and the patient's beliefs about nursing and the delivery of nursing care. This is perhaps a fundamental problem with the use of nursing models in UK nursing, in that the philosophies of the involved parties have not been explored. A nursing model is adopted for various reasons but if the basis of the model, the philosophy, is not recognizable by those who are to use the nursing model then problems may be ahead as all attempt to fit their understanding of nursing, and the delivery of care, into a framework that is in conflict with their fundamental beliefs about nursing.

A NURSING SYSTEM

By 1991 Orem had developed '. . . a theoretical concept of a nursing system' (p. 62). *System* was defined as comprising individuals, actions or other phenomena that were related to each other in some way. As a result of the

ship they acted and could be viewed as a whole. Therefore, any
nge to the components of the whole (individual, action to other) have an
impact on the whole; that is, the system. Nursing systems had an added
ingredient of self-organization. A nursing system would be produced through
nursing and patient action required to develop a relationship for the purpose
of the delivery of patient care. Timing of action was viewed as important.

> Nursing has no concrete existence except through persons in
> relationships of nurse and patient and through what they choose and
> proceed to do or not do within the relationship. (p. 63)

Orem viewed the nursing system as a product that would have a positive
influence on the patient.

Orem's conceptual (i.e. thinking) model considered the following:

- *Self care*: learned behaviour that is usually directed towards the
  development of goals that increase well being and health.
- *Dependant care*: performed by 'responsible adults for socially dependent
  individuals' (p. 62).
- *Nursing agency*: consists of the attributes of those prepared to be nurses
  and who are able to help others to realize their ability/lack of ability to
  behave in an appropriate manner to meet various needs at various times
  in certain situations. Such needs may be associated with the physical,
  psychological and sociological aspects of ill health and injury. To do this,
  nurses may use various technologies or other methods.
- *Self-care agency*: viewed as complex and is the ability for adults to
  recognize factors within themselves that can be managed so that various
  needs may be met and self-development may take place.

THE SELF-CARE DEFICIT THEORY OF NURSING

This model of nursing was further developed by way of consideration of
self-care, self-care deficits and nursing systems. The result of this was the
self-care deficit theory of nursing which explained the relationship between
what individuals do and '. . . their demands for self care or the care demands
of children or adults who are dependents' (p. 73). The term *deficit* is viewed
as a relationship that incorporates action and the ability of the individual
to seek self-care or dependent-care. Self-care deficits have their basis in the
structure and function of the person.

This model accepts that nursing responds to individuals that are unable
to act to meet needs in themselves because of a change in their health. Self-
care occurs when the individual is mature enough to understand the impact
of actions upon health and needs. Disabled persons or persons with chronic
illness may be unable to act in a manner to meet needs and maintain good
health and so require the assistance of nursing. Orem views the model as
being able to assist nurses in the delivery of structured nursing care, in the
development of nursing knowledge and in the teaching and preparation of
nurses to practice nursing.

There are eight functions:

- To determine the views of humans within society.
- To recognize the role of nursing in society.
- To establish a language of nursing and through this identify concepts, knowledge and practice.
- To develop nursing research and education.
- To 'reduce cognitive load' (p. 74) by the provision of a framework for the receipt of information and to consider nursing in relation to everyday situations.
- To 'allow inferences to be made' about the development of nursing within society and various communities.
- To increase 'a style of thinking' (p. 74) and communication in nursing.
- To increase the cohesion of nurses and to bring about consensus about various aspects of nursing work and care delivery.

It is also appreciated that nurses may wish to develop various practice styles within the theory. Nurses want to see persons as individuals and are aware of personal judgements, likes and dislikes. Nursing will develop within the system and will require evaluation. Documentation of nursing will improve and reflect the organization of nursing as set out by the theory. Referral between nurses and other agencies is increased; nurses are involved in nursing discharge procedures. Nursing boundaries are challenged and debated and the responsibilities of nurses are enhanced in relation to the delivery of patient and family care.

Denyes (1988) supports Orem's approach to health being maximized by the use of self-care. This is developed further and three categories are identified as prerequisites for self-caring. These are knowledge of self, self-awareness and knowledge of strategies to support health; ability to take responsibility by being motivated and recognizing the needs of others by doing no harm to others; finally, there is a need to value self. From the given information it may be suggested that for an individual (patient or nurse) to accept the idea of self-caring and then put it into practice they must recognize the above attributes.

These can be summarized below:

- knowledge of self and strategies to support health
- self-awareness
- ability to take responsibility
- motivation
- valuing others and doing no harm to others
- valuing self.

What has Orem's model of care to do with community nursing?

Orem's model of nursing provides a framework for the evaluation of other nursing models as follows:

(1) *Determine team (nurses and clients) philosophy*
- characteristics of nurses
- view of nursing

(2) *The model of care*
- theory of nursing
- obstacles to the development of theory
- development of nursing
- development of organization of work framework incorporating assessment, action and evaluation

(3) *Evaluation of the model*
- continuing development of theory
- evaluation and development of philosophy.

All of the above need to be considered within the community setting and specific application of the model of nursing within hospital and community settings needs to be thoroughly examined.

Therapeutic nursing: an alternative to nursing models in the community?

A development of frameworks for care may be considered to be therapeutic nursing. So the term therapeutic nursing may be seen as the answer, for it may offer a more holistic approach to care of the patient and therefore a more realistic framework for care (Wilson-Barnett, 1984; Pearson, 1989). This modern approach to frameworks for care is viewed as requiring nurse autonomy, skill, knowledge and the ability to communicate and solve problems (Pearson and Vaughan, 1986; McMahon, 1988).

This raises a number of problems, for, according to Pearson (1989), acute hospitals do not encourage nurse autonomy and tend to concentrate on the medical approach to care via crisis and symptom intervention. This leads to the meeting of physical needs only and the patient is not cared for holistically. Once again, all of this needs to be related to the meeting of needs of individuals in the community via established assessment processes that reflect various philosophies including the patient and nurse. The influence of the medical model and the work of other agencies in the community, such as social services, and their impact upon the assessment, delivery and evaluation of nursing care in the community should also be considered in detail.

McMahon and Pearson (1992) suggest that four areas of nursing may be considered therapeutic (p. 5): the nurse–patient relationship; nursing interventions; traditional and non-traditional; and patient teaching. Ersser (1988) viewed being therapeutic as providing comfort and a suitable environment. Muetzel (1988) considered partnership, intimacy and reciprocity as the ingredients of the nurse–patient relationship, which may then be considered therapeutic.

All the principle nursing models view health holistically, and see it as the objective of nursing care. In the past, nurses theorists have considered the therapeutic aspects of nursing from a number of different perspectives. (McMahon, 1992: 3)

A strategy for nursing care in the community:

- know your own philosophy
- know the philosophy of your colleagues
- know the philosophy of your clients.

Relate all to local and national philosophies and policies re community care:

- know the definition of assessment, planning, action and evaluation
- know how clients and families view these terms
- know how colleagues view these terms
- know how other agencies e.g. social workers view these terms
- know how hospital colleagues view these terms.

Put all this together to come up with a working definition of assessment, planning, action and evaluation that will form the basis of any protocols within the community setting:

- get to know the frameworks for care in the hospital, used by other agencies
- find out what your colleagues understand by various frameworks for care
- find out how the various components (e.g. assessment) fit into various frameworks
- consider how decisions about care are made by community staff, ask colleagues and managers.

Now, consider a suitable framework for care that compliments hospital and other agencies' approach to organization of care and decision making. The framework should be sensitive to the philosophies of those involved in its use and administration. Now get patients, clients and their families to evaluate the usefulness of any model for care put forward. The above strategy may be very difficult to execute in practice. If so, you need to consider why and how some of the issues of concern may be addressed. The initial approach may be through the patients you know in the community that form part of your caseload. You could always get them to evaluate aspects of the care given. The difficult part here is to design a tool that allows the patient freedom of thought and choice regarding the answers given to the questions raised. Not easy . . . but worth a try!

Pulling the issues together . . .

If you are a nurse working in the community you are in a good position to contribute to a local assessment of community care needs in your area. In particular you can:

- identify people with potential and actual nursing needs;
- develop a profile of your neighbourhood;
- analyse your workload/caseload; and
- talk to people and their carers to find out what their perceived needs are. (CCSF & RCN, 1993: 9)

This relates to the philosophy, collaboration and organization of care and may be a good starting point for community nurses. Community nurses could begin by asking persons in the community and their carers how, why and what they require. From this, the community nurse can consider what they believe is the direction the community care should take, taking into consideration the role of other agencies in the community, the direction of the assessment, the role of the hospital and the planning and delivery of care as done by nurses and community nurses.

Caseload is another important starting point, you need to know where you stand before you go anywhere else; that is, you need to evaluate what you are doing and your workload before you move on. The purpose of this chapter has not been to get you to change your work practices but to get you to think about alternative ways of working and organizing and to consider you role in care assessment, planning and delivery and evaluation of care in the community. The whole emphasis of the chapter has been to review the position of various nursing models in relation to the community but this cannot be done in isolation of what is happening in the community now.

This chapter has also raised issues relating to wider community nursing practice as community nurses are being asked to assess the needs of the community as a whole. Again, this comes back to the awareness, understanding and ability to assess various needs and problems in collaboration with others, in particular hospitals, social services and the patient and carers. The final question to be asked is – can frameworks for care help community nurses address such issues?

Some evaluations of Orem's model of care

When health was considered merely the absence of disease, the relationship was not upheld. This is an excellent example of differing results based upon changes in conceptualising one variable. How one views self-care is altered by the operational definition of the intervening variables and this type of influence needs to be identified. (Allen and Hayes 1989: 80)

A mechanism for intervention is an inherent part of Orem's model and Hartley (1988) tested the conceptualisation that there is a relationship between the nursing system and self care concepts. Based upon the proposition that a supportive–educative nursing system influences self care behaviour, it was found that regardless of the congruence between teaching and learning style, supportive–educative strategies were effective. (Allen and Hayes 1989: 80)

Allen and Hayes (1989) believe that the tools that have been used to develop and evaluate models need to be considered. Gulik (1987) developed the Activities of Daily Living Self-Care scale. This was developed 'using the activities of daily living inherent in the universal and developmental self-care requisites of Orem's model' (Allen and Hayes, 1989: 82). The tool was designed to be used with a specific group of patients, those with multiple sclerosis. According to Gulik (1987), the tool needs to be tested on various client groups before it may be used in general. This raises an important question about the use of a nursing model like Orem for all client groups. Is this realistic? In practice can one framework be useful for all client groups? The answer lies in its evaluation with various client groups and the evaluation should be done by community nurses involved with certain client groups. Dodd (1982, 1984, 1988) investigated one aspect of Orem's model – self-care behaviours, particularly in persons diagnosed as having cancer and in relation to treatment protocols.

. . . Bunting (1988) has identified that the concept of perception is used in various nursing models and notes that there are some differences from one model to another. Lang and Hamlin (1988) have also identified that self-concept is of great relevance in most of the models. Also, the notion that nursing is humanistic can be found in a number of models, or the model itself is described as humanistic (Fenton, 1987). (Allen and Hayes, 1989: 86)

Attention needs to be paid to the concepts that are used in more than one nursing model. Such concepts are often essential to understanding the models even though they are not specific to the model. (Allen and Hayes, 1989: 86)

References

Allen, M.N. and Hayes, P. 1989: Models of nursing: implications for nursing research. *Recent Advances in Nursing* **24** 77–92.
Benner, P. 1984: *From novice to expert: excellence and power in clinical nursing.* Belmont, CA: Addison-Wesley.
Blattner, B. 1981: *Holistic nursing.* Englewood Cliffs, NJ: Prentice-Hall.
Bunting, S.M. 1988: The concept of perception in selected nursing theories. *Nursing Science Quarterly* **1** 168–74.

Chinn, P.L. and Jacobs, M.K. 1987: *Theory and nursing: a systematic approach.* St Louis: CV Mosby.

Community Care Support Force and The Royal Collage of Nursing (CCSF & RCN) 1993: *Community care: what hospital and community nurses need to know.* London: HMSO.

Cookfair, J.M. 1991: *Nursing process and practice in the community.* St Louis: Mosby Year Book.

Denyes, M.J. 1988: Orem's model used for health promotion: directions from research. *Advances in Nursing Science* 11(1), 13–21.

Desmond, S.M. and Price, J.H. 1988: Self-efficacy and weight control. *Health Education* 19(1), 12–21.

Dodd, M.J. 1982: Assessing patient self-care for side effects of cancer chemotherapy. *Cancer Nursing* 5 447–51.

Dodd, M.J. 1984: Patterns of self-care in cancer patients receiving radiation therapy. *Oncology Nursing Forum* 11(3), 23–7.

Dodd, M.J. 1988: Patterns of self-care in patients with breast cancer. *Western Journal of Nursing Research* 10(1), 7–24.

DoH 1989: *Caring for people: community care in the next decade and beyond.* Cmd 849. London: HMSO.

Dingwall, R., Rafferty, A.M. and Webster, C. 1988: *An introduction to the social history of nursing.* London: Routledge.

Ersser, S. 1988: Nursing beds and nursing therapy. In Pearson, A. (ed.), *Primary nursing: nursing in the Burford and Oxford nursing development units.* London: Croom Helm.

Fenton, M.V. 1987: Development of a scale of humanistic nursing behaviours. *Nursing Research* 36, 82–7.

George, M. 1994: Two cheers for the changes. *Nursing Standard* 8(27), 18–20.

Gulik, E.E. 1987: Parsimony and model confirmation of the ADL self-care scale of multiple sclerosis persons. *Nursing Research* 36(5), 278–83.

Hardy, L.K. 1988: Excellence in nursing through debate – the case of nursing theory. *Advances in Nursing* 21, 1–13.

Hartley, L.A. 1988: Congruence between teaching and learning self-care. A pilot study. *Nursing Science Quarterly* 1, 161–7.

Hurst, K., Dean, A. and Trickey, S. 1991: The recognition and nonrecognition of problem solving strategies in nursing practice. *Journal of Advanced Nursing* 16, 1444–55.

Jolley, M. and Allan, P. (eds) 1989: *Current issues in nursing.* London: Chapman & Hall.

Kendrick, K. and Simpson, A. 1992: The nurses' reformation: philosophy and pragmatics of Project 2000. In Soothill, K., Henry, C. and Kendrick, K. (eds), *Themes and perspectives in nursing.* London: Chapman & Hall.

Lang, K.A. and Hamlin, C. 1988: Use of the Piers–Harris self concept scale with Indian children: cultural considerations. *Nursing Research* 37, 42–6.

MacFarlane, J. 1986: The value of models for care. In Kershaw, B. and Salvage, J. (eds), *Models for nursing.* Chichester: John Wiley.

Marriner, M. 1979: *Nursing management of the patient with pain,* 2nd edn. Philadelphia: J.B. Lippincott.

McCaugherty, D. 1992: The concepts of theory and practice. *Senior Nurse* 12(2), 29–33.

McMahon, R.A. 1988: Discharge planning: home truths. *Geriatric Nursing and Home Care* 8(9), 16–17.

McMahon, R. 1992: Therapeutic nursing: theory, issues and practice. In McMahon, R. and Pearson, A. (eds), *Nursing as therapy.* London: Chapman & Hall.

McMahon, R. and Pearson, A. (eds) 1992: *Nursing as therapy.* London: Chapman & Hall.

Muetzel, P. 1988: *Therapeutic nursing.* In Pearson, A. (ed), *Primary nursing: nursing in the Burford and Oxford nursing development units.* London: Croom Helm.

Nursing Standard Comment (1993) *Nursing Standard* **89**(3), 3.

Orem, D.E. 1991: *Nursing: concepts of practice*, 4th ed. St Louis: Mosby Year Book.

Pearson, A. 1989: Therapeutic nursing-transforming models and theories in action. *Recent Advances in Nursing* **24**, 123–51.

Pearson, A. and Vaughan, B.A. 1986: *Nursing models for practice*. London: Heinemann.

Roper, N., Logan, W.W. and Tierney, A. 1983: *Using a model for nursing*. Edinburgh: Churchill Livingstone.

Royal College of Nursing (RCN) 1992: *Powerhouse for change: a manifesto for community health nursing for the 1990s*. London: RCN.

Sbaih, L. 1992: *Accident and emergency nursing: a nursing model*. London: Chapman & Hall.

UKCC 1994: *Report on proposals for the future of community education and practice*. London: UKCC.

Walsh, M. and Ford, P. 1989: *Nursing rituals: research and rational actions*. London: Heinemann Nursing.

Wilson-Barnett, J. 1984: Key functions in nursing: the fourth Winifred Raphael memorial lecture. London: RCN.

PART TWO

Main ingredients

6 Paediatric care

Bernadette Carter

Paediatric nursing in the community appears to have been marginalized for some time. It has now, quite rightly, been recognized as a specialist branch of community nursing. Previously, those nurses working in this field had to rely on 'apprenticeships' or health visiting/school nurse training. The English Nursing Board (ENB) have subsequently made amends and it now stands alongside other branches in its own right.

Bernie Carter has a wealth of experience researching paediatric care. Here she utilizes her experience and knowledge to examine the community through the child's point of view. Models of care are also revisited, and I make no apology for this since they are viewed from a specific perspective: that of paediatric care. Useful guidelines are offered with regard to the assessment of needs.

The current emphasis on paediatric community nursing reflects both the changes within paediatric nursing as a whole and those occurring within nursing in general. It particularly reflects the changes occurring in the way that health care services are provided, funded and managed. Although fundamentally the development of paediatric community nursing can be seen as beneficial to both service users (the child and their family) and the service provider, there are some dangers in embracing this approach to care delivery too enthusiastically. At its most simple, community care provides psycho-social benefits (both short and long term) to the child and cost/resource benefits to the providers of the service. It could be argued simplisticly that paediatric community nursing is a panacea for some of the troubles afflicting the hospital-based provision of health care although this is not entirely the case. Within this chapter a number of key issues are addressed in an attempt to provide a comprehensive picture of the diversity of roles that paediatric community nurses (PCNs) undertake and the philosophies that underpin the care they deliver. The need for professional development, the rights of the child and their family within this framework of care and the boundaries which are imposed on the role by both internal and external constraints are also examined. Future directions and possibilities are also considered.

Children's nursing focuses on the fundamental need to care for and serve the child's best interests. This is achieved by basing nursing care and interventions on a number of fundamental principles. Underpinning these principles is the acknowledgement that children have both unique and special (physical, psychological, cultural, spiritual and social) needs and they have specific rights. The child is always the focus of care and, whenever appropriate, their family should be closely involved in their care. Whilst attempts have, and continue to be made, to ensure that the hospital environment is supportive and child and family friendly it is impossible for such an alien environment to provide the same type of familiarity and level of support networks that are available within the child's own home. This recognition led to a move towards developing an integrated, national paediatric community nursing service. The need to provide ongoing support and care in the community and indeed to reduce the need for some children to be hospitalized has been evident for a number of years. The Platt Report (1959) stated that:

> Children should only be admitted to hospital when medical treatment they require cannot be given in other ways without real disadvantage. (Ministry of Health, 1959)

This report highlighted and reiterated the findings of earlier work on the detrimental effect that periods of separation could have on children (Bowlby, 1953).

Although paediatric community nursing services have been established in some areas of the country since the 1950s (Whiting, 1994a) there has been no real concerted effort, either by successive governments or by children's nurses as a professional group to respond to the specific and complex needs of children (Taylor, 1994). Indeed as Burr (1990) points out, 'Paediatric nursing has had too low a profile both within and without the profession due to the ignorance of the nursing needs of children'. This has hampered the development of community nursing provision. A notable exception to this apathy was the work undertaken by the National Association for the Welfare of Children in Hospital (NAWCH) (now Action for Sick Children (ASC)) which continued to strive to ensure that children's rights were respected and fulfilled and that professionals acted to implement the recommendations of the Platt Report (Ministry of Health, 1959). Indeed by 1991 when the Department of Health published *The Welfare of Children and Young People in Hospital* an area still of concern was that of children languishing unnecessarily in hospital. This report mirrors some of the concerns and recommendations of the Platt Report published 32 years earlier when it recommends that:

> Good child health care is shared with partners/carers and they are closely involved in the care of their children at all times, unless exceptionally this is not in the best interests of their child. (Department of Health, 1991: 2)

and:

> Children are admitted to hospital only if the care they require cannot be as well provided at home, in a day clinic or on a day basis in hospital. (Department of Health, 1991)

The emphasis is clear in this report – children should, whenever possible, be nursed outside of the emotionally stressful hospital environment (Thomas, 1994). Whilst this is a laudable aim, some problems exist when the patchy, although developing, natures of paediatric community nursing services are considered. It is obviously too soon to move children out of hospitals into the community on a wholesale basis.

In trying to understand paediatric community nursing, consideration of both the child's community and paediatric nursing in general must be made so that the developments and innovations occurring within this new and dynamic area of practice can be fully appreciated.

The child's community

A central concept to paediatric community nursing is the notion of community itself. However, untangling the concept of community, yet alone community care, is tricky. Definitions of community have been offered, although Skidmore (1994) suggests that in terms of a person-centred approach a definition of community is irrelevant. Regardless of definition, the concepts of change, flux and dynamism are central to community. Community care can therefore be seen as quite a nebulous concept and as Skidmore (1994) discusses, community care is 'increasingly romanticized as a concept'. The notion of care in or by (or maybe both) is another area open to discussion and debate and Skidmore (1994) proposes that it includes the assumptions:

- that there is a community
- that the community cares
- that formal structures (such as hospitals) can be separated from the community
- that communities are safe and friendly places (p. xii).

These assumptions must be considered and challenged by the PCN if they are to provide an effective level of care. Simply seeing the mythical community as the best and only opportunity for the continuing care of the child is naive. The nurse must ensure that the community is going to be safe, supportive and caring and that it is seen as an integrated whole with the hospital forming just one part of the child's and family's community. Indeed, this does happen where an 'open access' arrangement is available for the family to bring their child into hospital if they feel they cannot manage at home.

Just as the individual's community changes over time so does the child's perception of their community. Their community extends beyond the walls of their home. For the sick child, community care should mean more than simply care at home – however beneficial or altruistic this may be. A child's community, even a very young child's community, extends beyond their home and is made up of people outside of their own immediate family. It is composed of their extended family, neighbours, the people they meet at the shops and local amenities. It involves their family's friends and contacts and other children they meet at playgroup, school, leisure activities, church, etc. A child's potential community is complex. For the sick child this rich and diverse network of social contacts and potential support can be lost or not accessible if the PCN does not try to ensure that care in the community provides the opportunity to integrate fully into their own society. A child's community reflects the cultural values, beliefs and attitudes of the family and again the PCN must try and ensure that the child being cared for at home is allowed to continue to be part of those beliefs, attitudes and values. With a family-centred approach to care, the nurse should attempt to ensure that not only are the risks of the child becoming isolated minimized but also that the family does not become isolated by its caring role. Child care for children without specific health needs is an all-consuming commitment and this is much more so for families caring for children with particular health needs. The 'routine' that may accompany meeting the child's needs can, if not careful, segregate families from social interaction and make it difficult for them to take part in their usual activities. It is the skill of the PCN that encourages integration, helps overcome obstacles and allows the family to establish a way of living their life (with appropriate professional support) that is acceptable to them. Scannell *et al.* (1993) highlight a number of problems which have been reported by families of sick children including:

> loss of privacy; loss of parental control over child client; lifestyle differences between professional and family caregivers; and difficulty in obtaining, retaining and reimbursing competent professional caregivers. (p. 70)

They go on to state that:

> ... while delivering service within the family's territory, the professional must clarify the definition of client with family members, must negotiate shared control of care/service resources and routines, and must negotiate rules for use of family space. (p. 71)

Paediatric nursing: philosophy of care, models and theories

Contemporary paediatric nursing aims to meet the health care needs and deficits of the child as an individual and to acknowledge their own special place within their community and to have their right to information about, and involvement in their care (see Table 6.1).

The general philosophy that guides child health care services is one which aims to reduce the potential short- and long-term impact of hospitalization to a minimum (Caring for Children in the Health Services Committee, 1987).

Table 6.1 The needs of the child as an individual. With permission RCN, 1994

In working towards the provision of appropriate facilities for sick children, nurses would:

Recognize each child as a unique, developing individual whose best interests must be paramount

Listen to children, attempt to understand their perspectives, opinions, and feelings and acknowledge their right to privacy

Consider the physical, psychological, social, cultural, and spiritual needs of children and their families

Respect the right of children, according to their age and understanding, to appropriate information and informed participation in decisions about their care

The intention or aim must be to ensure that, whenever appropriate, children should be nursed at home (Taylor, 1994). An overriding concern must be that there is a level of equity within service provision so that all children who could benefit from care at home have access to a suitable service. This is part of the challenge in developing care in the community for children (Gow and Ridgeway, 1993). The need to establish more services and develop links between existing services is seen as an aim of the Paediatric Community Nurses Forum (RCN PCNF, 1994a):

> . . . to ensure the provision of a paediatric community nursing service to be available to every sick child and its family throughout the United Kingdom.

Philosophies of child-centred care or family-centred care are becoming established with hospital-based care provision and fundamentally the principles can, should and are applied within the community setting (see Table 6.2). Community teams develop their own philosophies which reflect their own beliefs and values as practitioners and the type of service they wish to offer.

Table 6.2 Philosophy of nursing care at home (Stepping Hill Hospital, Stockport). (Marland, 1994)

The children's home care sisters view each child as an individual who has special needs and rights in regards to the provision of health care

Each child and family have the right to specialist nursing care within the home environment which can be facilitated by the team's holistic approach to care

The child and family will be adequately prepared for discharge into the community and feel confident and knowledgeable enough to continue the nursing care at home with the support of a named home care sister

The team aims to forge links between the hospital and community to provide an integrated care which enables the child and family to achieve an optimum level of well being

The ultimate aim is to provide an accessible and equitable service to all children in the Stockport Health Authority

The framework upon which family-centred care is established highlights the need to place a value on the family's contribution to the child's care and psycho-social well being. The family is seen as part of the child's natural environment and vice versa (Nethercott, 1993). Indeed, parental involvement is stated as a Standard of Care (RCN, 1994b). Campbell *et al.* (1993) propose that family centred care is a '... nursing defined and led concept within the UK'. In using a truly family-centred approach, parents are not only instrumental in being partners in their own child's care but also in determining the development of policy. Again this can and could be utilized in making parents active participants in developing paediatric community nursing services. The benefit of empowering and involving parents in these sorts of decisions is that the service truly responds to the parent's/children's needs rather than the professional's perspective or understanding of those needs. The service not only will *develop* in the community but will be *developed* by the community.

Table 6.3 Eight elements of the framework. (Shetton *et al.*, 1987) (commentary added)

1 Recognition that the family is the constant in the child's life while the service systems and personnel within those systems fluctuate

The provision of a PCN aims to support the family 'constant' and provide ongoing contact with named professionals

2 Facilitation of parent–professional collaboration at all levels of health care

The PCN is more likely to develop a truly collaborative relationship with the parents as interaction occurs within the parent's own home environment. Organizationally, the nurse has to fit in with family resources, and innovative care is stimulated to develop due to the unique situations the professional finds themselves in

3 Sharing of unbiased and complete information with parents about their child's care on an ongoing basis in an appropriate and supportive manner

Trust (reciprocal trust) is a vital component of care as delivered by the PCN and much of their role lies in support, education and exchange of information. Exchange is perhaps more likely to occur when a true partnership in care results – both parent and professional can develop together as a result of this equitable relationship

4 Implementation of appropriate policies and programmes that are comprehensive and provide emotional, spiritual, cultural and financial support to meet the needs of families

With the families remaining in their home environments assessment of the needs on a more comprehensive basis is more likely to provide a realistic appraisal upon which action can be taken

5 Recognition of family strengths and individuality, and respect for different methods of coping

Again assessment with the family of their strengths provides both the family and the nurse with a realistic picture of how the PCN can utilize professional skills. It will also facilitate joint strategy planning to build upon existing coping mechanisms and reduce the risk of maladaptive coping

Table 6.3 continued

6 Understanding and incorporating the developmental and emotional needs of infants, children and adolescents, and their families into health care delivery systems

Even if health care is being delivered within the child's own home/community setting the PCN must be still cognizant of the potential effects that health care intervention can have on the child's developing personhood. It can be disruptive for both the child and their family and its impact should not be discounted

7 Encouragement and facilitation of parent-to-child support

The PCN is in an ideal situation to develop a supportive relationship such that the parent–child relationship is fostered and develops appropriately. The PCN is always a guest (albeit often a welcome guest) in the child's home which means that visits and therapy should be timed, whenever possible, to fit in with the family's routines and schedules

8 Assurance that the design of health care delivery systems is flexible, accessible and responsive to family needs

Access to health care personnel and services is a vital part of supporting the family caring for their child at home. Efficient contact with the PCN out-of-hours services, and open access (for named children/families) to hospital support is paramount to reduce the potential for families feeling isolated and 'just left to get on with it'. An efficient communication system, which listens, responds and liaises, is essential

Campbell *et al.* (1993) see family-centred research based within the elements of the framework as a means of developing children's nursing (see Table 6.3). This framework acknowledges that the child is not a separate entity from their family or the community in which the family lives. As Wise (1994) states:

> The child's main need (which may not be the most urgent health-care need) is to be within the context of family membership. This is normality, this is the most health-effective, socially effective, psychologically effective and probably most cost-effective context within which to treat dependency situations. (p. 38)

Whyte (1990) discusses the concept of family health as being a holistic system that is dynamic and based on five dimensions – biological, sociological, psychological, cultural and spiritual. Family nursing aims to:

> ... promote, maintain and restore family health, it is concerned with the interactions between the family and society and among the family and individual family members. (pp. 22–3)

> The health of families is important to all levels of society, and nurses have the potential to be a valuable resource to families in difficulty due to health problems. (p. 23)

Wright and Leahey (1990) identify and describe three trends in nursing of families, '. . . increased diversity in clinical practice; increased family research; and increased family content in academic settings'. Within paediatric clinical practice two major trends in the nursing of families exist: family nursing and family systems nursing. Family nursing can occur in two main ways. One in which the individual is focused on, within the context of their family. Another approach is one in which the family is focused on, with the individual as context. Family systems nursing contrasts by considering the whole family as the unit of care. The focus is on both the individual and the family. Wright and Leahey (1990) predict that the different approaches to nursing of families will stimulate practitioners to 'analyse their own practice with families to either defend, expand or abandon it' (p. 150). It will provoke a reconsideration of the 'inter-connectedness between illness, the individual and the family' (p. 150) and an interactional perspective will dominate. This will encourage the nurse to look wider for solutions in terms of considering interactions at both a micro and macro level. Family research within clinical practice is minimal and an area that would greatly benefit from further consideration. Many questions need to be addressed including the 'reciprocal relationship between family functioning and the course and treatment of an illness' and the 'efficacy of family treatment'. Wright and Leahey (1990) acknowledge that family-focused care has always been a part of nursing but see the value of and urgent need to 'entrench itself in academic and clinical settings' (p. 153).

In paediatric nursing, the relationship between professional and patient goes beyond the interaction between the nurse and the child and especially in the case of the PCN it will involve parents, grandparents, siblings, friends, school teachers and members of a multi-disciplinary team. The family and the family's own support structures are involved in the relationship (Schultz, 1981).

Casey (1993) bases her Partnership Model of Nursing Care on a family-centred approach. The emphasis on partnership, consistency and promoting the value that parents place upon themselves as skilled care givers appears central to the model. Casey and Mobbs (1988) describe the partnership model of paediatric nursing as evolving from a description of nursing practice, based on nursing activities. The starting point of the model is one of partnership which is negotiated on an ongoing basis with the parents. The nurse remains accountable at all times for care, and all care, both family and nursing care, should be documented carefully. Primary nursing is advocated by Green (1986) as an appropriate means of care delivery and Casey and Mobbs (1988) endorse this as an ideal method of implementing the partnership model. Partnership is seen as essential within paediatric community nursing (Sidey, 1989). Equity and negotiated partnerships are ways for the PCN to develop their care and professional practice. Maximum health gain is thought to be achievable through partnership (RCN, 1993). Partnership, negotiated partnership anyway, places a duty on the nurse to ensure that the delegated carer is supported appropriately (Casey, 1993) in terms of resources, advice and information. Again this model was developed for use within the hospital context but can be applied within the home setting. Glasper (1990) highlights the value of partnership in care in which parents are seen as the providers of care with teams of PCNs providing assistance and support. Casey (1988) identified central features of the model which highlight the dynamic, ongoing nature of negotiated partnership (see Fig. 6.1)

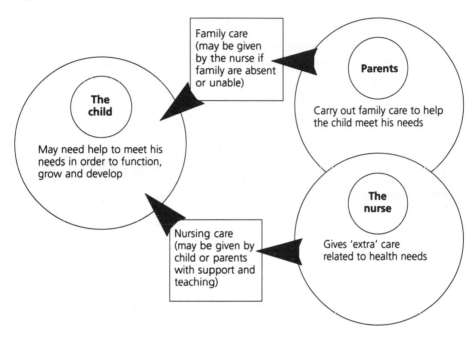

Figure 6.1 Casey's partnership model Casey, A. 1988. *Senior Nurse* **8**(4). Reproduced with kind permission of RCN Publications.

Casey sees the model as being flexible and able to evolve and respond to changes in paediatric practice and sees its strengths as an 'abstract–idealistic' model as a tool for '. . . describing, discussing and improving the care of sick children' (p. 193). There is no reason why it should not provide a strong model for care delivery in the community. It also provides a framework for audit which is vital for PCN teams which must be able to identify the benefits of their service (qualitative and quantitative, financial and economic) to the purchasers of the care packages they deliver.

King (1990) identifies that the concept of partnership is important in relation not only to both the nurse and the child/family but also with other members of the multidisciplinary team. She emphasizes the crucial role of the paediatric liaison nurse who aims to provide ongoing support for families needing help caring for their child. This role is one that is urged to be addressed by Thornes (1993) in *Bridging the Gap*. King (1990) sees the role of the liaison nurse as one which helps to provide a cohesive and supportive service for parents of chronically ill children and one which facilitates their learning to live with, rather than be dominated by, the chronic illness.

Casey (1993) identifies four paediatric nursing activities which underpin care (see Table 6.4). With paediatric community nursing being a relatively new and emerging aspect of children's nursing it does need to look towards establishing a theoretical basis from which to extend its knowledge basis. Using a family-centred/partnership approach appears to reflect those issues of importance to PCNs and engender an atmosphere in which to '... promote and support the art, science and practice of paediatric community nursing' (RCN PCNF, 1994a).

Table 6.4 Paediatric nursing activity. (Casey, 1993)

The paediatric nurse:

1 Carries out *family care* and *nursing care* to help meet the child's needs, so that he or she may achieve his/her full potential. (Family care is the care which the children themselves or their parents usually carry out to meet their needs. Nursing care is the 'extra' care he may need in relation to a health-related problem)

2 *Supports* the child and family by helping them to cope and continue to function

3 *Teaches* knowledge and skills to help the child and family towards independence from the health care team

4 *Refers* the child/family to, and consults with, other members of the caring team when appropriate

Provision of PCN services: issues and problems

Paediatric community nursing can be seen to act as a support to parents. It should be remembered that only a minority of sick children are admitted to hospital. Most sick children can, and are, cared for at home by their parents/families with or without support by PCNs or other community-based professionals (Taylor, 1994). However, nearly one million children are hospitalized annually (Caring for Children in the Health Services, 1987) although there is a change in the trend of hospitalization (shorter periods of stay in hospital, more use of day surgery and outpatient provision). In spite of the obvious benefits to the child and the family it seems frustrating that PCN provision on a national basis is patchy, although these gaps are being reduced. Whiting (1989a) found that only 12.6% of district health authorities had a community child care nursing team. Whiting (1989b) describes paediatric community nursing as, perhaps '... one of the quietest revolutions'. Whiting (1988) states that during his study there were over a million children discharged from hospital yearly in England and that there were less than 100 PCNs to meet their needs (compared with 13 170 district nurses, 3420 community psychiatric nurses and 1610 community mental handicap nurses). However, there has been considerable growth in provision in recent years and as Tatman (1994) suggests in many areas in the country home care teams '... occupy a niche which was previously empty'. Most professionals recognize the need for paediatric community services (Lane and Baker, 1994). Indeed they are no longer seen as a needless expense or 'luxury' but as an essential component of district health delivery (Gatford, 1992). Growth in service provision has occurred due to:

... long standing recognition of the need to enable sick children to be cared for at home instead of in hospital; changes in treatment of some illnesses; and technological advances which have made treatment in the home easier and safer. (Tatman, 1994)

Marland (1994) identifies three key themes in relation to the provision of care by PCNs:

1 Paediatric community teams bridge the gap between hospital and caring for the sick child at home.

2 Ongoing evaluation of such a service enhances the holistic approach to care of children.

3 The key to setting up such a service is good communication and support from managers. (p. 40)

Historically, it appears to be the needs of children in the community that have provided the stimulus for the development of services. Gillet (1954) describes the first 'modern' home care nursing scheme for children which developed in Rotherham in 1949 in response to the high infant mortality associated with the very severe winter of 1947. Two Queen's nurses were appointed to work with the general practitioners and to nurse appropriate infants at home – this service is accredited with reducing infant mortality from gastroenteritis. This success was thought to be due to a reduction of problems associated with cross-infection in hospitals. Further services were set up in Birmingham (Smellie, 1956) and Paddington (Lightwood, 1956). In 1957 St Mary's Hospital, London, developed a paediatric home care scheme which was set up to reduce the numbers of children being unnecessarily admitted to hospital and with an aim to reduce length of stay in hospital. The cost savings made by the introduction of the scheme seem impressive even though direct comparisons are difficult.

Although the early schemes seem to have produced impressive results even under quite difficult situations, and considering the context under which these schemes were being developed, it is striking to note that no further paediatric home care schemes were developed from 1954 to 1969 (At Home, 1994). However, service provision for sick children at home has developed in recent years. Whiting (1994a) highlights that in 1981 only eight generalist PCN schemes existed in the UK but that this number had increased to 61 by April 1993. The number continues to grow with 149 services established by 1995 (RCN PCNF, 1995a). However, it is still acknowledged that increased services should be made available and that less that one-third of health districts provide a PCN service (Cumberlege, 1994). Service provision is not uniform in relation to: the nature and extent of services provided; how children are referred to the service; who pays for the service; the relative autonomy of the nurses themselves; the hours the service is available; the range of skills and qualifications that PCNs hold; whether they are part of a team or working in isolation; or if a specialist or more generic service is offered. The range of professional practice initiatives is immense with innovations occurring within the care of children with constipation (Manchester); diabetes and enteral feeding needs (Birmingham); gastroenteritis (Waltham Forest); liaison with day surgery unit (Southampton); cystic fibrosis (Kettering), the dying child (Nottingham) and oxygen-dependent babies (London) (RCN, 1993). The contribution that the PCN can make to the lives of sick children and their families is potentially vast (see Table 6.5).

Table 6.5 Contributions that paediatric community nurses (PCNs) can make (RCN, 1993)

- Assess the particular needs of a family which has a sick child within it

- Enable children to be nursed in all community settings, for example playgroup, nurseries, residential homes, respite care facilities and their homes

- Enable children with a debilitating disease to fulfil their potential, enhancing their quality of life

- Provide opportunistic health promotion for the whole family

- Plan, in co-operation with the family, the special nursing needs of the ill child

- At the end of life, enable the child to die with dignity in the place of their choice

- Provide crisis intervention, thus offering continual support to families who live with a high level of stress associated with caring for a child with a chronic illness

- Enable parents to feel confident and competent when caring for their child

- Teach families to carry out specific nursing procedures, including high-tech procedures

- Act as an interface between community, hospital and all other agencies, for example cubs, school camps or sport camps, providing continuity of care and facilitating the normal activities of childhood and adolescence

- Help families network with others, reducing feelings of isolation and despair

- Offer appropriate support and help following bereavement

- Prevent hospital admission and attendance. PCNs can also facilitate early discharge while the option of day care is made more available

- Teach student nurses, community nurses, medical students, GP trainees and others

- Act as a specialist resource for all health care workers

- In common with district nurses and health visitors, paediatric community nurses will be able to prescribe certain medicines once the regulations are in place

The NHS Management Executive Report *Building a Stronger Team: the nursing contribution to purchasing* (1993) highlights a pilot PCN scheme that was set up to 'explore nursing and rehabilitation needs of children with learning disabilities, long-term conditions and recurring acute needs for whom care in the community was thought appropriate and possible'. After six months trial the scheme was evaluated and conclusions reached were that:

> ... the service had been innovative and beneficial to the client group, identifying needs that had not previously been met. The pilot scheme had shown where and how care could be more appropriately delivered in the community. Most important of all, it had been regarded with appreciation ... .(p. 9).

This scheme was developed, monitored and evaluated by a steering group of provider nurses, purchasing authority representatives and consultant paediatricians who decided to make the pilot scheme a substantive one after positive evaluation.

Gow and Yerrell (1989) highlight the range of services that can be offered by PCNs including bereavement visits, care of children with malignant disease, terminal illness, oxygen-dependent babies and postoperatively.

Arnfield (1990) highlights that even children who are terminally ill benefit by being cared for at home as it is usually the preferred setting for children and their families.

Quality health services for children require that their physical and emotional well being needs are met. This involves ensuring that there are strong links between hospital services and community services (Thomas, 1994). In the *Bridging the Gap* report (Thornes, 1993) a number of key issues were identified including improving 'reception' and 'transfer of care' of children and their family through the interfaces (i.e. points of contact with different elements of the health service). The concepts underlying this report have relevance to the work of the PCN and can guide some care delivery (see Tables 6.6 and 6.7).

Robbins (1987) again endorses the need for developing PCN services as a means of providing comprehensive and ongoing care of the child/family. Family-centred care and partnership are seen as integral to the role of the paediatric nurse.

Another way in which PCNs can play a part in proactive, modern health care delivery is identified with the *Health of the Nation* document (DoH 1992) which highlights continuity of care between hospital and community as a theme of 'good nursing practice' (p. 14). Whilst paediatric nurses may have traditionally associated their role as caring for the sick child, the focus is changing to one in which a health promotion role is seen as increasingly important (see Table 6.8). Clinical specialists are also noted. Health promotion is a key issue for all nurses (see Chapter 4) and should be an integral part of their role. As members of a multidisciplinary team, PCNs may well have an opportunity to play an integral role in promoting

Table 6.6 Four concepts underpinning the *Bridging the Gap* report (Thornes, 1993, p. 10, pt 2.1)

- Parents have the main responsibility for their child's health care at all times

- The traditional divisions between primary and secondary care are no longer appropriate as a basis for planning and can hinder the move towards a seamless service

- The relationship between the primary health carers and a family continues as a child moves in and out of specialist care and the GP remains pivotal in care and support

- Specialist care can be given in many settings and involves staff who are expert in both the particular condition and in the care of children

Table 6.7 Nine principles for the delivery of care at interfaces Thornes, 1993

A Knowledge and information should be shared between professionals and families, so that the parents, and children when they are able, are in a strong position to take part in planning and decision making

B There should be equity in access to, and quality of, service. Particular care should be taken to ensure that vulnerable families receive appropriate services

C Consultations, tests and treatment should be provided as close as possible to each child's home. If a child has to travel to a distant hospital, attention should be paid to practical help for the family

D Referrals to specialist services, especially those provided by community health agencies, can be made by a range of health professionals who should work to agreed criteria to ensure that the care is integrated

E The boundary between primary and specialist care, and thus the point of referral, varies from place to place, according to the facilities and expertise available in the primary setting. The important criterion is for all concerned to accept an agreed standard of care and to ensure that the child is in the right place to receive it

F The boundary between care in the hospital and at home, and thus the point of referral back to the primary carers, should vary from place to place according to the facilities and expertise available in the primary team and the home. The important criterion is for all concerned to work to a recognised standard of care and to ensure that the child's family has appropriate support to provide it

G The steps taken to ensure continuation of the pattern of care should be made explicit to families, so that the parents know who is managing their child's clinical care at every stage and where to go for clinical help

H Parents should be quite clear about the care they are expected to provide and at what point to seek clinical help

I Communications should be organized in such a way that the professional managing a child's care has sufficient, timely information to continue the care

Table 6.8 Principles of good nursing , midwifery and health visiting: developed from *Targeting Practice: the Contribution of Nurses, Midwives and Health Visitors* (DoH, 1993a)

Characteristics of good nursing, midwifery and health visiting practice.

- Good practice embraces both existing and new practice (extended or otherwise), that is 'done well'

- Practice can describe any activity in which nurses, midwives and health visitors are engaged and therefore includes all activities of management, leadership and organisation and care delivery

- Good practice cannot be applied globally to specific activities. Activities considered good practice in one area are not necessarily good practice in another

- Good practice can be applied to quite different activities addressing the same issue. 'Good' does not equate with the single 'right' approach (p. 94–5)

children's health, for example, in relation to the 'Accident Target' which aims to reduce ill health, disability and death caused by accidents. Children are given specific attention in the *Target Practicing* document through service developments aimed at reducing head injuries among children and campaigning to prevent accidents. PCN services must not only reflect identified health needs in the community but also be proactive in assessing and identifying new needs and then in meeting them. These new services should meet the needs of the public (RCN PCNF, 1994b).

Development of a PCN team should be based on a needs assessment which will provide a profile of needs of children, services required, resources available, and the use made of existing services. It should also generate opinions on proposed services, and numbers of children/families likely to use the service. Needs assessment aims:

to develop an accurate picture
to help avoid operational conflicts
to raise staff awareness
to assist in obtaining funding
to identify resources (RCN PCNF, 1994b).

Needs assessment can be achieved by: reviewing literature, reports and guidance notes; defining catchment population; defining age range to be covered; defining target groups; defining available resources within proposed team and community; defining numbers of children in target group(s); assessing other relevant services; defining types of service to be offered and the type of home care team to provide care (e.g. hospital-based home care team, community-based home care team, resource nurse, nurse specialists).

PCN services are an essential part of the patchwork of community care provision even if some purchasers do not recognize their value or worth. Managers must be convinced of the need to re-evaluate priorities in providing care. The profile of PCN teams must be heightened so that their services are purchased and utilized effectively by the providers (RCN, 1993). However, funding remains a constant bugbear for practitioners wishing to set up and/or develop services. An issue of critical importance is funding, especially in relation to who actually bears the cost when a child is transferred/discharged from hospital care to ongoing community care. Often two different providers are involved (hospital and community) and a level of wrangling occurs as to whose budget the child's ongoing care will be deducted from. Whiting (1994b), arguing the concerns he feels about transfers of highly dependent children from hospital to community, illustrates three areas of concern in relation to resourcing situations such as transfer:

resources to fund one to one nursing care which will allow a patient to be transferred from hospital to community;

resources to fund the purchase of an expensive item of equipment which will allow a patient to be transferred from hospital to community;

resources to underwrite the cost of drugs, a cost which is already being picked up by an overstretched hospital pharmacy budget, but which a General Practitioner says he simply can't afford . . . and so a patient cannot be transferred from hospital to community.

PCNs face dilemmas such as this every day along with other ethical and moral issues. Despite a commitment to negotiated partnership, the nurse may in reality face situations where they may disagree with some decisions or actions taken by the child's parents. The problem in this situation relates not so much whether the parents know best but what is in the best interests of the child. It may be difficult for the nurse to separate their own personal feelings and opinions from the issue so that they can view it in an objective manner or be able to provide a forum for discussion with the parents, which is ultimately the most important route to solving the problem. Ultimately, it is the parent's (and the child's where appropriate) right to choose – even if the nurse may not completely agree with the decision. Moving care into the community and away from the disempowering environment of the hospital reflects the higher expectations of an increasingly well-informed public. Fradd (1994) discusses the need for paediatric nurses to empower themselves if they are to be truly able to empower the families they work with. This will ultimately result in parents exercising their rights, duties and responsibilities to their children and making informed decisions.

Swanwick and Barlow (1993/4) discuss some of the contentious issues surrounding delivering quality care in respect to how to define quality, what should be measured and which perspectives should be considered. Central to the delivery of quality care is the involvement of the family. Quality is determined not only by quality from the practitioners but also from the setting and context in which care is delivered. Quality care is dynamic and reflects not only the beliefs and values of society as a whole but particularly the beliefs, values and attitudes of the paediatric nursing profession. Quality care can only be delivered if all factors that impinge on care delivery are taken into consideration. Within an evolving area of practice such as paediatric community nursing, quality is a concept that cannot be ignored. Quality is important as it may well be the means of developing and evolving service provision. Swanwick and Barlow (1993/4) highlight a number of issues that contribute to the concept of quality (see Table 6.9). The need for developing quality audit tools is highlighted and the need for these to be appropriate to the specific care delivery context is reinforced

Table 6.9 Issues contributing to quality. Modified from Swanwick and Barlow (1993/4)

Specific to paediatrics	*Socio-political milieu*
advocacy	quality assurance
child and family centred care	resources
physical and psycho-social safety	
changing needs of developing child	
The professional	*The consumer – child and family*
skills	acceptability
knowledge	accessibility
attitudes	efficiency
perceptual awareness	appropriate care
	effectiveness

The profession
  research minded
  philosophical foundations
  management
  ethical framework
  standards

(Swanwick & Barlow 1993/4). Preparing PCNs for their role is not easy and until relatively recently specific educational preparation has been somewhat *ad hoc*. Scannell *et al.* (1993) interviewed home care nurses about the meaning of their work and identified differences between their professional role in hospital and in the community. A number of issues were highlighted for consideration, particularly the need to adjust personally to the role of community nurse. Although the nurses reported enjoying the one-to-one contact with the child, they were surprised by the way that parents validated their practice through evaluating the effectiveness of their interventions. This level of scrutiny can be expected when the professional moves into practice within the family home. Some nurses reported that they found it difficult to determine what exactly their role was since they were neither 'servant nor guest' – role clarification was clearly an important issue for the nurses in the study. In some instances PCNs have not been identified as a separate group with specific educational and practice needs (UKCC, 1994a). This lack of awareness on the part of the UKCC proved a disappointment for PCNs (Dryden, 1992).

Historically, PCNs have been poorly served in terms of educational opportunities. Little has been available that has been specifically tailored to their needs. Many, in order to gain a community health qualification, have undertaken district nurse courses or health visiting courses which, whilst providing a level of enlightenment for hospital time-served nurses about the workings of the community, has done little to develop or foster a specific understanding of the child's community and their professional role within it. Whiting (1994b) reports the repeated representations made by the RCN PCN Forum to the ENB and UKCC highlighting the need to develop specific courses suitable for PCN practitioners. A modified district nurse course resulted which goes some way to meeting needs but there is a degree of wariness as to how effectively it is in doing so. Langlands (1994) highlights the UKCC's acknowledgement of the desirability of appropriate education to allow a quality service to be provided. The proposals put forward in the PREP document (UKCC, 1994a, b) (see Table 6.10) state that all community health care nursing courses will be at first degree level, equally divided between theory and practice, have common core learning with other health care nursing programmes, have a period (12 weeks) of supervised practice and involve a system of credit accumulation and transfer (Langlands, 1994). Specific issues looked at within the specialist programme will focus on management, practice and leadership.

Table 6.10 Specific learning outcomes. With permission UKCC (1994a)

The nurse should achieve the following specific outcomes applied to the care of community nursing practice:

Clinical nursing practice

- assess, plan, provide and evaluate specialist clinical nursing care to meet care needs of acutely and chronically ill children at home

---

Care and programme management

- initiate and contribute to strategies designed to promote and improve health and prevent disease in children, their families and the wider community

- initiate action to identify and minimize risk to children and ensure child protection and safety and

- initiate management of potential or actual physical or psychological abuse of children and potentially violent situations and settings (UKCC, 1994a: 43)

Whilst programmes may be student centred, modular, flexible and allow choice, it is difficult (although not impossible) to determine how such courses can meet the diverse professional needs of the students. The PCN's role involves communication, play, education, health promotion, supporting hands-on caring over a wide range of specialities and requiring a wide range of nursing and technical skills, advocacy and liaison to name but a few.

Fradd (1994) highlights the high level of skill and judgement required by PCNs in relation to treatment options for particular children in their care. The autonomy, knowledge and responsibility/accountability are possible to implement due to the Scope of Professional Practice (UKCC, 1992). The future of all aspects of paediatric practice including paediatric community nursing lies in examining both the skills and knowledge required to drive practice forward in a creative, flexible and innovative way (Fradd, 1994).

Supporting the parents/families of chronically sick children

One area of expertise that all PCNs must develop lies in relation to supporting parents. Whilst the number of medically fragile/chronically ill babies and children discharged into the community has risen, very little has been done in terms of researching and evaluating the effect that this has on parental stress and the effect it has on the parent's own quality of life. In the USA the costs of home care for medically fragile/technologically dependent children is reported as being exorbitant and the savings made when home care is seen to be a viable option are significant. However, Leonard *et al.* (1993) report that much of the success of home care of these children is dependent on the parent's psychological status. The physical and psychological demands placed on parents who willingly and lovingly care for their children at home must be a paramount concern for the PCN. Part of a family-centred strategy of care must involve caring for the parents, who should not feel imprisoned in their own homes by their child's needs. Technology is both a blessing and a curse. Technological developments have allowed even the critically ill child to be nursed at home, and have encouraged increasingly early discharge of infants and children who require monitoring and technological support. Although many parents feel relaxed whilst the monitor is keeping an additional eye on their child (Smith, 1984), some parents find the technology itself a source of stress and one that requires strategies to cope with (Stevens, 1994). Stevens' (1994) study shows the crucial need for adequate information, presented in a variety of formats (video, print, telephone contact) and a co-ordinated support network to reduce the potential social isolation experienced by mothers.

The effect on the family of having to cope with highly dependent children has been studied in the USA (where financial considerations necessitate the transfer of chronically sick children back to their homes as soon as feasibly possible) (Scharer & Dixon, 1989). Factors that influence the stressfulness for parents coping with their chronically ill child have also been the focus of research. The two types of home care that researchers have focused upon as areas of high stress are home ventilation and home apnoea monitoring – these situations require the parents to be continually 'on-call' and alert to their child's potentially changing needs. The level of vigilance required is thought to have a negative effect on the family care givers. Ray and Ritchie (1993), in their study of factors affecting parents' coping, found that the level of integration, support and co-operation within the family were important. Additionally, maintaining an optimistic outlook (emphasizing positive aspects and making positive and/or selective comparisons) was supportive of coping and maintaining hope. Finally, the perceived care-giving burden was a factor in how much stress parents perceived they felt. Implications from this research highlight the need for nurses to work with the families, minimize the restrictions imposed by caring for the child and assess and promote family supportiveness. This is supported by work by Teague *et al.* (1993) who highlight the need for a holistic and active approach to family support. Interestingly, in a study undertaken by Mueller and Leviton (1986), families of developmentally disabled children found that they experienced greater care control problems with health professionals in the context of home rather than clinical-based care delivery. The need to assess the impact of the technologically dependent child on family life is vital (Blum, 1984). Fleming *et al.*'s (1994) study again demonstrated the most important role of the nurse in meeting the family's needs by providing support, information and help. Other areas of input by the PCN are equally vital and perhaps form the bulk of care delivery.

The sterility of hospital settings in terms of real-life experiences has been noted by Kielhofner *et al.*, (1983), and the difficulties in introducing a programme to support the needs of children growing up in hospital is evident in Wells *et al.* (1994), who identify the need for creating innovative methods for supporting the child's physical and psycho-social needs. They highlight the importance of introducing effective programmes since these may have 'lifelong implications'. Again the need for PCNs to ensure that care in the community occurs in an atraumatic manner with appropriate support is highlighted. Research may well be necessary to determine how 'home-like' home-care of a child with specific and high-level needs is for both the child and their family. There is a risk that care at home may simply be a cosmetic response to an intractable problem. One of the most important aspects of care at home lies in the appropriateness and effectiveness of discharge planning. This is a key issue, not only in the highly dependent child, but also in the more 'routine', low-tech child. However, it must be acknowledged that the highly dependent child does obviously present special and particularly complex planning problems. Lewis *et al.* (1992) cite that the most 'nurturing environment' for the child is usually the child's natural family home. They further state that in highly dependent children a case management approach is probably the most appropriate approach to meeting the child's needs. The preparedness of the child and their family to go home as well as the community to receive them must be clearly defined and guaranteed (although guarantees are almost impossible to give). Collaboration is vital throughout all stages of planning and implementation (Donar, 1988; Rogers *et al.*, 1991; Lewis *et al.*, 1992).

Harris (1988) describes two situations in which, despite rigorous discharge planning, home care of the child simply did not prove successful. She reports that the most obvious reason for failure of home care is 'lack of community and family resources'. However, within this broad umbrella term she identifies 'emotional depletion', 'incongruent priorities' and 'inadequate financial resources'. Although health and welfare provision may be different in the UK compared with the USA, inadequate financial resources are still an issue in first determining whether home care is appropriate and possible and in relation to its ongoing support. Families who are financially overstretched are already under stress and home care may be another part of that burden. Emotional depletion is described as the response to dealing with the ongoing, and unremitting burden of care which can result in family burn-out. Nurses need to be aware of signs of family stress or distress and offer appropriate care and support. Incongruent priorities can sometimes occur when the child, their family and the health professionals have different expectations and goals. The child's best interests should always have priority, although the beliefs and values of the family (and the health professionals) are important and need to be valued and respected. Harris (1988) concludes her discussion by identifying a number of factors that need consideration when home care is starting to fail (see Fig. 6.2).

The importance of play as a therapeutic mode to help hospitalized children cope with the trauma associated with medical procedures, strange environments and changes in routine has been well established (Betz and Poster, 1984; Bolig, 1990; Hall and Cleary, 1988; Vessey and Mahon, 1990). Jessee (1992) argues that despite the acknowledgement that play is important, '. . . the degree to which nurses actively initiate therapeutic play

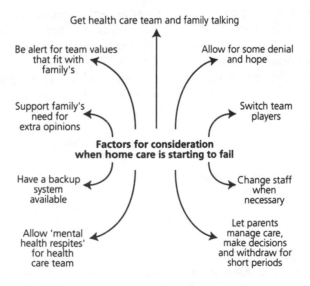

Figure 6.2 Failing home care (adapted from Harris, 1988)

in the hospital setting is minimal'. This may also be true for paediatric nurses working within a community setting and is an area that should receive active consideration. Jessee (1992) cites Thompson and Stanford (1981) who identified four discrete functions of hospital play which could also provide guidance for community-based play for the sick child: to prepare for medical procedures; to enhance communication; to master developmental skills; and to cope with negative emotions and stress. Again this is an area that PCNs can and should be developing in partnership with parents. It would be simplistic to suggest that simply removing a child from an institutional setting to their own home environment also removes any fears, worries, concerns and distress from the child. A change of setting does not obviate the need for psychological support – indeed the child's psycho-social needs may perhaps be masked by them being at home.

Peterson (1990) identifies a number of reasons why play is important for children during a hospital admission, including improving the child's coping strategies and developing their communication and relationship skills. She goes on to propose the value of parents playing with their child as it can give them confidence in other aspects of their child's care. Peterson highlights the intrinsic value of play to the child's emotional well being when stating, 'The right to play is truly a basic right for each child, whatever the social or economic situation may be. Indeed, the fostering of play is clearly part of preventative medicine' (p. 41).

Schemes developed to meet specific needs/range of provision

Schemes have developed to support a number of needs and deficits, some of which will be discussed in more detail. Stainer (1992) reports the development of a scheme to support babies requiring supplemental oxygen with bronchopulmonary dysplasia (BPD) in the community, thus reducing the necessity for prolonged hospital admission. The scheme appears successful in meeting the needs of the babies and parents, and professionals feel confident with the scheme. The cost savings between hospital and community are significant although no formal evaluation of the service appears to have been undertaken. Bishop et al. (1994) highlight the move towards increasingly technical/technological nursing care being entrusted to PCNs; this type of care they term 'hospital-at-home'. The need for careful discharge planning and ongoing communication between hospital and community practitioners is emphasized in their case history of an adolescent girl in the terminal stages of leukaemia. An issue of particular interest in this paper is the child's confidence in being, and determination to be, nursed at home. The importance of involving the child in decisions that affect them is thus emphasized and it is part of the PCN role to prevent erosion of the child's right to autonomy and self-determination (Peace, 1994; Franklin, 1994).

Home care schemes have also proved to be a valuable source of support to children with cystic fibrosis requiring long term, repeated courses of intravenous antibiotics. In this situation the PCNs in conjunction with hospital-based staff are responsible for developing and maintaining an education and support programme for parents, or children where appropriate, administering intravenous antibiotics often through central venous cannulae (although percutaneous cannulae are used in some situations). The PCN facilitates the care given by the parents or carers and gradually the role will often change from educator to supporter as the parent or child becomes increasingly proficient, competent and confident. Parents who have been given appropriate education and support can often see intravenous administration as simply an extension to their existing role as care giver (Sidey, 1989; Kendrick, 1993).

Conclusion

In conclusion, therefore, paediatric community nursing can be seen not so much as a means of removing children from the hospital to the community but rather obviating the need for removing sick children from the community into hospital. Paediatric community nursing initiatives would seem to be responding not only to existing needs and health care challenges but also by being proactive in terms of moving towards practice in the twenty-first century. The document *The Challenges for Nursing and Midwifery in the 21st Century* (DoH, 1993b) identifies not only the drivers of change (societal expectations, technological innovations, the demands for health care, policy initiatives such as the emphasis on community and primary care), but identifies areas that PCNs are already either trying to meet or utilizing in their everyday practice. Although a number of issues still need to be addressed, such as research focused on parent's and children's views and opinions of the service and auditing the effectiveness and quality of the services offered, much has already been established. High-quality, innovative care is being provided within the community and children's health needs are now being met more appropriately than ever before. Progress is perhaps slower than many practitioners would desire but very real constraints (mostly financial) exist which limit the development of care strategies. However, progress is being made and the political and professional climate is now more conducive to fostering initiatives.

References

Arnfield, A. 1990: Oncology in the 1990s. *Nursing Standard* 4(22), 53–4.
At Home 1994: *At home: the newsletter for homecare therapy initiatives*, Issue 7. Caremark: Harlow.
Atwell, J.D. and Gow, M.A. 1985: Paediatric trained district nurse in the community: expensive luxury or economic necessity? *British Medical Journal* 291, 227–9.
Betz, C. and Poster, E. 1984: Incorporating play in the care of the hospitalized child.

Issues in Comprehensive Paediatric Nursing **7**, 343–55.

Bishop, J., Anderson, A and McCulloch, J. 1994: Hospital-at-home: a critical analysis. *Paediatric Nursing* **6**(6), 12–15.

Blum, R. 1984: *Chronic illness and disabilities in childhood and adolescence*. Philadelphia: Grune & Stratton.

Bolig, R. 1990: Play in health care settings. A challenge for the 1990s. *Children's Health Care* **19**(4), 229–33.

Bowlby, J. 1953: *Child care and the growth of love*. Penguin: Harmondsworth.

Burr, S. 1990: Change in the 1990s. *Nursing Standard* **4**(22), 50–1.

Campbell, S., Kelly, P. and Summersgill, P. 1993: Putting the family first. Interpreting a framework for family centred care. *Child Health* **1**(1), 59–63.

Caring for Children in the Health Services Committee 1987: *Parents staying overnight with their children*. London: CCHS Committee.

Casey, A. 1988: A partnership with child and family. *Senior Nurse* **8**(4), 8–9.

Casey, A. 1993: Development and use of the partnership model of nursing care. In Glasper, E.A. and Tucker, A. (ed.), *Advances in child health nursing*. Harrow: Scutari Press, 183–93.

Casey, A. and Mobbs, S. 1988: Partnership and practice. *Nursing Times* **84**(44), 67–8.

Cumberlege, J. 1994: It's time to put children first. *Paediatric Nursing* **4**(8), 4.

Department of Health 1991: *The welfare of children and young people in hospital*. London: HMSO.

Department of Health 1992: *The health of the nation: a strategy for health in England*. Cmd 1986. London: HMSO.

Department of Health 1993a: *Targeting practice: the contribution of nurses, midwives and health visitors* [*The health of the nation*]. London: HMSO.

Department of Health 1993b: *The challenges of nursing and midwifery in the 21st century. The Heathrow debate*. London: HMSO.

Donar, M.E. 1988: Community care: paediatric home mechanical ventilations. *Holistic Nursing Practice* **2**(2), 68–80.

Dryden, S. 1992: Strong feelings. *Paediatric Nursing* **May**, 5.

Fleming, J., Challala, M., Eland, J. *et al.* 1994: Impact on the family of children who are technology dependent and cared for at home. *Pediatric Nursing* **20**(4), 379–88.

Fradd, E. 1994: A broader scope to practice. Professional development in paediatric nursing. *Child Health* **Apr/May**, 233–8.

Franklin, P. 1994: Straight talking. *Nursing Times* **90**(8), 33–4.

Gatford, A. 1992: Keeping the sick child out of hospital. *Professional Care of Mother and Child* **March**, 84–5.

Gillet, J. 1954: Domiciliary treatment of sick children. *Practitioner* **172**, 281.

Glasper, A. 1990: Emancipation of parents. *Nursing Standard* **4**(22), 55.

Gow, P. and Ridgeway, G 1993: The development of a paediatric community service. In: Glasper, E.A. and Tucker, A. (ed), *Advances in child health nursing*. Harrow: Scutari Press, 269–76.

Gow, M. and Yerrell, P. 1989: A family friend. *Nursing Times* **85**(4), 63–5.

Gray, R. 1993: Defining roles for today. Community development and health visitors. *Child Health* **Aug/Sep**, 79–82.

Green, L. 1986: A special friend. *Nursing Times* **82**(36): 32–3.

Hall, D. and Cleary, J. 1988: The development of play for children in hospitals: British and European perspectives. *Children's Health Care* **16**(3), 223–30.

Harris, P. 1988: Sometimes pediatric home care doesn't work. *American Journal of Nursing* **June**, 851–4.

Jessee, P.O. 1992: Nurses, children and play. *Issues in Comprehensive Pediatric Nursing* **15**, 261–9.

Jessop, D.J. and Stein, R.E. 1991: Who benefits from a pediatric home care program? *Pediatrics* **88**, 497–505.

Kendrick, R. 1993: Teaching children with cystic fibrosis and their families to give IV therapy. *Paediatric Nursing* **5**(1), 22–4.

Kielhofner, G., Barris, R., Bauer, D., Shoestock B. and Walker, L. 1983: A comparison of play behavior in nonhospitalized hosiptalized children. *The American Journal of Occupational Therapy* **37**(5), 305–12.

King, A. 1990: The role of the paediatric nurse. *Nursing Standard* **4**(33), 35–7.

Lane, M. and Baker, S. 1994: Mentoring in the community. *Paediatric Nursing* **6**(6), 10–11.

Langlands, T. 1994: Looking to the future. *Paediatric Nursing* **6**(6), 8–9.

Leonard, B.J., Brust, J.D. and Nelson, R.P. 1993: Parental distress: caring for medically fragile children at home. *Journal of Pediatric Nursing* **8**(1), 22–30.

Lewis, C.C., Alford-Winston, A., Billy-Kornas, M., McCaustland, M.D. and Tachman, C.P. 1992: Care management for children who are medically fragile/technologically dependent. *Issues in Comprehensive Pediatric Nursing* **15**, 73–91.

Lightwood, R. 1956: The home care of sick children. *Practitioner* **177**(July), 10–14.

Lindsay, B. 1994: The child and family: contemporary nursing issues in child health care. London: Ballière Tindall.

Marland, J. 1994: Back where they belong. Caring for sick children at home. *Child Health* **2**(1), 40–2.

Ministry of Health 1959: *Report of the Platt Committee. The welfare of children in hospital.* London: HMSO.

Mueller, M. and Leviton, A. 1986: In-home versus clinic-based services for developmentally disabled child: who is the primary client – parent or child? *Social Work in Health Care* **11**, 75–88.

NHS Management Executive 1993: *Building a Stronger Team: the nursing contribution to purchasing.* Department of Health. London: HMSO.

Nethercott, S. 1993: A concept for all the family. Family centred care: a concept analysis. *Professional Nurse* **Sept**, 794–7.

Peace, G. 1994: Sensitive choices. *Nursing Times* **90**(8), 35–6.

Peterson, G. 1990: Let the children play. *Nursing* **3**(41), 22–5.

Ray, L.D. and Ritchie, J.A. 1993: Caring for chronically ill children at home: factors that influence parents' coping. *Journal of Pediatric Nursing* **8**(4), 217–25.

Robbins, M.E. 1987: The role of the nurse. *Nursing* **24**, 905–7.

Rogers, M., Riordan J., and Swindle, D. 1991: Community-based nursing care management pays off. *Nursing Management* **22**(3), 30–4.

Royal College of Nursing 1993: *Buying Paediatric Community Nursing: An RCN guide for purchasers and commissioners of health care*, **December**. London: RCN.

Royal College of Nursing 1994a: *Paediatric nursing – a philosophy of care: Issues in nursing and health* **10**. London: RCN.

Royal College of Nursing 1994b: *Protecting children: a Royal College of Nursing guide for nurses* **April**. London: RCN.

Royal College of Nursing 1994c: *Nursing and child protection: an RCN survey*, **March**. London: RCN.

Royal College of Nursing 1994d: *Newsline* **19**, 8. London: RCN.

Royal College of Nursing, Paediatric Community Nursing Forum (RCN PCNF) 1994a: *Paediatric Community Nurses New Members Information Pack*, **April**. London: RCN, 4.

Royal College of Nursing Paediatric Community Nurse's Forum (RCNPCNF) 1995: *Directory of Paediatric Community Nursing Services*, 12th edn. London, RCN.

Royal College of Nursing Paediatric Community Nurse's Forum (RCN PCNF) 1994b: *Wise decisions: developing paediatric home care teams.* London: RCN.

Royal College of Nursing Society of Paediatric Nursing 1994: *Standards of care for paediatric nursing*, 2nd edn. London: Scutari Press.

Scharer, K. and Dixon, D.M. 1989: Managing chronic illness: parents with a ventilator dependent child. *Journal of Paediatric Nursing* **4**, 236–47.

Scannell, S., Gillies, D.A., Biordi, D. and Child, D.A. 1993: Negotiating nurse–patient authority in pediatric home health care. *Journal of Pediatric Nursing.* **Apr**, 70–8.

Schultz, P.R. 1981: When the client means more than one: extending the foundational concept of person. *Advances in Nursing Science* **10**(1), 71.

Sidey, A. 1989: Intravenous home care. *Paediatric Nursing* **May**, 14–15.

Shetton, T. *et al.* 1987: Family Centred Care for Children with Special Healthcare Needs. Association for the Care of Children's Health, Washington.

Skidmore, D. 1994: An ideology of community care. London: Chapman & Hall.

Smellie, J.M. 1956: Domiciliary nursing service for infants and children. *British Medical Journal* **5**, 256.

Smith, J. 1984: Psychosocial aspects of infantile apnea and home monitoring. *Pediatric Annals* **13**, 219–23.

Stainer, A. 1992: Recent advances 3: home O_2 therapy. Home oxygen therapy for preterm babies. *Professional Care of Mother and Child* **June**, 174–7.

Stevens, M.S. 1994: Parents coping with infants requiring home cardiorespiratory monitoring. *Journal of Pediatric Nursing* **9**(1), 2–12.

Swanwick, M. and Barlow, S. 1993/4: A caring definition. Defining quality care in paediatric nursing. *Child Health* **Dec/Jan**, 137–41.

Tatman, M. 1994: 'Wise Decisions': setting up paediatric home care services. Conference Paper Abstract. RCN PCN Conference April.

Tatman, M.A., Woodroffe, C., Kelly, P.J., Harris, R.J. 1992: Paediatric home care in Tower Hamlets: a working partnership with parents. *Quality in Health Care* **1**, 98–103.

Taylor, J. 1994: *The continuum of care. The child and family. Contemporary nursing issues in child health and care.* London: Ballière Tindall, 174–96.

Teague, B.R., Fleming, J.W., Castle, A., Kiernan, B.S., Lobo, M.L., Riggs, S., and Wolfe, J.G. 1993: 'High-Tech' home care for children with chronic health conditions: a pilot study. *Journal of Pediatric Nursing* **8**(4), 226–32.

Thomas, S. 1994: Child's Play? *Nursing Times* **90**(3), 42–4.

Thompson, R. and Stanford, G. 1981: *Child life in hospitals.* Springfield, IL: Charles C Thomas.

Thornes, R. 1993: [On behalf of Caring for Children in the Health Services] *Bridging the gap: an exploratory study of the interfaces between primary and specialist care for children within the health services.* London: Action for Sick Children.

United Kingdom Central Council 1992: *The scope of professional practice.* London: UKCC.

United Kingdom Central Council 1994a: *Report on proposals for future of community education and practice.* UKCC: London.

United Kingdom Central Council 1994b: *The future of professional Practice. The UKCC standards for education and practice following registration.* London: UKCC.

Vessey, J.A. and Mahon, M.M. 1990: Therapeutic play and the hospitalized child. *Journal of Pediatric Nursing* **5**(5), 328–33.

Wells, P.W., DeBoard-Burns, M.B., Charles Cook, R. and Mitchell, J. 1994: Growing up in hospital: Part 1, Let's focus on the child. *Journal of Pediatric Nursing* **9**(2), 66–73.

Whiting, M. 1988: Community pediatric nursing in England in 1988. Unpublished MSc thesis, University of London.

Whiting, M. 1989a: Home truths. *Nursing Times* **85**(14), 74–5.

Whiting, M. 1989b: Home care for children. *Nursing Standard* **4**(22), 52–3.

Whiting, M. 1994a: Meeting needs: RSCNs in the community. *Paediatric Nursing* **6**(1), 9–11.

Whiting, M. 1994b: *Funding of community care.* Abstract of paper delivered at RCN Congress, April.

Whyte, D. 1990: The family with a chronically-ill child. *Paediatric Nursing* **Nov**, 21–3.

Wise, G. 1994: The changing family. In: Lindsay, B. (ed.), *The child and family. Contemporary nursing issues in child health care* London: Ballière Tindall.

Wright, L.M. and Leahey, M. 1990: Trends in nursing of families. *Journal of Advanced Nursing* **15**, 148–54.

7 Adult care

Eileen Groves

With more and more emphasis on care in the community for adults, general practitioner (GP) fundholders and a shift in responsibility for care means that this branch of nursing, along with the practice nurse, is 'blessed' with increasing responsibility. The incorporation of nurse prescribing (if and when this receives approval) will also see them under pressure to make significant savings in the use of the accoutrements of care delivery (e.g. dressings). Eileen Groves locates this specialism within nursing by taking the reader through the history of district nursing and then examining implications for the future. The name of this specialism has changed several times but the importance of the role has remained prominent.

District nursing

The district nurse is a registered nurse who has successfully completed a district nursing course within an institute of higher education. This education, with integrated taught and supervised practice, enables the nurse to give skilled research-based nursing care to patients within a community setting (home or residential home), and to offer appropriate support to relatives and carers. The district nurse is professionally accountable for assessing the needs of the patient and family, for initiating programmes of care, ensuring their implementation and for the continual evaluation and reassessment of such programmes. They are also responsible for monitoring the quality of the care given by themselves or others in their team.

Along with all other health care professionals, district nurses are working in an environment of major change with significant developments in the demands for community health care. At the same time, ideologies of the welfare state are shifting towards a free market economy within the health care services, and challenges are being made to health care managers, both hospital and community, to improve efficiency and provide a cost-effective service. Alongside this shift, there has been an emphasis towards individual accountability for health status, the introduction of new technology, changes in demographic trends and new diseases such as acquired immune deficiency syndrome (AIDS), all of which have implications for nurses working in the community.

The shifts in political thinking have led to a move towards community-based rather than hospital-based care for all but the acutely ill, resulting in a greater workload being placed on community health and social services.

The Government recognises that achieving the aim of ensuring that more people are looked after in their own homes for a longer period is likely to involve greater demands on the community health services. Community nursing care, therapy services, and services such as chiropody all have a part to play in enabling people to remain in the community. (DoH, 1990)

Yet the ideology of community based care is not a new concept. In the UK as long ago as 1962, the 'Hospital Plan' recommended cuts of 50% in bed occupancy of so-called 'long-term patients', those in institutionalized care (i.e. those with psychiatric illness or mental handicap or the frail elderly or physically disabled, those who needed continuing care).

In drawing up the hospital plan, it has been assumed that the first concern of the health and welfare services will continue to forestall illness and disability by preventative measures; and that where illness or disability nevertheless occurs, the aim will be to provide care at home and in the community for all who do not require the special types of diagnosis and treatment which only a hospital can provide. (NHS, 1962)

Community care then is the realization of a long-term plan towards long-stay hospital retraction requiring the provision of services and support to people who need extra help to be able to live as independently as possible in their own homes or in a smaller homely setting in their local community.

The Government White Paper, *Caring for People* (DoH, 1990), outlining community health strategies for the 1990s is concerned with the general mechanisms through which community care ought to be delivered. Essentially, for community care to be effective, both health and social services should be included in the provision of care, and it is crucial that both work effectively together to plan and implement their respective responsibilities to patients and clients. The effective operation of community care depends on how successfully such collaboration between health and social services in providing flexible packages of care to meet individual needs can be achieved, and in identifying joint strategic objectives. The practical and logistical problems in devising and implementing collaborative packages of care involving both health and social services in terms of defining who does what, and the boundaries of responsibility and accountability between what is considered to be social care and what is considered to be health care, are immense and the subject of much discussion and debate at the time of writing.

The introduction of the *Patient's Charter* (DoH, 1995) adds the further dimension of patient choice to decisions regarding how and where and in what way patients and clients may wish to be cared for. Nurses working in the community setting have a unique opportunity to move away from the traditional medical model of care commonly used as a basis for hospital-based care, and implement individualized holistic programmes of care which take account of the patient's lifestyle and family situation and which require knowledgeable application of the social sciences. The development of the primary health care team approach to care in the late 1970s and 1980s helped to develop a clearer understanding of the role, function and skills of all involved in the maintenance of the long-term sick in the community (i.e. district nurses, GP, health visitor), either working together from a health centre or with named 'attached' contacts, thus facilitating the provision of holistic care. Many primary health care teams also had the attachment of a social worker and community psychiatric nurse, so the idea of working together to benefit patient/client care is not new to community.

The World Health Organization in its Alma Ata declaration (WHO, 1978) noted the importance of primary health care in achieving its strategy of health for all by the year 2000, and defines primary health care as:

> essential health care made universally acceptable to individuals and families in the community by means acceptable to them, through their full participation and at a cost that the community and the country can afford. It forms an integral part of both the country's health system of which it is the central function and main focus and of the overall social and economic development of the community.

Effective primary health care requires elements of primary medical care and treatment and preventative services from a multidiciplinary team of health care workers each with their own discrete area of expertise yet working together to contribute to the health and welfare of the population it serves.

District nursing is an integral part of primary health care and has a specific role to play within the multidisciplinary provision of community-based client-centred care. The role and development of the district nursing service is well documented in other texts (Stocks, 1960; Baly, 1981), therefore it is the intention within this chapter to give only a brief overview of that role and development, but then to look at it in context within the new-style market-led Health Service and Community Care Act implemented in 1993, and consider the implications of these changes to district nursing practice.

History and development of the district nursing service – overview

Visiting the sick and caring for them in their own homes has existed since time immemorial. As with hospital nursing, district nursing increasingly became associated with various religious orders, with women (nuns) and sometimes monks belonging to such orders undertaking a caring role. For example, in the seventeenth century the Order of St Vincent de Paul formed the Sisters of Charity who would attend people in their own homes to make a meal, wash the patient and make him or her comfortable.

Prior to the amended Poor Law Act 1834, (the New Poor Law which introduced the workhouse to care for the poor sick), many of the old Poor Law committees employed parish nurses to care for the pauper sick in their own homes, a practice which was to continue after the Act as it was found to be a cheaper way of providing care than admitting the patient to the workhouse. (Compare with the philosophy of the Community Care Act 1995!) Needless to say the diversity of the tasks undertaken and the standard of care provided was very dependent upon the individual nurse and it was not until the mid-nineteenth century that efforts were made to introduce a higher calibre of woman with some basic training and nursing skills to take on the caring role. Until then, between the latter part of the seventeenth century to the mid-nineteenth century, nursing in general was made up of a female workforce with work undertaken simply for financial gain or goods 'in kind', as portrayed in Dickens' notorious character, Sarah Gamp.

In 1840, Elizabeth Fry, usually associated with prison reform, made an attempt to provide a practical nursing service in the home for which a small salary was paid. The women had to be protestant and of good character. Things continued in that way until 1859 when William Rathbone, a wealthy Liverpool merchant ship owner and a Quaker, employed a nurse Robinson who had been trained at St Thomas's Hospital London, to look after his ailing wife who was in the terminal stages of consumption (tuberculosis). The work was so much appreciated that he contacted Miss Nightingale with a view to providing this type of service to all the sick at home. It must also be said that as an employer he no doubt recognized the value and advantages which would result in the early return to work or service following illness. 'A nice example of charity going hand in hand with nineteenth century utilitarianism' (Baly, 1981). A training scheme was set up at Liverpool Royal Infirmary. Miss Nightingale stressed that the women had to be of good education, have hospital training and have a knowledge of public health matters.

The first trained district nurses were allocated to the districts of Liverpool in 1863 (Baly, 1981). Each district was run by a Ladies Voluntary Committee which dealt with the financing of the service and appointed a superintendent to deal with the day to day organization and administration and the organization of the nurses' work load. Unfortunately, it was not thought necessary for the superintendent to have undertaken district training herself, or even to be a nurse. Compare this with some of today's management strategies where often it is not nurses who are managing nurses. It has to be said that this state of affairs was not one that Miss Nightingale condoned.

1887 saw the Jubilee year of Queen Victoria. This was marked by the donation of £70 000 collected by women towards the founding of an institute for training district nurses. This became known as the Queen's Institute and supported locally with voluntary funds was to be responsible for the education and development of district nursing for the best part of the next 100 years. It is interesting to note that it was felt necessary to have a district nurse certificate to practice as a district nurse 30 years before state registration for nurses was established in 1919. The National Health Service Act of 1946 made the district nursing service a statutory provision which was to be available to all people when necessary.

As in its beginnings, a major part of the district nurse's caseload today continues to be the care of those highly dependent patients, often with a multiplicity of health problems, who require general nursing care and attention. However, modern medical technology and treatments leading to shorter hospital stay, the increase in the numbers of elderly infirm, the continuing developments in day case surgery, and the ability to install computerized technical equipment in the home setting, have all had implications for the service and the education and preparation of district nurses for practice to meet these demands.

Service provision for district nursing

Local policy and local need determine the nature of the service, some providing a 24-hour cover seven days a week, others only until 10 or 11 p.m. Patients will normally have been referred to the district nurse by the GP or may have been discharged from hospital and referred via the district nurse liaison service for follow-up care. Patients may be visited just once, for example for removal of sutures from a small surgical wound, or require visits for many years in the case of chronic illness or disability.

The varied nature of the district nurse's work requires the nurse to have good all-round generalist skills with practice firmly rooted in up-to-date research-based care and the ability to be a proactive, reflective practitioner, responsive to need and change. A typical daily case load for a district nurse is likely to comprise of:

- visits to administer insulin to patients who through disability or advancing age are not able to administer their own insulin;
- general nursing care to the acute and long-term sick, the terminally ill and the disabled;
- adminstration of a wide range of injections, e.g. antibiotics, controlled drugs, and other prescribed drugs;
- a variety of wound dressings ranging from surgical dressings to dressing of leg ulcers;
- administration of eye drops;
- health education and health promotion activities;
- health assessments for the over 75s.

For many years district nurses, like health visitors, worked within small geographical areas. This had the advantage that the nurse became a well-known and respected member of that local community and as a result was in a position to assess the health needs of a particular area with some accuracy and initiate wherever possible strategies for meeting those needs. The disadvantage was the problem of having to communicate and liaise with a number of other professionals and agencies who might be connected with that geographical patch; for example, on a large housing estate there may be people registered with GPs representing every practice within a particular catchment area, making it difficult for the nurse to be able to form good working relationships with all.

As referred to above, the 1970s saw the development of the primary health care team concept and the advent of large purpose-built health centres with group attachment of GP, district nurse, health visitor and midwife forming the team. This had the advantage of all the professionals who may be dealing with a patient/client being under one roof, thus enabling communication and liaison regarding treatment strategies and case conferences to discuss care planning to take place with all concerned in the care of that particular patient/client and their carers.

The role of the district nurse in the 1990s

Since 1981, possession of the ENB award of district nurse, in addition to being on Part 1 of the Register, has been mandatory in order to practice the full range of district nursing duties, including admission and discharge of patients to and from the care of the district nursing service. This award is currently at Dip HE level 11, but the introduction of the UKCC Community Prepp in 1996 will see a unified discipline of Community Health Care nursing at level 111. There will continue to be discrete specialist disciplines contained within such an award, and district nursing will be retitled, Nursing in The Home – District Nursing.

The district nursing service is comprised of some 18 000 nurses in total (DoH, 1992), a figure which includes a range from qualified district nurse to nursing auxiliary. Figures show that of these numbers some 9119 were qualified district nurses (DoH, 1988). The introduction of skill mix into the community arena is likely to see this number remaining static or even falling, as the number of district nurses undertaking the district nurse award continues to fall (DoH, 1989) despite the increased numbers of referrals for community-based care as early discharge and relocation of the elderly and chronically sick and disabled to community settings continues to accelerate.

The district nurse's role has been defined in the Chief Nursing Officer's statement:

> The district nurse is the leader of the district nursing team within the primary health care services. Working with her may be RGNs, ENs and nursing auxilliaries. It is the district nurse who is professionally accountable for assessing and reassessing the needs of the patient and

family, and for monitoring the quality of care. It is her responsibility to ensure that help, including financial help and social help is made available as appropriate. (DHSS, 1977)

This statement was reaffirmed and brought into line with current health care policy in 1991 when a seminar comprising members of the District Nursing Association stated as part of the key issues in district nursing:

Activities of district nursing practice will be carried out in collaboration with other practitioners in primary health care, including practice nurses, health visitors, general practitioners, social workers, care managers and will require the district nurses to:

- participate at policy level by active involvement with agencies concerned with health care, and where appropriate, social care;
- analyse health care needs at case load and local population level, identify priorities and maximise available resources;
- participate actively in the measurement of quality health care in relation to consumer satisfaction, practitioner and team effectiveness, and efficient utilisation of resources;
- prepare and utilise information that will contribute to the provision of health care;
- undertake initial diagnosis and assume therapeutic responsibilities for episodic and continuing care;
- accept direct referrals from members of the local community and from other professionals, ensuring accessibility of community nursing services to the consumer;
- teach self-assessment skills and health promotion activities to enable people to influence their own health;
- establish and maintain the effective working of the nursing team, determining the competencies and skill mix of the team within the multidisciplinary setting of primary health care;
- provide nursing expertise to the primary health care team and act as a source of specialist and expert advice on nursing and health promotion to the nursing team and to others working within primary health care;
- co-ordinate the contributions of all providers of care – statutory, lay and voluntary – across primary and secondary care;
- recognise specific interests and abilities of individual members of the team, motivating them in professional development and advising on staff development programmes;
- initiate and contribute to research, as well as drawing on research to extend the knowledge base of district nursing practice and community nursing;
- manage any budgetary resource, making a case for resources to meet the health needs of the neighbourhood and the community. (DNA, 1992)

It has also been stated that District nurses have a vital role to play in ensuring that *Health of the Nation* (DoH, 1992) targets are met and as such are seen as a key to the successful implementation of *Caring for People* (DoH, 1990). Quite a tall order!

However, district nurses are finding increasingly that many aspects of their role outlined above are becoming more difficult to achieve or have been taken out of their hands with the new community trusts, GP fund holding, the development of skill mix strategies in the community and in some areas the demand for provision of a Hospital at Home service.

Skill mix

As in all other areas of health care work, skill mix is now an integral part of health service management policy in the community affecting all branches of community care. The overall aim of skill mix initiatives was said to relate to creating a balance of assorted skills, from unqualified care assistants to highly skilled practitioners, in such a way as to provide a quality service at a cost efficient rate – value for money.

> Skill mix is concerned with ensuring that appropriate skills are available to meet identified needs. It helps to promote the flexibility and creativity that is necessary for cost-effective and responsive practice and starts from a health needs based assessment of the local population. (DNA, 1993)

However, as Sturdy (1991) points out, such flexibility should be founded solely on the basis of practice which is responsive to need and should not rely simply on a mix of grades without consideration of the skills required to meet needs. It is essential that patients and clients receive quality care delivered at the point of need by the most appropriately qualified health care professional.

It may appear to be relatively easy to view the district nurse's workload in terms of tasks, and as such delegate those seemingly low-skilled tasks, for example bathing, to unqualified members of the team, yet is is difficult to quantify the amount of valuable information which may be gained in such activity through skilled observation and carefully directed conversation.

The nurse specialist in the community

Since the mid-1970s there has been a steady increase in the numbers of nurse specialist working in the community, for example, stoma therapists, diabetes specialists, continence promotion nurses, most of whom work in an advisory capacity as resource persons rather than being involved in actual hands-on care. They provide a useful back-up service for the district nurse and supply up-to-date information and advice to community nurses, patients and clients relating to the control and management of their particular health problem.

The McMillan nursing service is also now well established in most areas providing support and counselling for the terminally ill cancer patient and family and liaising with and advising the GP and district nurse on effective pain and symptom control.

GP fundholding

As yet, it is uncertain just what effects GP fundholding may have in the long term to the contracting and managing of district nursing services. It is envisaged that there will probably be a mix of those practices which employ district nurses directly and those who will contract a district nursing service from a commissioning agency, for example a community trust unit. GPs will be looking to purchase a quality, efficient and effective district nursing service within the limitations of their practice budget, and a service which is sufficiently flexible to meet the needs of a particular practice population. This may in reality mean purchasing a range of community services and resources from a variety of sources not necessarily locally based.

What is certain is that the work of the district nurse is likely to increase dramatically as the political shift towards care in the community widens and develops in the 1990s. The continuing changes in demographic trends, with changing patterns of health and disease and with links between poverty and ill-health becoming well recognized and documented, will continue to bring many challenges for all health care professionals in the community as they strive towards meeting the demands of a needs-based service and working towards the goal of *Health for All* by the year 2000 (WHO, 1991) and targets for *Health of the Nations* (DoH, 1992).

References

Baly, M.E. 1984: *A new approach to district nursing*. London: Heinemann.

District Nursing Association (DNA) 1990: *Key issues in district nursing*. London: DNA Publications (UK).

District Nursing Association (DNA) 1992: *District nursing practice*. Edinburgh: DNA Publications (UK).

District Nursing Association (DNA) 1993: *Skill mix and GP fundholding*. Edinburgh: DNA Publications (UK).

DHSS 1977: *Nursing in primary health care*. Circ. CNO (77)8. London: HMSO.

DoH 1988: *Health and personal social service statistics*. London: HMSO.

DoH 1989: *NHS workforce in England and Wales*. London: HMSO.

DoH 1990: *Caring for people – community care in the next decade and beyond*. London: HMSO.

DoH 1992: *Health of the nation*. London: HMSO.

DoH 1995: NHS, *the patient's charter and you*. London: HMSO.

DoH 1995: NHS responsibilities for meeting continuing health care needs. London: HMSO.

NHS, 1962: *A hospital plan for England and Wales*. London: HMSO.

Stocks, M. 1960: *Nursing and social change*. London: Heinemann.

Sturdy, C. 1991: *A guide to skillmix for managers*. Cited in *District Nursing Association UK Newsletter* **X**(1) Spring 1993.

UKCC 1994: *The future of professional practice*. London: UKCC.

World Health Organization 1978: *Report on the primary health care conference*. Alma-Ata: WHO.

World Health Organization 1991: *Targets for health for all by the year 2000*. Geneva: WHO.

8 Elder care

Susan Moore

In the Introduction to this book mention was made of the consequences of demographic change, Susan Moore explores these issues further in relation to the elder care in the community. This is another marginalized and yet important field of community nursing. This chapter highlights the importance of this specialism and exposes some of the assumptions about community care. The inevitability of growing old is explored alongside the politics of caring. Whilst elder care is viewed in its own right, Susan Moore recognizes the special skills that other community workers can contribute within this field.

It could be argued that most of us look forward to 'growing up', experiencing new freedoms, developing increasing confidence in our own abilities and valuing our independence. However, in contrast we often dread 'growing old', of becoming increasingly frail and, worst of all, losing our independence and becoming dependent on others for our daily needs.

The common stereotype of the elderly person as frail and dependent which, as Victor (1991) points out, is prevalent in many countries, both developed and developing, is likely to be due to the '. . . interplay between several key factors'. One factor is that research into aging, for example has mainly concentrated on the 'problems' associated with old age, for example, sickness and disability, rather than examining normal ageing, where the majority of older people live happily and independently within the limits of their physical functioning.

From an analysis of data, collected for the 1985 OPCS General Household Survey, Victor (1991) showed that 60 per cent of the population 65 years and over rated their health as 'good', 30 per cent as 'fair' and only 10 per cent as 'poor'. This is in stark contrast to the myth that the elderly are much less healthy (and, therefore, more dependent) than younger age groups. However, it is true that Britain has an increasingly ageing population. The average life-expectancy is 72 years for men and 77 years for women and in 1985, 15.8 per cent of the British population were age 65+ years. This is projected to rise to 21.6 per cent of the total population by the year 2036, with a rapid expansion in the numbers of people aged 85 years and over (Laing and Hall, 1991).

Although many people do remain fit and relatively healthy, during the last three to four years of life they become more vulnerable to the major illnesses of cancer, heart disease and stroke. Also, degenerative conditions such as Parkinson's disease and rheumatoid arthritis seem to become more acute during these later years of life (Laing and Hall, 1991).

Moreover, increasing age also increases the risk of having to live alone due to the death of a partner or close relative. In 1988, The OPCS General Household Survey (cited by Laing and Hall, 1991), showed that there were 17 per cent of men and 36 per cent of women aged 65–74 years living alone, increasing to 29 per cent of men and 61 per cent of women aged 75 years or older.

Elderly women, therefore, are more likely to be living alone than elderly men (who die earlier). It has also been found that living alone for an elderly person increases the likelihood of them being admitted to hospital or other residential care. It is also recognized that elderly people are heavy users of health services, being the main consumers of most medical specialisms (Victor, 1991). It is the age group 85+ years who account for the highest cost of health services, including prescriptions.

Inpatient admissions are only a part of the overall usage of health-related services by elderly people. Reductions in the length of hospital stay mean that many elderly people are discharged from hospital needing continuing care, follow-up care or rehabilitation.

Hospital discharge and the elderly

A study undertaken by Neill and Williams (1992), concerning the discharge of elderly people from hospital to community care, demonstrated that there was often pressure on old people to move out of hospital 'quicker and sicker'; furthermore lack of appropriate support often led to readmission.

They also identified that some older people needed a period of recovery and 'special care'. Those elderly people who had been admitted under the care of a geriatrician were more likely to experience a successful planned discharge, including a predischarge home assessment and follow-up care. Other patients who had been on general medical or surgical wards, were more likely to have been discharged with minimal support, increasing the risk of readmission.

The *Patient's Charter* (DoH, 1992) stresses the importance of a planned discharge and the setting up in advance of appropriate community services. It also stresses the importance of patient and carer consultation in the planning processes.

Neill and Williams (1992) found that the most successful discharge schemes, operated by hospitals, were those where hospital-based and community nurses worked closely together to plan the discharge and follow-up. They also felt that there should be a screening of patients on admission, to identify those elderly people who were the most vulnerable (i.e. those who had an emergency admission or who were living alone) who might require additional services on discharge home which were not currently being provided. Where the elderly person is going to be discharged into the care of another elderly person, there should be an assessment of the health and social care needs of both, not just the pat.

Another important feature of discharge planning that needs to considered is that where relatives and friends take an active part 1 postdischarge care initially, it cannot be taken for granted in the long term. Nor should they be used as a cheap alternative to professional care, where this would be more appropriate.

The Community Care Act

One of the major aims of the Community Care Act (DoH, 1990) was to help people to: '. . . live as independently as possible in their own homes, or in "homely" settings in the community'. It was acknowledged that the majority of care for elderly people was provided by relatives (often elderly themselves), friends or neighbours, with little or no professional help.

Following the full implementation of the Act in April 1993, local authority social service departments, in collaboration with health authorities, have become responsible for assessing the individual needs of elderly people, designing 'packages of care' and ensuring their delivery within available resources. Care managers (often social workers), are to be appointed by the social service departments to monitor the effectiveness of these 'packages'. The costs of nursing and other medically related care will remain the responsibility of the health authority, whilst the costs of social care and places within residential and nursing homes which cannot be met by the elderly person's own resources are now to be met within the local authority social service budgets.

The government has directed that the majority of the social service budget (made up of a revenue support grant and local charges including council tax) should be spent in the private sector, which essentially in the long term will transfer most of the residential provision for the elderly from public to private organizations, thus reducing the need for local authority accommodation. Local authorities have also been directed to use, wherever possible, voluntary providers of services (e.g. transport, day centres etc.) to reduce costs. These might be organizations such as Cross Roads, the Red Cross or local voluntary organizations.

An additional requirement under the Act, is for local authorities to monitor and inspect care homes and to be involved in new joint planning activities with health authorities. These might involve discussion on policies of hospital closure and discharges to continuing care in the community (George, 1994).

According to George (1994), because of the community care reforms and other NHS-related changes, there could be several purchasers/providers of health and social care for an elderly person, which could lead to confusion about 'who should be doing what' and as a result, an unsatisfactory service for the client. Dimond (1993) has also predicted that there will not be adequate resources to meet all assessed needs. Therefore, resources must be allocated according to well-defined and agreed priorities. The effectiveness of the resource allocation for community services must be closely monitored and priorities redefined as appropriate.

Hancock (1993) has observed that the effective assessment and delivery of services for elderly people will require close collaboration between local authorities, health authorities and other agencies, including the voluntary sector. In particular, she believes that the assessment of an elderly person's needs should be a 'multidisciplinary exercise', which recognizes the responsibilities and contribution of each agency in providing the most appropriate services.

For the elderly person who needs both nursing and social care, nurses and social workers could both be involved in assessing needs within joint assessment visits, commissioning the services from the appropriate providers, co-ordinating and evaluating the effectiveness of the 'care package'. Although the overall care manager would often be a social worker appointed by social services, where the elderly person had mainly nursing or other health-care related needs, the care manager could be a community nurse (e.g. a district nurse or health visitor).

The care manager would not normally provide the client's services themselves but would 'commission' the required health and social care services from the health authorities, community health trusts, social services and private and voluntary agencies. As Dimond (1993) points out the provision of community health services varies, with some NHS trusts separating community care from acute services and some combining inpatient and community services for single specialities like the elderly.

Fundholding GPs can now buy some community services (e.g. district nursing) from the health authorities. At the moment GPs cannot directly employ them, but this is likely to become a possibility in the near future. Cost effectiveness will increasingly be a major consideration for the care manager in the 'commissioning of services' for the elderly person. In particular, they have been directed to make use of the voluntary and private sectors as providers of services where they are a cheaper option but also to remove as much dependency as possible on 'state' provision.

Essentially, all social care services provided to the elderly person in their own home are 'means tested' (e.g. the home help service), as are places in local authority or private residential homes. If the elderly person has sufficient funds, they will have to contribute financially to the cost of their social care and they may also be asked to contribute to the cost of providing aids and adaptations required in their own home.

Some local authorities, in an attempt to keep their council tax low, have had to increase their charges for social care services. Simmons (1994) reports how a pensioner living in the London borough of Wandsworth has received a bill for £600 for home help services. If he had been living in nearby Lambeth, his home help service would have been free. This shows clearly how there can be inequity in charges for social care, which are not directly related to the person's ability to pay.

Worth (1994) has identified that problems with provision of aids and adaptations to the home were one of the major areas of concern in the discharge of elderly people from hospital to the community. This was one of the main features of 'unsatisfactory discharges' cited by the community nurses, in Worth's study, and was also reported to increase the likelihood of that elderly person being readmitted.

George (1994) reports that despite the recent community care reforms, there are still problems with home adaptations and aids. The government has actually reduced the amount of money given to local authorities for such facilities. Lack of the required facilities for the elderly person to maintain their independence at home may delay their discharge from hospital or increase the burden for their carer. Delayed discharge may increase the waiting times for other patients to be admitted and may increase the pressure on the elderly person to go into long-term residential care, rather than back to their own home.

The British Medical Association reported that there was pressure being put on doctors to move elderly people out of hospital and into residential or nursing homes, in order to 'free up' hospital beds (BMA, 1992). Many Health Authorities are entering into contracts with the private sector to take their elderly patients with continuing care needs into private residential care, so that long-stay wards can be closed. It was a matter for concern for the BMA that elderly people could be 'caught in the cross-fire' as health authorities and social services debate whose responsibility it should be to fund those care needs. The fear is that the increased costs of providing residential care for growing numbers of elderly people predicted to need such care in the future will mean that 'state' provision is likely to be available 'on a means tested basis for only the poorest members of the elderly population'.

The role of the community nurse

For many years district nurses and to a lesser extent health visitors have provided much of the professional support for the elderly person and their carers in the community setting. As part of the 1990 GP contract (NAHA, 1989), all elderly people over the age of 75 years are entitled to a yearly home visit. The visit would include: an assessment of the home environment; lifestyle and significant relationships, including whether there was a supportive carer involved; a mobility and mental assessment; assessment of hearing and vision; a general functional assessment; and a review of medication. The aim of such a visit is to provide a health-screening service to ensure that the health-related needs of the elderly person are being met appropriately. It is also an opportunity to assess whether the needs of that person's informal carer are also being met.

Many of these screening procedures could be carried out by a suitably qualified community nurse on behalf of the GP. The UKCC (1990), identified district nurses and health visitors as being the most suitable community nurses to carry out these procedures. However, because of the very heavy workload that these community nurses already carry, in reality it is often the practice nurse (see Chapter 10) who is carrying out most of these procedures, but this requires much closer supervision by the GP. In some areas, there are small numbers of health visitors who are employed specifically for the elderly and they will carry out these assessments but most health visitors are still working mainly with the 0–5 age group and their families. This health surveillance of elderly people was one of the priorities set out in *Caring For People* (DoH, 1989) to reduce the need for hospital and residential care and to: '... encourage and prolong independent living'.

The Royal College of Nursing (RCN, 1993) published a guide for fundholding GPs entitled *Buying Community Nursing* to highlight the benefits of the community nursing service for the practice and their patients.

One of the important contributions that qualified district nurses could make to the care of patients within a practice population (including the elderly) is their ability to accurately assess patients' needs and plan appropriate individualized care (see Chapter 7). Health visitors could also make a valuable contribution in the production of a health needs profile, so that services could be targeted more appropriately and, therefore, more cost effectively (see Chapter 12).

These benefits also included 'an opportunity to integrate the work of practice nurses and community nurses', which was felt would improve the health care service to patients. The RCN quoted research which indicated that care by qualified nursing staff was more likely to increase patient satisfaction and produce a shorter length of patient dependency. However, increasingly fundholding GPs will be looking for cost effectiveness in the provision of community nursing services for their elderly patients. Community nurses will need to continue to demonstrate that they provide the best option. Otherwise, GPs are likely to look for alternative cheaper sources of support, perhaps from private care agencies, or from social services. These support staff are likely to be much less qualified than district nurses or health visitors, perhaps having only National Vocational Qualifications in Health and Social Care. Therefore, they are unlikely to be able to provide as detailed an assessment of health care needs as a district nurse or health visitor, or provide the same level of support.

Support for carers

Atkin (1993) investigated community nurses' effectiveness in supporting informal carers of elderly people. He found that support fell into two broad categories:

1 First of all: community nurses gave practical help such as changing dressings, giving injections and help with personal hygiene. Some carers

particularly welcomed this practical help as a relief from tasks which they otherwise might have found difficult or embarrassing to do themselves.

2   A second type of help that community nurses were reported to give to carers was that of emotional support. Carers valued the opportunity to have someone else to talk to and discuss their worries with. It was also an opportunity for the community nurse to give information about benefits and services available to the carer and where required, make the necessary referrals for those services.

Atkin (1993) also found that many carers did not have any contact with community nurses on a regular basis so that the support that they were receiving was often minimal. Increasing demand for community nursing services, particularly district nursing and the reduction in the numbers of qualified staff following the recent 'skill-mix reviews', has meant that the emotional support of carers has often had to 'take a back seat' to the more technical nursing tasks that can be legitimized in workload audits.

According to Atkin (1993), the problems associated with the actual support of carers have meant that the potential for their support by community nurses has yet to be fully realized. Just as the elderly are not one homogeneous group, there are also different types of informal carers. Many elderly people are supported by their partners (Victor, 1991). However, as mentioned above, women are more likely to live longer than men, so many elderly women have no partner to care for them. From a review of the available data, Victor (1991) concluded that of the carers who were not partners, many were women, particularly daughters and daughters-in-law. However, there were also increasing numbers of men acting as carers so that informal caring cannot be seen as a predominately female activity. Many of these carers were themselves elderly, often reporting loss of other social contacts as a consequence of their caring role. This was an aspect of being a carer which they found particularly stressful.

Some carers are well supported by a network of relatives and friends, or through organizations such as the Carer's National Association and Age Concern but many are coping alone without outside support. Laczko (1993), points out that many carers of elderly people are still in employment and are trying to combine work with the demands of their caring role and as a result, they have significantly less weekly income from all sources (including benefits) than non-carers.

Benefits for elderly people and their carers

Because of the frequency of changes to the state system of benefits, it is not possible within this chapter to give a comprehensive review of all the benefits available to men and women over retirement age and their carers. However, it is intended to give a brief overview of the main benefits payable.

RETIREMENT PENSION

At the time of writing, women aged 60 years and men aged 65 years are entitled to a weekly retirement pension. The amount payable is variable, depending on previous national insurance contributions and is taxable. The amount payable reduces if an individual has other income; for example, if they carry on working or have an occupational or private pension.

In 1993, the basic retirement pension for a married couple under 80 years was £89.80 per week.

INCOME SUPPORT

If the state pension is not enough to live on, it may be possible for the elderly person to claim income support. This is a means-tested benefit made up of a personal allowance, a premium for being a pensioner but less the retirement pension. For example, in 1993 a retired couple aged 68 and 75 years would be entitled to an extra £8.20 per week calculated as follows:

Couple's personal allowance		£69.00
Pensioner premium		£29.00
	Total	£98.00
Less Retirement Pension		£89.80
Income Support Entitlement		£8.20

(Source: Benefits' Agency, 1993)

Although the couple would get only an extra £8.20 per week, entitlement to income support would mean that the couple would get help also with glasses and dental costs and possibly some help with rebate of council tax. People with savings of over £8000 cannot claim income support and people with more than £3000 in savings may get only limited support.

From April 1993, an elderly person who was receiving income support in their own home and who entered a residential or nursing home, would continue to receive it to help with their accommodation costs. People living in residential or nursing homes before April 1993 will continue to receive income support at a higher level. The new funding arrangements from April 1993 have removed any financial incentive to move into residential care, as the elderly person would receive only the same level of income support as they had received in their own home.

ATTENDANCE ALLOWANCE

This is a tax free weekly benefit for people age 65+ years who need help with personal care. This can be used by the elderly person to buy extra care from a care agency, or it could be paid to their informal carer to provide those services. There are two rates of attendance allowance payable:

The lower rate of £30.00 per week is payable for people who need help during the day or night.

The higher rate of £44.00 per week is payable for people who need help during the day *and* night.

Elderly people who move into residential or nursing homes are still entitled to attendance allowance if they are meeting the full costs themselves and are not receiving income support. For those elderly people who are receiving financial help from their local authority towards the cost of their residential care, or receiving income support, they will lose their attendance allowance after four weeks.

INVALID CARE ALLOWANCE (ICA)

This is a taxable benefit for carers under retirement age, who provide care for the elderly person for more than 35 hours per week. In order to get ICA the elderly person who is being cared for would have to be eligible for attendance allowance (i.e. needing help by day or night). If the carer was receiving any other benefits, such as income support or housing benefit, these would be taken into account in the calculations for ICA eligibility. The basic rate of ICA is £33.70 per week but ICA may be cancelled out by other benefits already claimed.

Whilst the carer is receiving ICA, national insurance credits are put on the carer's national insurance record without charge. This helps to preserve the carer's retirement pension entitlement.

FINANCIAL SUPPORT FOR RESIDENTIAL CARE

From April 1993 people entering residential care, for the first time, would have their care needs assessed by their local authority social services department and their requirement for either residential or nursing home identified.

Where an elderly person is likely to have a need for nursing care, the assessment of needs would be undertaken together with a qualified nurse. Social Services would also assess whether the elderly person would qualify for financial help from them to meet the home fees. For people who qualify for full financial help, it would be made up of income support and help from the social service budget up to an agreed limit. If the costs of the home are above the limit set by social services, then the deficit would have to be made up from the elderly person's own funds or by contributions from relatives.

As stated above, some health authorities have entered into contracts with private nursing homes to provide continuing care facilities and are willing to pay 'top-up' fees to make up any shortfall.

Increasingly, private insurance companies are targeting the middle-aged, to encourage them to take out policies to provide for care in retirement, including residential care. It is clear that there will not be enough 'public' funds to meet the majority of residential care needs for the large numbers of elderly people predicted to be living to extreme old age in the future and so individuals will need to make adequate provision for their old age much earlier during their working lives.

Moving into residential care

The government's proposals for care in the community assumes that large numbers of people will still be available in the future to act as informal carers for the increasingly elderly population. Victor (1991) poses the question as to whether there will be an adequate supply, as factors such as increased divorce rates, the reduction in family size and the increased financial need for women to work outside the home are likely to reduce the number of people available. Also, even if there are people willing to take on the role of informal carer, should these volunteers be exploited as a cheap alternative to 'state' support?

Victor (1991) believes that the government's community care 'reforms' are actually masking the truth that for many of the elderly, care in the community means 'care by the community' and in particular, care by informal carers (see Chapter 3).

Although many elderly people do manage to live independently in their own homes, or with support by informal or formal carers, there comes a time for some when they need to consider moving into residential care. Sometimes this is because the elderly person has become too physically or mentally frail to care for themselves. They may have had an illness, such as heart disease or stroke, which has left them more disabled than they were before. They may be too frail to live alone, even with community nursing services or the support of an informal carer. Their care needs may have become too much for their carer to support, even with community services. Often the need to consider residential care is precipitated by the loss of a partner, or other carer.

Following the implementation of the Community Care Act, local authority social service departments are responsible for assessing the elderly person's needs for alternative residential care if they cannot continue to be maintained at home and assessing whether they need sheltered housing, a residential or nursing home.

Local authorities are required to use private or voluntary providers of residential accommodation, to reduce the need for local authority provision. In recent years there has been a rapid growth in private residential care for the elderly and although local authorities are required to monitor these homes and ensure that legal requirements are being met, there is still great variation in what is provided for the elderly person which will affect the quality of the resident's experience. Many people are concerned about the quality of the service that will be provided for elderly people in these private homes.

It is proposed to consider a case study example to illustrate how one large provider of housing and care for the elderly (Anchor Housing) is working towards ensuring that the highest possible standards are achieved, through improving their operational systems and procedures, ultimately to achieving the British Standard 5750 of 'quality systems'. Anchor, formally a registered charity, was founded in 1968 and is the largest provider of housing and care for the elderly in the UK.

Within England, Anchor has 600 sheltered housing schemes, 70 residential and nursing schemes and 31 schemes which allow people to 'stay put' in their own homes with assistance.

Their community nursing home schemes provide residents with 24-hour care in a 'homely' setting. Partnerships also exist with some local health authorities to provide continuing care facilities in community nursing homes, for elderly people who would otherwise have had to remain in hospital.

Anchor, in their 'mission statement', state a commitment to 'increase the quality of life and personal contentment of elderly people living within their schemes' (Anchor Housing, 1992).

In order to be able to achieve the above and to ensure a high quality of care provision, Anchor examined its organizational and management of care systems, to develop operational policies of 'core' and 'local' procedures that would be open to both internal and external audit and meet the quality standard of BS 5750. One of the key aims of the quality system that Anchor developed was to ensure that all staff fully understood their roles and the roles of others in order to ensure that the required service standards were being achieved, especially that the needs of residents were being met appropriately.

The development of the quality system has involved staff from the highest levels of management, down to the maintenance support staff in comprehensive staff training and development programmes.

All staff have been asked to examine their current working practices and suggest ways of improving them and have been invited to comment on the feasibility of suggested core and local procedures. Residents' and relatives' views have also been sought and taken into account in the development of procedures. An example of a 'core' procedure that would be used within all of the Anchor schemes, is the 'key worker' system.

Part of Anchor's philosophy is that every resident should have a named member of staff responsible for their care planning and overall welfare, including social activities. In their nursing home schemes, a first level nurse would be responsible for 'overseeing' individual care plans where the key worker was not themselves a first level nurse. The key worker would be involved in any preadmission visits to the elderly person whether at home or in hospital, to establish an initial rapport with the intending resident and their family and be involved in the preadmission assessment of needs.

When the elderly person is admitted to the scheme, the key worker will spend time enabling the new resident to 'settle in', introducing them to the other residents and the facilities available. During the resident's stay, the key worker will continue to 'befriend' the resident and monitor their needs, ensuring that they are met appropriately.

All procedures and operational policies have had to take account of relevant legislation (e.g. the Registered Homes Act, the Health and Safety at Work Act, the Food Safety Act and COSHH Regulations). Additionally, nursing procedures have had to meet UKCC regulations and be based on a sound research rationale. These procedures and their effectiveness are kept under review and where they do not appear to be meeting what is required, requests for 'corrective action' are made and procedures changed where necessary.

A system of internal and external audit is undertaken to ensure that staff are working to the agreed procedures and that the quality system as a whole, is maintaining the necessary standards. An annual quality report is prepared, which contains a review of the residents' stated needs, their feelings about the quality of the service being provided, the views of the staff and an evaluation of the quality system as a whole. This is an opportunity also to identify areas for further development or improvement.

Conclusion

As has been discussed above, growing older is inevitable. There are increasing numbers of old people living to extreme old age (80+ years) and who are likely to be living alone, or supported by carers who are themselves elderly.

More people are being cared for in the community with higher levels of dependency than before the recent NHS and community care reforms. This has resulted in an increased demand particularly for district nursing services; and district nurses are finding it increasingly difficult to give the necessary 'emotional support' to elderly people and their carers because of their increased workload and the decreased numbers of fully qualified staff following 'skill-mix reviews'.

In many areas, local authorities are being forced to cut back on, or increase the cost of the social care services that they provide in order to keep the council tax low as the government's revenue support grant may be insufficient to provide services to meet all assessed needs.

Retired people may find that, despite state benefits, they may still have insufficient funds to meet their needs and there is a danger that the need to balance the social service budget will mean that care will be purchased from the cheapest provider, which may affect the quality of that care.

The growth of private care agencies providing home-based services and residential care could, in theory, widen the choice for elderly people and their carers. In reality, choice is often narrowed down to cost.

If the elderly person needs specialized nursing care which only the district nurse can provide, then the cost of this service will be met by the health authority or fundholding GP where appropriate. However, if the needs are mainly for social care (e.g. help with personal hygiene or dressing and shopping), then the elderly person will have to pay the full cost, or a contribution assessed by social services.

The increased use of private agencies to provide social and residential care facilities for elderly people and the decrease in local authority provision, may narrow the choices available. As the growth in private care agencies and private residential and nursing homes expands, there will be an increasing need for social service departments to monitor accurately the quality of care provided, including the quality of life experience for those elderly people involved.

It has been shown how one large private provider of residential and nursing home care is committed to ensuring high standards of care which are open to outside scrutiny. However, many homes which are not run by charitable organizations are run on purely business lines. As Nazarko (1994) points out, increasingly more heavily dependent elderly people are being admitted into nursing homes and some homes are struggling to provide the levels of qualified nursing staff required within the fees limit that social service departments are able to pay.

In contrast, some local authorities are able to pay a 'premium' for the provision of extra care facilities. This is possible because some areas get a higher level of revenue support grant than others.

Inadequacy and inequality in funding for community services, remains the major obstacle to achieving the aim of 'living as independently as possible in their own homes' for many elderly people or 'living in "homely" settings in the community', which was one of the main aims of the 1990 Community Care Act. Lack of appropriate levels of benefit for elderly people and their carers is likely to 'impoverish' the quality of their lives further, as they struggle to meet the costs of caring.

Community nurses and social service staff do have a vital role to play in assessing needs and implementing appropriate care 'packages'. But unless adequate funding is made available and priorities for allocation of resources take into account 'quality of life' issues, then the aims of care in the community for the elderly will remain just empty promises.

References

Anchor Housing 1992: *Quality assurance manual*. Oxford: Anchor Housing.
Atkin, K. 1993: Nurses's effectiveness in supporting carers. *Nursing Standard* **42**(7), 38–9.
British Medical Association (BMA) 1992: *Priorities for community care*. London: BMA.
Benefits' Agency 1993: *Caring for someone*. London: HMSO.
Dimond, B. 1993: Who cares for the future? *Elderly Care* **5**(3), 11–16.
DOH 1989: *Caring for people*. London: HMSO.
DOH 1990: *Community Care Act*. London: HMSO.
DOH 1992: *The patient's charter*. London: HMSO.
George, M. 1994: Two cheers for the changes. *Nursing Standard* **27**(8), 10–11.
Hancock, C. 1993: New dimensions in caring. *Elderly Care* **3**(1), 18–19.
Laczko, F. 1993: Combining paid work with elder care: the implications for social policy. In Luker, K.A. (ed.), *Health & Social Care* **1**(2), 81–9.
Laing, W. and Hall, M. 1991: *The challenges of ageing*. London: BPI.
NAHA 1989: *The 1990 general medical practitioner's contract*. Briefing document. London: NAHA.
Nazarko, L. 1994: Out with the old. *Nursing Standard* **25**(8), 46.

Neill, J. and Williams, J. 1992: *Leaving hospital: elderly people and their discharge to community care*. London: HMSO.

OPCS 1985: General household survey. In Victor, C.R. (1991) *Health & Health care in later life*. Milton Keynes: OU Press.

OPCS 1988: General household survey. In Laing, W. and Hall, M. (1991) *The challenges of ageing*. London: BPI, p. 6.

Royal College of Nursing (RCN) 1993: *Buying community nursing: A guide for GPs*. London: RCN.

Simmons, M. 1994: Flagship is sailing in choppy waters. *The Guardian* **April 20th** p. 6.

UKCC 1990: *Statement on practice nurses & the new GP contract*. London: UKCC.

Victor, C.R. 1991: *Health & health care in later life*. Milton Keynes: OU Press.

Worth, A. 1994: Community nurses & discharge planning. *Nursing Standard* **21(8)**, 29–30.

PART THREE

Add a touch of environment

The school

Jennie Humphries

School is, for most of us, our first experience of communal life. Here too, apart from the formal lessons, we learn much about that which society expects of us. There is, also, evidence that we start to develop ideas about health and illness during this period of life (Richman and Skidmore, 1984). Jennie Humphries effectively explores how the community nurse relates to the school environment. She revisits the notions of health promotion and empowerment whilst maintaining a nursing focus. This chapter initiates the section on environment and reinforces many of the issues raised within other chapters.

Introduction

The term *school nurse* can be simply described as a nurse who works in schools; but this belies the diverse and intricate nature of the role and function of this branch of the nursing profession. The primary function is working with school age children though this naturally involves close collaboration with parents (or carers) of the children and with other professionals.

The school nurse is a specialist practitioner in primary health care and is the key health professional for children at school (Tyrrell, 1984; British Paediatric Association, 1995). Whether based within a school or a health centre, the role is significant in that it involves being an active member of both the school team and the primary health care team. This is not a juggling of roles, rather it is a significant development towards working to encourage collaboration in the promotion of health of the schoolchild.

School nurses are part of the NHS and are employed by health authorities or NHS Trusts. The immediate management varies, some school nurses are part of a community unit whilst others are attached to a paediatric unit.

School nursing is one of the few areas within the nursing profession that focuses almost entirely on health maintenance and health promotion (see Chapter 4). It is unique in that the client group are all children and are predominantly healthy. The caseload consists of children attending schools within a defined area so all children who are being educated in a state school have a school nurse, regardless of their health, educational or social status. Most independent schools also employ a school nurse and, in the case of residential schools, the role may also involve a variety of clinical duties (Allen, 1992).

The school nurse is the named nurse for usually between 1000 and 2000 children with ages ranging from three years to 18 years. The majority of these children are healthy and school nurses actively search out and respond to the health needs of the school age population to whom they are responsible.

The practical working role of the school nurse varies throughout the country depending upon the employing authority, the school and to some extent upon the school nurse themselves. Typically, a school nurse may work from a local health centre or clinic base and have two or three primary 'feeder' schools and one or two high schools together with perhaps a school for children with special needs. In some parts of the country secondary schools have a nurse 'on site'. This system is popular with school nurses because it permits a useful working relationship to be built up with the school team and, as they are part of the whole school system, it enables them to develop close relationships with the pupils.

Unless the health of children is accounted for, the full benefits of education provision cannot be gained. It was this realization that prompted the establishment of the school health service in 1907. The present service regards the achievement of optimum health as a right for all children of school age (BPA, 1995). The promotion of the health and well being of the child in the present and of the adult in the future are vital aims of the service. The school nurse has been part of the school health service since its inception and the role has developed considerably over recent years, reflecting changes within society and adaptation to account for legislative reforms that affect both health and education provision. To some extent these changes have meant that school nurses have been obliged to alter and refine their function. However, many new and innovative practices have occurred as a result of the nurses themselves, who have had the vision of a school nursing service that could meet the health needs of school age children.

The fundamental function of the contemporary school nursing service is that of health promotion. What this term actually means has prompted much debate (Ewles and Simnett, 1992) though a widely accepted definition is that provided by the World Health Organization (1984), 'Health promotion is the process of enabling people to increase control over, and to improve their health'.

Tannahill (1985) considers that the definition requires clarification both on a theoretical level and for practical purposes. He has devised a model to indicate how the essential ingredients of health promotion combine with the overall intention to emphasize the enhancement of positive health and the prevention of ill-health. The model (Fig. 9.1) incorporates three overlapping spheres of activity of health promotion: prevention, health protection and health education. A central principle is one of the empowerment of individuals, groups and communities. It follows, therefore, that it is this that should permeate throughout any and all health-promoting activities, from one-to-one teaching to community development initiatives. In fulfilling the function of health promotion, the school nurse undertakes a variety of roles:

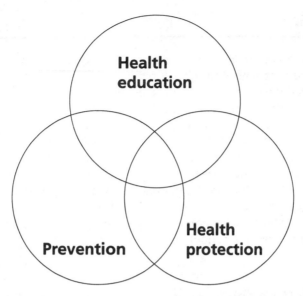

Figure 9.1 A model of health promotion. With permission Health Education Authority (copyright holder).

- a health education facilitator/adviser to pupils, and their parents and teachers, both in groups and on a one-to-one basis;
- a public health nurse, contributing to the development of school and community programmes and other initiatives that aim to promote health;
- a counsellor to school children (and their parents) of all ages;
- a clinical nurse, with responsibility for health interviews and screening procedures. They may assist the doctor with medical examinations and immunization and vaccination programmes within their designated schools. The clinical role also involves the care and management of children who have special needs because of health problems, illness or disability;
- a liaison officer, especially between the health and education sectors, but also the social services and voluntary agencies.

Though most of the work of the school nurse is within the school situation they also do home visits if the child has particular health needs or sometimes routinely prior to school entry. In addition, they may work within specialist clinics, such as those for children with asthma or eneuresis or in teenage family planning clinics. Involvement in running groups, for example those for children with eating disorders or those experiencing difficulties with self-image or relationships, means working with other professionals in both the voluntary and statutory services. In these cases the location varies and thus the school nurse is very much a community health specialist.

Prevention

The prevention sphere is perhaps the one that equates most easily with the traditional view of school nursing functions. Since the role was developed, school nurses have been involved in screening and surveillance programmes that fall within the realms of prevention. However, this particular aspect of work has witnessed several changes that have resulted in the development of the health interview as the health assessment technique undertaken by most school nurses (Fletcher and Balding, 1992; RCN, 1992). The health interview maintains the prevention aspect of health promotion but it also encompasses the other two spheres of health education and health protection. Health interviews reach all children, provide a link between screening and health education and highlight particular areas of need, of individuals and also the school and wider community.

The health interview

When the school health service was first established, its cornerstone was the school medical examination. Until 1959, statutory regulations stipulated the number and timing of the medical examinations each child had to have during the period of compulsory education. The role of the school nurse developed around these regulations and was primarily to ensure the smooth running of the medical examinations. For example, it was their job to ensure there was minimal disruption to class work by liaising with the teachers (Ottewill and Wall, 1990). The major part of the work, however, was as accessory to the role performed by the doctor. This was both for the purposes of the examination itself, including the preparation of room, records, equipment and the children, assisting during the actual examination and also afterwards, in following up non-attenders and referrals. They also supplemented this aspect of the service by providing their own assessment programme, including vision and hearing screening, growth monitoring and hygiene inspections. The emphasis on the routine and regular health screening and surveillance of school children restricted the school health service's ability to develop a more responsive service that addressed the changing needs and wants of the children, their parents and their teachers (Ottewill and Wall, 1990).

Although a more selective system of medical inspection occurred during the 1960s, it was not until 1974 that medical examinations ceased to be obligatory. This coincided with the transfer of the school health service from the responsibility of the education authorities to become part of the NHS. Impetus for the trend towards a selective approach to the medical examination of school children came from the Court Report (1976) and a report by the National Children's Bureau (1987), which suggested that routine medicals were unnecessary and that medical time and skills would be better targeted towards those children who had, or were at risk of developing, health problems. Both reports advocated the retention of the school entry medical and the continuation of routine health screening for all children by the school nurse. This focused the school nurse as the major health professional in the screening and surveillance of most ordinary children after their initial school medical examination at age 5 years. Nevertheless, it became apparent that the mechanistic approach to the school nurse health assessment of children was inappropriate. The task-oriented and rigid programme (Bagnall, 1991) did not allow a holistic approach to be adopted. School nurses recognized the inappropriateness of the format and also the potential for developing screening procedures into a system of health assessment that catered for the needs of the client and provided them with an increase in job satisfaction. The present system, the health interview, evolved. This encompasses a more dynamic search for health needs rather than merely a screening for problems and it involves the child as an active participant.

The approach is not a mini-medical, nor is it an attempt to duplicate the doctor's medical examination. Rather, it is seen as a more appropriate method of combining routine screening with a discussion of health-related issues that are of relevance to the child and, in the case of the young child, to his or her parents.

> It (the health interview) will include a comprehensive assessment of the child's physical, emotional and developmental health. It may include physical examination such as the measurement of height and weight and/or screening tests such as vision or hearing. It will provide an opportunity for the child to raise any health concerns he or she may have. The assessment may be carried out on an individual or group basis and in a range of settings: home, school, health centre. (HVA, 1991: 3)

Because health interviews give children an opportunity to voice their own needs and concerns about health they are a significant step towards empowering the individual; the focus is on what the child feels to be important, not what the health professional sees as relevant.

The results of the interviews can form the basis for planning health education for individuals, groups or the whole school. They also serve to indicate the needs and wants of the school, and the wider community, and can enable the nurse to explore initiatives and plan interventions that reflect these.

The health interview is now regarded as an essential part of the school nurse's role (HVA, 1991). Evaluation of the system suggests that they are well received by the consumers (Inglis, 1989; Fahey and Cutting, 1992; Williamson, 1992). The pupils benefit because the emphasis is a client-centred health promotion approach. Nurses are becoming increasingly aware of the need to pass responsibility for health on to their clients. School nurses are no exception. Even very young school children can learn how to protect and enhance their health. In a one-to-one or small group setting, children can explore their own feelings and attitudes towards health. This enables the child to recognize the importance of health and the responsibility that is required to maintain and improve health status by health-enhancing activities. Thus, there is emphasis, not only on specific health-related topics but also on those attitudes and behaviours that contribute to good health. Health behaviours that are forged in childhood can do much to sustain health-enhancing attitudes and beliefs in the future.

Allowing children to take responsibility for their own health is a way of telling them that their feelings and perceptions are important. This alone can result in a raising of self-esteem and a positive self-image. Kalnins *et al.* (1992) note that empowerment, where children are concerned, often relates more to the theoretical than the practical, to the policies rather than the action. The Children's Act 1989 (DoH, 1991) is a policy document that emphasizes the right of children to be consulted in matters that concern them. This associates with interactions in health care. Jane Naish of the Health Visitor's Association raises an important question:

> . . . how much do they (Community Nurses) talk to the child, and that includes five year olds, and listen to what they say? (Thompson, 1991)

The health interview represents practical action in promoting children's rights. The health interview also serves to illustrate the relevance of the health services in assisting individuals and groups towards good health. It illustrates that health services can be responsive to the needs and wants of individuals. This is an important health-promoting activity; the accessibility, approachability and responsiveness of the health services are vital parts of primary health care (Vuori, 1984). For many children, the major contact that they have with the health service is that with the school health service. A favourable impression can influence their future use of the health services; if they feel empowered by the contact, and not merely a passive recipient, it may instigate the development of active participation in the health services as they grow up.

The shift towards health interviews rather than the medical examination of children is now being extended to include the child at school entry. The stimulus for this came in 1989 following a report about the child health services, *Health for all Children* (Hall, 1989). This suggests that the provision of universal school entry medicals are unnecessary for the majority of children. The emphasis of the report is on empowering parents to take responsibility for their children's health. Since they are closest to the child, listening to parents' concerns will be as likely to detect those problems that can be treated as would a medical examination. It also has to be considered that this approach is likely to result in a more cost-effective service, since medical skills and time can then be directed towards those children with, or at risk of developing, health problems. Two years later a second edition of *Health for all Children* (Hall, 1991) reiterated the recommendations for the core programme of child health surveillance in the preschool years. The report acknowledges that the responsibility for child health surveillance moves to the school health service when the child is 5 years but it is suggested that the comprehensive preschool surveillance should eliminate the need for a medical examination at school entry. This suggestion is supported by a later report specifically about the health services for school aged children (BPA, 1995). The recommended approach to health assessment at school entry is a universal health interview by the school nurse, together with height and weight assessment and vision and hearing screening. Medical examination can then be provided on the basis of the school nurse interview, because health records are incomplete or indicate actual or potential problems or because of parental concern. This report stresses the role of the school nurse as 'the key figure in carrying out the care programme' (p. 44).

In practice, there are those school health services that remain in favour of universal school entry medicals (Whitmore and Bax, 1990; Elliott *et al.*, 1994) whilst others opt for a nurse-led approach and selective medical examination (Richman and Miles, 1990; Mattock, 1991; Broomfield and Tew, 1992; Bolton, 1994). The school-entry health interview takes a different perspective to that of the interview with older children. The child is encouraged to participate in the health discussion, but there are obvious limitations to the contribution a 5 year old can make as to the assessment of his or her health (Waldron and Brown, 1992). Also, because a comprehensive health and development picture is required, it is the parents (or carers) who are normally the major participants in the school-entry health interview. The focus remains client centred but both the parent and the child occupy the position. This is useful in promoting the school health service and in establishing relationships with parents as well as the children (Waldron and Brown, 1992). Evaluation of the school-entry health interview in terms of satisfaction for clients and practitioners appears to be favourable (Richman and Miles, 1990; Waldron and Brown, 1992; Bolton, 1994). Richman and Miles (1990) state:

> It now seems that there is no longer a place for routine medical examination of all children at school entry. A health interview with the school nurse maintains the direct contact that parents prefer and allows efficient screening. Those children that do have problems benefit from the extra medical time available to them. There is an increased opportunity for health education by the school nurse.

Children in need

A vital function of the health interview is to detect those health problems that could be detrimental to the health and development of the child, especially within the educational setting. Identifying children in need is important because only if they are identified can appropriate assistance be provided. Children in need are defined within the Children Act (1989) as:

> he is unlikely to achieve or maintain, or to have the opportunity of achieving or maintaining, a reasonable standard of health or

development without the provision for him of services by a local authority: his health or development is likely to be significantly impaired, or further impaired without the provision for him of such services, he is disabled. (section 17(10))

The Children Act (1989) lays down responsibilities for the local authorities in relation to children in need. However, whilst some special needs are clearly identified in infancy there are others that are less clear cut and these may not be determined until a child reaches school:

> Surveys have shown that the known prevalence of most types of disability increases once the child has gone to school. This may be because the extra rigours of school life bring to light the minor disabilities. It may also be because more of them are brought to the attention of the services within schools, such as the school medical service. (Pickin and St Leger, 1993: 93)

School nurses may be the first to identify children in need because of their surveillance programme. Ní Bhrolcháin's (1993) review of some of the recent research into school entry assessments suggests that approximately 40 per cent of children at school entry have health problems. Some of these will be detected or dealt with for the first time.

In addition to identifying the needs of children, the school nurse is instrumental in helping to meet these needs. It has been estimated that 20 per cent of all children will require some support in school (DES, 1978; Broomfield and Tew, 1992). Since the 1981 Education Act, many more children with learning difficulties and with physical disabilities and chronic illness are educated in ordinary schools. The Children Act (1989) places emphasis on the local authorities to provide services that aim to keep the child in the community with their family and to help those children with disabilities to lead as fulfilling a life as possible. The NHS and Community Care Act (1990) also stresses that people with special needs should be provided with services that enable them to live in their own homes and that their carers should receive practical support (DoH, 1989). School nurses can make important contributions towards the care that children with special needs may require. They will often conduct preschool visits to nursery schools or to homes to help establish relationships with families and to discuss the particular health or developmental needs of the child. Children with medical conditions, special dietary or treatment needs and those with learning disabilities or developmental delays may require extra help and support from the school health service. Parents are the major source of information and need to be aware of how this part of the health service can best serve the interests of their child.

Within mainstream education it is only rarely that the school nurse is involved with any clinical procedures that the children require. Usually the children are able to perform these functions themselves, for example giving medication or emptying catheter bags. In more complex cases, assistants are employed to be with the child throughout the day, for example a child with a tracheostomy or severe impairments of mobility. Nevertheless, the school nurse is important in assisting with the management of chronic disease, such as asthma, diabetes and cystic fibrosis (UKCC, 1994). Liaison with other agencies and providing support to the child, family and the school are necessary if the child is to gain optimum benefit from education provision. A range of nursing skills is required to assess and monitor the child's health and development, within the educational establishment. School nurses who work at schools for children with specific needs are usually involved to some extent in clinical nursing care, though children are always encouraged to self-care as much as they are able.

Regardless of where a child with special health and/or educational needs receives schooling, the school nurse has a part to play as a resource person for parents and teachers. Their nursing expertise and experience are prerequisites in ensuring that factors such as environmental conditions, both physical and social, are conducive to the child with special needs learning and developing to his or her potential.

Drop-in clinics

A service provided by the school nurse that is closely affiliated to the health interview is the drop-in clinic. As the name suggests, these sessions allow pupils to see the school nurse on an informal and unannounced basis. They are normally set up at lunchtime so that they provide an opportunity for the child to have access to a health professional without asking anyone's permission. This acknowledges the children's responsibilities for their own health and their right of access to the health service. These are important principles in the quest towards empowering children. Any issue may be discussed and these sessions can be especially useful in allowing children an opportunity to discuss emotional problems for example those regarding relationships and self-esteem (Turner, 1994).

Health education

Education and health are closely connected (see Chapter 4). The term 'health education' implies that people benefit from learning about health. In the past decade there has been a shift from the traditional approaches of health education (such as information giving and steering people towards behaviour change) towards a more general approach that utilizes a holistic view of health and the concept of empowerment.

For most of the history of health education within the school curriculum there has been the involvement of health professionals (Tones et al., 1990). Part of the 'standard' school nursing duties between 1948 and 1974 described by Ottewill and Wall (1990) are '. . . taking health education classes on a variety of subjects, such as hygiene, exercise, menstruation and other aspects of growing up, smoking and, from the late 1960s, drug abuse' (p. 183).

This reflects the content of early health education within schools, which focused on physical health and hygiene, and also the process of health education, with the concentration being primarily on the provision of health knowledge (Tones *et al.*, 1990). By the 1980s there was a broadening of the concept of health and a recognition that certain processes and methods of health education were more effective than others. Whitehead (1989) notes that three key principles have emerged concerning effective health education in schools.

- That attention has to be paid to how children make decisions about health. Health education is not merely giving the children information but helping them to clarify their ideas, values and attitudes. It is also about allowing children the opportunity to practice making health choices by utilizing active learning methods.
- That learning and health behaviour are closely connected to a person's self esteem and self image, thus methods need to be directed at enhancing these.
- That health education requires more than single lessons on isolated topics. Key themes need to be revisited in ways that match a child's level of maturity.

Although most school nurses are involved in formal health education lessons within schools, this aspect of the role has to be viewed in context with the other functions of school nursing and with the prevailing philosophy that integrates health education within the school curriculum. School nurses are now more actively involved in the planning of health education using their skills and expertise to advise teachers about health topics. They collaborate with teachers in devising and delivering lessons and may also work in teams with other school nurses so that small group work can be facilitated. Health education sessions can provide an ideal opportunity to allow the children to take the initiative, both about the topic and the method of delivery. The childrens' perception of health education topics and the strategies employed to deliver them are important. Igoe (1993) suggests that some methods can seem boring to children and Moon (1987) points out that children bring knowledge and information to the learning arena and advises that this resource should be capitalized on. She also notes that if children are keen to learn about their concerns about health the messages are much more likely to be successful. In order to utilize this approach there is the need ask the pupils about their concerns. The health interviews provide a forum for discussion and small groups are often used to inform children about what they can expect of the interview (Bagnall, 1991) or as follow-up sessions to address health topics that seem to be of particular interest.

Several strategies of health education have been developed with the intention of giving children the initiative in their own health education. One such approach is the child-to-child movement that was introduced following the Alma Ata declaration on Primary Health Care (WHO, 1978). The basic ideas are not new, and the approaches have their roots in traditional family teaching. But the co-ordinated and planned activities represent the 'new' type of health-promotion activity that concentrates on both the rights of the child and the child as a resource. In other words, there is emphasis placed on empowering the child.

THE IDEAS

- Health is viewed as a holistic concept and as an essential ingredient in the child benefiting from education.
- Children are regarded as responsible beings who can help both themselves and others to stay healthy and become healthy.
- Knowledge and understanding about health is seen as important, as is the development of ideas and skills to enhance good health and prevent ill-health.

THE APPROACHES

Children are encouraged to take action on health-related issues so that learning in school can be linked with the home and the community. The approaches are concerned with the present but are intended to be developed so that they will also apply in the future. Also, they are very much concerned with children learning from each other and teaching each other (Bonati and Hawes, 1992).

Another child-centred approach to health education is Kidscape (Elliot, 1992). The focus is child protection but due to the multifaceted nature of this, many of the experiences provided within the sessions transfer to other situations. Once again there is emphasis on empowering children, both within the learning arena, and in enabling them to develop life skills.

There has long been expectation that school health education should address contemporary health problems and social ills (Lewis, 1993). Lewis notes that this 'principle of the curriculum being used as a vehicle to respond to national needs' can be seen regarding smoking, drugs, school age pregnancies, child abuse, HIV and AIDS. The targets of the *Health of the Nation* report (DoH, 1992) apply to young people, notably in relation to diet, smoking, sexual health, accidents and suicides. These set out interesting agendas for school health education programmes and can be used to raise awareness about health inequalities and about the social and economic factors that contribute to ill-health.

An important development in health education within schools is that of the health-promoting school.The concept was first introduced in 1983 by the WHO (Moon, 1993). The proposal heralded a move from traditional health education approaches towards a philosophy of health promotion. This involves all the people within the school, the local community (including parents) and also the environmental factors (social and physical) that impinge upon them. The features of the health-promoting school emphasize the interdependence of school, home and the community; the necessity for consultation and collaboration is acknowledged. Empowerment of individuals and groups is regarded as vital. In the individual, this may be the development of social skills or improving self-image. For groups, the level is that of development of the social setting; pupils can be encouraged and supported in the organization and teaching of lessons about health and can institute organizational change within the school by devising policies and programmes that affect health. Parents are consulted to establish what they see as priority health issues but frequently it is the children who encourage their families to consider health in a wider sense.

For the community, the intention is to cultivate attitudes and beliefs that can promote community development. The health-promoting school fosters links with the community to ensure a consistency of health messages given to the children. Collaboration between school and community is regarded as a two-way process so that outside agencies contribute to health-related activities within the school and for the community. Pupils become part of the health-promoting community and are involved in initiatives outside of school boundaries, for example litter campaigns or cleaning up graffiti. The concept of the health-promoting school involves appropriate teaching of health-related issues that are encompassed within the whole school curriculum. It also means that the school environment is developed in order that the principles taught are reflected within the whole environment. School nurses contribute to the health-promoting school philosophy in their work in teaching, counselling and surveillance. There is also the potential for school nurses to expand their role to include occupational health. There is strong support for this progression in order that a comprehensive service for the whole school can be provided (Staunton, 1983; Strehlow, 1987; HVA, 1991). Although there are school nurses who do provide a health advisory and/or counselling service to school staff (Hawes, 1989), this is often on an informal basis. The HVA (1991) recommends a higher profile and an extension of this aspect of the school nurse role:

> The school nurse also has an occupational health role within the school community, providing support and advice to teachers on coping with their own needs in addition to those of children. Recognition should be given to the skills and responsibilities of the school nurse (HVA, 1991: 9).

Health protection

The focus of this sphere stems from traditional public health measures that directly and indirectly affect the environment where people live and work. This encompasses legal and fiscal controls, regulations, policies and codes of practice that aim to enhance positive health and prevent ill-health (Downie *et al.*, 1990).

The role of the school nurse as a public health nurse has recently gained prominence. The 'new' public health movement which began in the late 1980s recognizes a need for close collaboration between public and voluntary agencies in all matters that affect the health of the public. In 1988 the Acheson Report defined public health as '. . . the science and art of preventing disease, prolonging life and promoting health through organised efforts of society'.

The *Health of the Nation* (DoH, 1992) also emphasizes that the health of the public requires a concerted effort by individuals, groups and organizations. Reid (1991) considers that there is a need for a clearer public health approach to the needs of the school-age population and sees school nurses as ideally placed to fulfil this function. The UKCC (1994: 55.22) states 'Community school nursing specialists have a critical contribution to make to the wider public health function'.

A major contribution that nurses can make to public health is to adopt a population perspective regarding health status and health needs; that is, to regard the community as a client (Higgs and Gustafson,1985; Anderson and McFarlane, 1988). For school nurses this entails the compilation of a school profile. This is the collection and analysis of data in order to assess, plan and implement strategies to address the health needs of the whole school. The school profile should provide a balance between primary and secondary data and between qualitative and quantitative methods of data collection and analysis (see Chapters 2 and 16). A systematic and professional approach is required in compiling the profile because it is used to enable services to be targeted at identified need (BPA, 1995) and in determining future practice and intervention strategies (HVA ,1991; Poulton, 1992). It also has the potential for influencing policy decisions within the school, within the local health services and within the community.

As both primary and secondary data are used this allows a sharing of information between others who may be undertaking school, practice or community profiles. This is especially useful because it means that the time and effort required for the collection of secondary data can also be shared. It can contribute to a more comprehensive community assessment and can indicate how different organizations, groups and individuals can work together to promote the health of the community.

In addition to determining the health needs of the school, the school profile is beneficial in ensuring that the wider policy decisions reflect both the needs and wants of the community. They can be especially effective in illustrating what services can be developed. It allows the school nurse to target developments within both school and the wider locality. The need for a teenage family-planning service, or a support group for children with eating disorders, requires efforts from other professionals and presenting the facts can do much to assist the development of such services. Within the school it may be seen that a policy about conflict resolution is necessary or that a snacking policy would assist in limiting the amount of dental caries.

The collection of data for the school profile has the potential to become a health-promoting activity in its own right. As Hawtin *et al.* (1994) point out, the active involvement of community members is likely to produce a more accurate and complete description of that community.

It could also be argued that involving pupils is a direct contribution to empowerment. Igoe (1993) notes that children function in a variety of social contexts that frequently thwart empowerment. By asking the pupils to contribute in the collection of information for their school profile, a message is sent that says they, and their ideas, are important. Encouraging pupils to devise data collection techniques may not always fulfil absolute methodological criteria but it can serve to instil refreshing perspectives about the health of the school. Both pupils and teachers can also be used as respondents in surveys and subjects in interviews to enable their opinions about the school to be documented.

The development of the school nursing service has occurred to a large extent because of the nurses' commitment to promote the health of the young. This development and commitment must continue. School nurses have to raise their profile to ensure that the pupils, parents and teachers recognize the value of health promotion and the role that the school nurse has in this vital area of care of young people.

References

Acheson, D. 1988: *Public health in England: the report of the Committee inquiry into the future development of public health function.* London: HMSO.
Allen, D. 1992: More than a mother substitute. *Nursing Standard* 6(15/16), 16–17.
Anderson, E.T. and McFarlane, J.M. 1988: *Community as a client.* Philadelphia: J.B. Lippincott.
Bagnall, P. 1991: The way forward for school nursing. *Health Education Journal* **50**(3), 115–18.
Bolton, P. 1994: School entry screening by the school nurse. *Health Visitor* 67(4), 135–6.
Bonati, G. and Hawes, H. 1992: *Child-to-child: a resource book.* London: Child-To-Child Trust.
British Paediatric Association (BPA) 1995: *Health needs of school age children.* London: BPA.
Broomfield, D.M. and Tew, J. 1992: Selective medicals at school entry. *Public Health* **106**, 149–54.
Court Report 1976: *Fit for the future.* London: HMSO.
Department of Health (DoH) 1989: *Caring for people: community care in the next decade and beyond.* London: HMSO.
Department of Health (DoH) 1991: *The Children Act 1989: an introductory guide for the NHS.* London: HMSO.
Department of Health (DoH) 1992: *Health of the nation: a strategy for health in England.* London: HMSO.
DES 1978: *Special educational needs.* Report of the committee of enquiry into the education of handicapped young people (Warnock report). London: HMSO.

Downie, R.S., Fyfe, C. and Tannahill, A. 1990: *Health promotion: models and values.* Oxford: Oxford University Press.

Elliot, M. 1992: *Protecting children, training pack for front line carers.* London: HMSO.

Elliott, M., Jones, J.C., Jones, R. *et al.* 1994: An inter-district audit of the school entry medical examination in Cheshire. *Public Health* **108**, 203–10.

Ewles, L. and Simnett, I. 1992: *Promoting health: a practical guide*, 2nd edn. London: Scutari Press.

Fahey, W. and Cutting, E. 1992: Pupils' views of school nurses. *Community Outlook* **March**, 29–31.

Fletcher, K. and Balding, J. 1992: *School nurses do it in schools!* Huntingdon: Amalgamated School Nurses Association.

Hall, D.M.B. (ed.) 1989: *Health for all children.* Oxford: Oxford University Press.

Hall, D.M.B. (ed.) 1991: *Health for all children*, 2nd edn. Oxford: Oxford University Press.

Hawes, M. 1989: School nursing in Norwich Health Authority. *Health Visitor* **62**(11), 351–2.

Hawtin, M., Hughes, G. and Percy-Smith, J. 1994: *Community profiling: auditing social needs.* Buckingham: OUP.

Health Visitors Association (HVA) 1991: *Project health.* London: HVA.

Higgs, Z.R. and Gustafson, D.D. 1985: *Community as client.* Philadelphia: F Davis.

Igoe, J.B. 1993: Healthier children through empowerment. In Wilson-Barnett, J, and Macleod Clark, J. (eds), *Research in health promoting and nursing.* Basingstoke: Macmillan.

Inglis, J. 1989: Health interviews for school children. *Midwife Health Visitor & Community Nurse* **25**(5), 202–4.

Kalnins, I., McQueen, D.V., Backett, K.C. *et al.* 1992: Children, empowerment and health promotion: some new directions in research and practice. *Health Promotion International* **7**(1), 53–9.

Lewis, D.F. 1993: Oh for those halcyon days! A review of the development of school health education over 50 years. *Health Education Journal* **52**(3), 161–71.

Mattock, C. 1991: Stepping off the medical treadmill. *Health Visitor* **64**(5), 154–7.

Moon, A. 1987: Pictures of health. *Nursing Times* **43**(1), 49–50.

Moon, A. 1993: Promoting the health promoting school. *Health Visitor* **66**(11), 416–7.

National Children's Bureau (NCB) 1987: *Investing in the future. Child health ten years after the Court Report.* London: NCB.

Ní Bhrolchaín, C.M. 1993: Routine or selective school entry medicals: a review of current literature. *Public Health* **107**, 37–43.

Ottewill, R. and Wall, A. 1990: *The growth and development of the community health services.* Sunderland: Business Education Publishers.

Pickin, C. and St Leger, S. 1993: *Assessing health need using the life cycle framework.* Buckingham: Open University Press.

Poulton, B.C. 1992: School nursing: more than bumps and bruises (RCN Nursing Update) *Nursing Standard* **7**(2), 9–14.

Reid, J.A. 1991: Developing the role of the school nurse in public health. *Health Education Journal* **5**(3), 118–22.

Richman, S. and Miles, M. 1990: Selective medical examinations for school entrants: the way forward. *Archives of Disease in Childhood* **65**, 1177–81.

Richman, J. and Skidmore, D. 1984: Children's perceptions of health and illness. Unpublished research report, Manchester Polytechnic.

Royal College of Nursing (RCN) 1992: *Survey of school nursing 1992.* London: RCN.

Staunton, P. 1983: Does the school nurse have an occupational health role? *Health Visitor* **56**(2), 49–50.

Strehlow, M.S. 1987: *Nursing in educational settings.* London: Harper & Row.

Tannahill, A. 1985: What is health promotion? *Health Education Journal* **44**(4), 167–8.

Thompson, A. 1991: Caught in the act. *Nursing Standard* **6**(3), 22–3.

Tones, K., Tilford, S. and Robinson, Y.K. 1990: *Health education: effectiveness and efficiency.* London: Chapman & Hall.

Turner, T. 1994: A message for Mrs Bottomley. *Health Visitor* **67**(4), 121–2.

Tyrrell, S. 1984: Community child health: a big step forward. *Lancet* **i**, 725–7.

United Kingdom Central Council (UKCC) for Nursing Midwifery and Health Visiting 1994: *The future of professional practice – the Council's standards for education and practice following registration.* London: UKCC.

Vuori, H. 1984: Primary health care in Europe – problems and solutions *Community Medicine* **6**, 221–31.

Waldron, S. and Brown, H. 1992: Involving parents in school health checks *Nursing Standard* **6**(18), 37–40.

Whitehead, M. 1989: *Swimming upstream.* London: King's Fund Institute.

Whitmore, K. and Bax, M.C.O. 1990: Checking the health of school entrants. *Archives of Disease in Childhood* **65**, 320–6.

Williamson, T. 1992: Health care interviews by school nurses *Health Visitor* **65**(11), 402–4.

World Health Organization 1978: *Report on the primary health care conference, Alma-Ata.* Geneva: WHO.

World Health Organization 1984: *Health promotion. A discussion document on the concept and principles.* Copenhagen: WHO.

10 Primary health care

Joyce Green and Bobbie Saltman

This chapter examines the history and development of the practice nurse. This should prove to be a key role when, and if, nurse prescribing is realized. Certainly, the English National Board (ENB) have now recognized this role as a discipline that stands alone and should have a recognised training. It could be argued that the practice nurse is well placed to co-ordinate the roles of all other primary health care workers for the benefit of the client. In many ways they are at the front-line of community care, being the first professional that the client encounters. However, as Joyce Green and Bobbie Saltman point out, defining the role, per se, is fraught with complications; the role differs from practice to practice and depends upon the health care needs of a specific community. Health needs are influenced by the environment and here is a health care professional who, perhaps more than most, is required to respond to local needs.

Introduction.

The Royal College of Nursing Practice Nurse Forum states that, although practice nursing has existed for more than a century, its acknowledgement as a leading force in community health nursing is relatively recent. The role and function of the practice nurse has been highlighted by the implementation of the new general practitioner (GP) contract in 1990 and the rapid increase in the number of practice nurses in the last decade. According to Knight (1992) there is no doubt that the role of the practice nurse has evolved explosively and is gaining momentum as practices take on board the many facets of the GP contract and community care developments.

In March 1993, the Department of Health published the report of the task group (set up by Baroness Cumberlege, Parliamentary Under Secretary of State for Health) entitled *New World, New Opportunities: Nursing in Primary Health Care* (NHS Management Executive, 1993a), which looked at the role and scope of primary health services in the National Health Service (NHS), including the contribution made by nurses. The report emphasizes that the most direct way of ensuring that patients' needs are met is by focusing services on the people registered with each general practice. The task group envisages the development of comprehensive primary care services organized around general practice and having a full range of nursing provision. The report also stresses the importance of teamwork as providing the best and most cost-effective outcomes for patients and clients. The practice nurse is a vital member of this team and it is beholden on Family Health Service Authorities (FHSAs) to ensure that there are adequate resources for the education, support and supervision of practice employed nursing staff.

A historical overview of the development of practice nursing

In 1920 the Dawson report advocated health centres, where doctors and nurses could work together to establish a primary health care service (MoH, 1920). However, it was not until the 1950s that this idea came to fruition and the first nurses were attached to general practice to work in collaboration with their doctor colleagues to provide an improved service for patients in the community. According to Bolden and Takle (1989), health visitors were amongst the first personnel to be attached to group practices followed by district nurses in the early 1960s.

The GPs soon became aware of the benefits of having nursing assistance in the practice but many were disenchanted by the restrictions put on health authority employed nursing staff by their employers, both in terms of the time available to them, to devote to working in the practice premises, and in the ways in which they were permitted to develop their clinical role within the practice setting. In the late 1950s and early 1960s some of the more far-sighted GPs began employing, privately, their own nursing staff to work in the practice and thus the practice nurse was born. In 1966, the NHS Terms of Service for GPs radically altered the way in which they were paid and reimbursed thus encouraging them to improve their premises and employ more ancillary staff. This resulted in more practice nurses being employed.

The title *practice nurse* has evolved from: treatment room nurse, clinic nurse, group practice nurse, family practice nurse and many others, but it is now generally accepted that:

> ... the Practice Nurse is a registered general nurse who is employed by the General Practitioner to work within the treatment room and is a member of the team responsible for the clinical care of the practice population together with the district nursing team of the health authority. (ENB, 1985)

However, many practice nurses have additional qualifications and as their role has developed their work has extended into the field of health promotion and they work closely with all members of the primary health care team. In some practices with the introduction of skill mix, state enrolled nurses are also employed as members of the nursing team.

Early studies showed that patients readily accepted the nurse in their new capacity (Reedy, 1972), but there is little evidence of what the attractions were for the nurse. The first of these must be personal choice; the practice nurse is not seconded or attached and has chosen to work in general practice and the reasons for doing so are varied. They may be disenchanted with the health service and nursing management; part-time hours may be easier to arrange; they may prefer to have the choice in who they work with and where and may enjoy the responsibility of a more autonomous role, as upheld by the joint working party on nursing in general practice in the reorganized health service (RCN and RCGP, 1974).

The path has not been smooth for practice nurses as many of their community nursing colleagues have seen them as a threat and much criticism has been levelled at them. In a study done in the 1980s, practice nurses were considered by many other nurses in the community as blacklegs (Batchelor, 1985).

Regardless of this, the number of practice nurses employed had risen to over 5000 by 1985. In 1986, the *Report of the Community Nursing Review Neighbourhood Nursing – A Focus for Care* was published (DHSS, 1986a). The review team chaired by Cumberlege recommended that:

> . . . subsidies to general practitioners enabling them to employ staff to perform nursing duties should be phased out and the provision of nursing services in the community should remain the responsiblity of district health authorities.

The practice nurses' response to this was angry and vociferous, particularly when the Royal College of Nursing (RCN) backed the Cumberlege recommendations. For the first time, practice nurses banded together and made their feelings known both individually and through practice nurse interest groups and the RCN practice nurse forum. The Royal College of General Practitioners pledged their full support to the practice nurses and eventually the RCN backtracked in support of members when many threatened to resign from the college. The recommendations relating to practice nurses were duly quashed!

However, there was a very positive outcome to this unrest. Practice nurses had left the nursing hierarchy in no doubt that as a group they were a force to be reckoned with; that they enjoyed their autonomous status and that they were prepared to stand together and fight for their rights.

One of the major valid criticisms of practice nursing was the lack of formalized postregistration training. This had, however, been recognized by the RCN working group (RCN, 1984) on whose report the national boards for nursing, midwifery and health visiting based the practice nurse training outline curriculum. The latter was enthusiastically received as a starting point but had many practice nurse critics who felt that it was not sufficiently advanced for experienced practitioners. Practice nurses were disappointed that it was only a certificate of attendance course and were also concerned at the lack of practice nurse input on some of the early courses. This prompted the Royal College of General Practitioners to set up a task force, with practice nurse input, to investigate the training needs of practice nurses (RCGP Task Force Report,1988).

It now became obvious to many people that practice nurse training should be on a par with that of their community nursing colleagues (e.g. district nurses and health visitors), and a specialist recordable qualification was required to enable them to take their place as equal members of the primary health care team.

By the late 1980s, practice nurses were being acknowledged by the profession and were represented nationally on both the United Kingdom Central Council for Nursing, Midwifery and Health Visiting (UKCC) and the English National Board (ENB). Following the introduction of the GP contract in 1990, which specifically mentioned practice nurses, the ENB included a practice nurse representative on the Primary Care Committee and in 1993 four practice nurses were elected to the UKCC.

The numbers of nurses employed in general practice has continued to rise and the most current estimate is in the region of 15 000. According to Bolden and Takle (1989):

> . . . the rapid expansion of practice nurse numbers over the past ten years has led to many new ideas and role perceptions and these need to be developed. Research explores these boundaries and teaching establishes the body of knowledge required to practice the discipline.

The next section of this chapter considers the development of practice nurse education and training and whether the needs of practice nurses are being met.

The development of practice nurse education and training

BACKGROUND INFORMATION

In 1980, the RCN Society of Primary Health Care Nursing set up a working group to review the development of practice nursing in the United Kingdom which concluded that practice nurses required further specific preparation for the duties that they undertake. A steering group was subsequently formed, which included representatives from the Council for the Education and Training of Health Visitors, the Panel of Assessors for District Nurse Training, the Royal College of General Practitioners and the British Medical Association (RCN, 1984). The composition of the group ensured that the views of practice nurses and general practitioners were well represented alongside those of district nurses and health visitors. The following terms of reference were agreed:

... to examine the training needs of practice nurses and other nurses employed to work in the treatment rooms of general practice or other health centre premises and to make recommendations.

The steering group recognized that many practice nurses had already had the opportunity to attend study days and courses in addition to some in-service training, but stated that:

... what is needed is a properly structured programme designed to bring these various factors together to meet the needs of the practice nurse. (RCN, 1984)

However, they stated that it would be unrealistic to suggest that every practice nurse would require or be in a position to receive the full range of training as set out in the report.

Between 1981 and 83, the steering group met on several occasions and detailed work was undertaken between meetings. The publication *Training Needs of Practice Nurses* (RCN, 1984) contained the report of the findings of the steering group and an outline curriculum for the recommended 10-day course.

The four national boards agreed to adopt the outline course as recommended by the steering group and to review the courses in three years. The course regulations state that:

... courses should be planned in collaboration with local general practitioners and, whenever possible, should be held alongside courses for district nursing and health visiting. If this is not possible courses can only be established when there is a 'satelliting ' arrangement with a district nurse/health visitor course. (The National Boards for England, Scotland and Northern Ireland, August 1985).

By siting these courses in institutions of higher education, it was hoped that this would facilitate shared learning with others also preparing to be members of the primary health care team.

By 1989, 32 courses had been approved in England, four in Scotland and one in Wales. Since then further courses have been approved by the National Boards as appropriate, to meet the training requirements of this group of nurses.

The national boards outline course curriculum

The course is aimed at registered general nurses on Part 1 of the UKCC professional register and is designed:

... to prepare the practice nurse to work as a member of the primary health care team, confident and competent to provide skilled nursing care within the health centre or practice setting. (National Boards, 1985)

The suggested course content is divided into three broad areas of study:

- professional role development
- procedures and techniques to be used in the treatment room/health centre
- management of the treatment room/health centre.

On successful completion of the course a statement of attendance was issued by the national board, initially; this has since been replaced by the National Board's Award in Practice Nursing.

Practice nurses are from a variety of nursing backgrounds with different levels of experience and expectations of what the job is all about, so it is vital that courses are flexible and allow for individual learning needs. As Knight (1992) states, we must ensure that practice nurses are given opportunities to be appropriately and adequately qualified, up-to-date and competent to a consistent standard. The implementation of the National Board's Curriculum was certainly an important first step.

A review of ongoing developments in practice nurse education

Within three years of the inception of practice nurse courses approved by the national boards, an evaluation was undertaken by the ENB. In spite of some difficulty in arranging courses to suit the needs of such a diverse group as practice nurses, who on the early courses varied considerably in terms of length of time in employment as practice nurses and were working to differing job descriptions, there was general satisfaction with the courses overall, although some students commented that there should be more emphasis on skills-related topics and were less interested in the socio-psychological aspects of the course. Those who advocated a longer course were unable to specify the desirable length but were of the opinion that a longer course would enable students to study new knowledge in more depth.

Although, at this stage, it was difficult to justify a recommendation for major changes, in view of the implications of the White Paper *Primary Health Care – An Agenda for Discussion* (DHSS, 1986b), which stated that the further development of the role of the practice nurse is central to the future of primary health care, it seemed appropriate to review their educational needs in the light of their expanding role. This review was undertaken by the ENB in 1989 with the co-operation of the other statutory bodies (Damant, 1990). The review group, under the chairmanship of Margaret Damant (project officer), recommended that practice nurse education should comprise of an employer-led induction programme in practice nursing as an initial preparation for the work as a practice nurse, to be followed by a course in practice nursing. The length of this course should ensure the award of a qualification which is recordable on the professional register maintained by the UKCC and the content capable of being awarded academic credit. There should also be opportunities for continuing education and further professional and academic study (Damant, 1990).

> The Report informed the general debate on community nursing and was explored further in discussions on the post-registration education required for community practice, which will result in new programmes of preparation for all community practitioners. (ENB, 1993)

However, since the first courses were implemented in 1986 there have been continual developments in practice nurse education. Most of the national board courses, if not all, have been extended and have been accredited with level two (i.e. Diploma level; based on the notional honours degree: level one = one years full time study, post 'A' level, level two = two years and level three = three years) CATS (Credit Accumulation and Transfer – a national scheme for recognizing academic achievement) points and some practice nurse courses are already fully incorporated within the Diploma in Higher Education framework.

Distance learning packages have been specifically designed for practice nurses and the ENB commissioned a project which resulted in the development of Accrediting Open Learning for Nurses in General Practice, published in 1992. This relates to the ENB's open learning packages on health promotion (ENB, 1993).

Some of these initiatives have been brought about as a result of the efforts of practice nurses themselves. They have been a most proactive group in drawing the attention of the statutory nursing bodies and institutes of further and higher education to their educational needs, and, in organizing an annual conference for practice nurses.

What of the future?

At the time of writing, the UKCC's recommendations for the implementation of the proposed changes in community postregistration education and practice preparation, are eagerly awaited. These changes will bring practice nurses into the mainstream of community nurse education and ensure that their training is on a par with that of other community practitioners.

According to Jeffree (1990) practice nurses have an individual responsibility to maintain and improve professional knowledge and experience. She states that 'such knowledge, experience, and professional competence might be gained through continuing education or research'. Opportunities are now available for practice nurses to study at both diploma and degree level and, as stated by Kirkham (1993), the national boards have also developed comprehensive and flexible systems of progressional education, aimed at enhancing the practice of nursing and meeting educational needs.

This decade, practice nurses have experienced many changes with the introduction of the GP contract in April 1990 and more recently the introduction of the New Guidelines on Health Promotion in General Practice from July 1993 (NHSME, 1993b). With the increasing emphasis on primary care services, it is important that practice nurses are adequately prepared for community practice and that their education and training reflect contemporary healthcare needs and the needs of the health services to enable them to meet these challenges.

The role and function of the practice nurse

Defining the role of the practice nurse is extremely difficult as the way the nurse's skills are utilized varies tremendously from practice to practice. Even in the same practice where more than one nurse is employed there can be differences dependent upon the needs of the practice population and the individual nurse's qualifications and experience.

Originally, the practice nurse was employed to carry out nursing procedures such as dressings, routine injections, ear syringing and immunization/vaccination of children and adults, leaving the doctors more time to concentrate on patient's medical problems. This, unfairly, earned them criticism from some primary health care colleagues that they were doctors' handmaidens. Many of the critics were themselves working to doctor's instructions as well as being controlled in what they could do by their employing health authorities.

Long before the GP contract in 1990, many practice nurses had extended their role to include venepuncture, taking cervical smears, teaching women breast self-examination, chronic disease management of asthma and diabetes and counselling. The practice nurse's role developed in response to the needs of patients. One of the most frequently reported findings in all studies is that patients see the practice nurse as having more time to spend with them than the GP (Sobal, 1982).

Health education and disease prevention have always been an integral part of the practice nurse's role but this was further emphasized with the introduction of the GP contract in 1990. Nurse-run clinics became the norm as GPs were paid a fee for all clinics approved by the FHSA. The number and range of clinics held in many GP practices increased (e.g. asthma, diabetes, coronary heart screening, well person, travel vaccination, hormone replacement therapy (HRT), menopause, lifestyle, quit smoking and obesity). This proved to be not a very cost-effective way of organizing the health promotion and screening functions of general practice.

Therefore, in July 1993, some of the aspects of the GP contract were changed and health promotion banding was introduced. Many clinics were discontinued as the FHSAs now under the new regulations only reimburse the GP for asthma, diabetes and coronary heart disease screening. This led to a reduction in hours for some practice nurses.

In addition to treatment room work and running the remaining clinics, practice nurses may do home visits and be responsible for managerial and administrative duties within the practice. These may include ordering and maintainence of stock, drugs and equipment, writing protocols, updating computer-held information, follow-up of patients requiring further treatment, audit, research and management of other nurses in the practice employ. In some practices, the practice nurse has input to practice policy making and may also have a teaching role in the training practices both for trainee GPs and other nurses.

Where a practice nurse is suitably trained, they may undertake a counselling role in specialist areas such as management of patients diagnosed as having a drink problem, a weight problem or those wishing to give up smoking. Practice nurses must keep clinically updated in all relevant areas of their work, for example those running well woman clinics must have current knowledge of the advantages and disadvantages of HRT.

As a member of the primary health care team, the practice nurse must be aware of their own limitations and referral of patients to other members of the team is important in areas where their expertise is more appropriate. Referrals may vary from practice to practice depending on qualifications and expertise of team members. In most practices, the team comprises of GPs, district nurses, midwives, health visitors and practice nurses but some health centres also employ specialists in alternative therapies and the team may also include chiropodists, physiotherapists, dieticians and psychologists. Within general practice, administrative and clerical support is provided by the practice manager, receptionists and clerical assistants.

The practice nurse's role has been the source of some controversy and has been debated extensively. The amount of work carried out by practice nurses varies according to the amount of time they spend in the surgery and the health needs of the practice population. There is no doubt that with the increased emphasis on promoting health and preventing ill health that the practice nurse has a valuable part to play in the primary health care team. According to Jeffree (1990), it is important to provide a health service that is accessible, affordable and acceptable and the emphasis on primary care services presents a challenge not only to those in a clinical capacity but also to those managing the service.

Community care and general practice

The NHS Management Executive (1992) state in their guidance booklet for GPs that:

> ... the White Paper 'Caring for People' and the NHS and Community Care Act 1990 set out a policy framework for developing community care by building on the best of existing good practice. The aim is to

enable people to lead an independent and dignified life at home or in locally based residential units or elsewhere in the community for as long as they are able and willing to do so.

The White Paper (DoH, 1989) recognizes that health in its broadest sense is an essential component of the range of services which may be needed to enable people to continue to live in their own homes for as long as possible. Interagency collaboration is, therefore, vital if the health, social and psychological needs of patients and clients are to be met. There is no doubt that the importance of the GP's role in community care is highlighted and the White Paper states that 'GPs are well placed to ensure that factors other than medical ones which affect the quality of life are taken into consideration'. The contribution made by community nursing staff is also recognized and the value of the nurse's and health visitor's contribution is identified as an important resource.

Assumptions have been made in central policy and guidance documents about the willingness of GPs to contribute to the formal assessment procedures and the design of care packages for people wishing to be cared for in the community. Henderson (1992) states that:

GPs want to be involved in deciding what should happen to patients in terms of their location and treatment. However, it cannot be taken for granted that all GPs will necessarily be willing or able to afford the time commitment to participate in multi-agency assessment procedures and design of care packages. They would prefer to be consulted, particularly on medical implications, so that their advice can be fed into the assessment procedures.

None the less the importance of collaborative working practices and a team approach to community care is recognized by many GPs who have established effective working relationships with the social services authorities in their locality.

What does this mean for the practice nurse?

According to Young (1993): 'Practice Nurses now form an expanding and increasingly important group of nurses in today's community health workforce'. Therefore, as members of the primary health care team, practice nurses should be able to play a key role in identifying those people registered with the practice who may be 'at risk' or have special needs and require assistance to continue to function in a community setting, for example elderly people, especially those who live alone, those who are chronically sick or have a physical or mental disability and those people on the practice list who are acting as carers. Practice nurses must recognize the value of a team approach and as Young (1993) states '. . . work closely with colleagues in both hospital and community settings so that people with complex and diverse needs on their practice list receive the range of services to which they are entitled'.

The primary health care team has a valuable contribution to make to the delivery of health care in the community and according to Ovretveit (1993): '. . . it is one of the few types of team which bring together different professions for a number of client groups, rather than for the special needs of one group in the community'. Current developments in community care build on the GP's existing role and those of other members of the primary health care team. From April 1993, local authorities have become the lead 'community care agency', with Social Services Departments (SSDs) being responsible for assessing individuals' social care needs. It is also the SSD's responsibility to ensure that an appropriate 'care package' of services is organized to meet those needs identified. GPs and community nurses are skilled in referring patients/clients for social care and in advising patients and carers how to obtain the services of other health and social care agencies so should play an important part in this process.

The practice nurse is in a key position to contribute, along with other community nursing colleagues, to the development of more patient-centred and better co-ordinated community services. Such services should be based on the medical, nursing and social needs of the patients, clients and their carers. This can be achieved by involvement with the GP in the assessment process and by providing or validating relevant information where a health problem contributes to the patient's overall needs.

The practice nurse also comes into contact with a wide range of client groups in the course of their work and should therefore utilize all available opportunities for health promotion and to give social advice. By collaborating with other community nurses, the practice nurse participates in a team approach to community care and helps to ensure that the diverse needs of individuals are met appropriately. The contribution that the practice nurse makes to the annual assessment of patients over the age of 75 years is important, as it is one area of work where unmet health and/or social needs of this client group may be identified and subsequently dealt with by referral to the appropriate agencies. The implementation of the Community Care Act has training implications for practice nurses for if they are to act as advocates for patients, clients and carers and enable them to make informed choices, practice nurses must be adequately and appropriately trained to make the assessments, give the relevant advice and be fully conversant with the health and social care provision and resources available in the locality served by the practice. As Young (1993) states: '. . . ensuring that the Community Care Act is a success will be just one of the many issues which must be taken on board by practice nurses in the 1990s'.

Conclusion

Practice nurses are now well established members of the primary health care team and part of their role is to collaborate with other team members to build a cohesive team of health care professionals who share common goals and are committed to planning and implementing care based on the health needs assessment of the practice population. Nursing is facing an uncertain and challenging future and it is important that community nursing services are flexible in their approach in order to meet the everchanging needs of patients and clients. Practice nurses have an integral part to play in the future development of the primary care led services. There is a tremendous opportunity for proactive health care professionals to develop the potential for new ways of delivering primary health care and the specialism of practice nursing is very much needed in meeting this challenge.

References

Batchelor, Sir I. 1985: *Hospital medicine and nursing in the 1980s* London: Duncans McLachlan.

Bolden, K.J. and Takle, B.A. 1989: *Practice nurse handbook.* London: Blackwell.

Damant, M. 1990: *The challenges of primary health care in the 1990s: a review of education and training for practice nursing, the substantive report.* London: English National Board for Nursing, Midwifery and Health Visiting (ENB).

Department of Health (DoH) 1989: *Caring for people: community care in the next decade and beyond.* London: HMSO.

Department of Health and Social Security (DHSS) 1986a: *Neighbourhood nursing – a focus for care.* Report of the Community Nursing Review (Cumberlege Report). London: HMSO.

Department of Health and Social Security (DHSS) 1986b: *Primary health care – an agenda for discussion.* London: HMSO.

English National Board (ENB) 1985: *The national boards for England, Scotland and Northern Ireland – practice nurse training – outline curriculum.* London: ENB.

English National Board (ENB) 1993: *A decade of quality education for quality care – the first ten years of achievement 1983–1993.* London: ENB.

Henderson, J. 1992: To lead or not to lead? The GP's role in community care. *Primary Health Care Management* 2(10), 9–10.

Jeffree, P (ed.) 1990: *The practice nurse – theory and practice.* London: Chapman & Hall.

Kirkham, C. 1993: Surveying post basic education. *Practice Nurse* 6(12), 750–3.

Knight, J. 1992: Overskill or underskill?: The training dilemma for practice nurses. *Primary Health Care Management* 2(5), 10–11.

MoH, 1920: Consultative council on medical and allied services. Interim report on the future provision of medical and allied services [Dawson report]. Cmd 693. London: MoH.

NHS Management Executive 1992: *General practitioners and 'Caring for People'.* London: DoH.

NHS Management Executive 1993a: *New world, new opportunities – nursing in primary health care.* London: HMSO.

NHS Management Executive 1993b: *New guidelines on health promotion.* London: DoH.

Ovretveit, J. 1993: *Co-ordinating community care. Multidisciplinary teams and care management.* Buckingham: Open University Press.

Reedy, B.L.E.C. 1972: The general practice nurse. *Update* 5(6), 571–6.

Royal College of General Practitioners (RCGP) 1988: *Task force report*. London: RCGP.
Royal College of Nursing (RCN) 1984: *Training needs of practice nurses*. London: RCN.
Royal College of Nursing and Royal College of General Practitioners (RCN and RCGP) 1974: *Report of the joint working party on nursing in general practice in the reorganised National Health Service*. London: RCN.
Sobal, J. 1982: Patient expectations and acceptance of a nurse practitioner. *Family Practice Research Journal* 2(2), 125–31.
The National Boards for England, Scotland and Northern Ireland 1985: *Practice nurse training – outline curriculum*. London: ENB.
Young, L 1993: The Community Care Act. *Practice Nursing* **19th January**, 8.

The work place

James Garvey

James Garvey brings work into the community, illustrating, succinctly, that what a person does offers many symbols to all observers. He also offers an effective argument as to why it is important to have a specialist practitioner in the field of occupational health, an area that has been losing political significance over the last 30 years. Garvey starts at the beginning with Flowerday (1878) and brings us up to date with the current state of the art. He flags up the need to be an effective practitioner–researcher in order to extend practice; a message all practitioners should heed. Other models of practice are explored which will, usefully, add to those discussed by Sbaih (Chapter 5). Like Richman (Chapter 1) he also recognizes the future, suggesting that occupational health nurses would do well to surf the super highway, or at least enter cyberspace. Garvey offers an optimistic and encouraging view of the future for this specialist branch of nursing; but, quite rightly, places the onus of progress on the practitioner.

Micro to macro – the exciting evolution of the OHN

Introduction

Since the dawn of mankind man has had to work by the sweat of his brow. Working practices and their outcomes have always been fundamental to his being and have played an important role in the evolution of societies throughout the world. Of course not everyone enjoys working, some prefer to do no work at all, perhaps by choice, others find themselves unemployed through no fault of their own and still others find themselves in work, either enjoying the experience or being dissatisfied with it. Whichever way we look, work and its effects have a major role to play in our lives. Nearly 2000 years ago St Paul wrote a letter to the Thessalonians and in it he had to remind the more indolent members of that community that they should work and if they didn't 'not to let anyone have any food if he refused to do any work' (*The Jerusalem Bible*, 1966). Perhaps these were rather drastic measures to take but such was the thought of the day, that hard work should be rewarded. He went on to say, 'we order and call on people . . . to go on quietly working and earning the food that they eat' (*ibid*). Working life was part of the total harmony of one's existence. To work was to live; the two were synonymous even in the days of St Paul. That ideal has not been lost with the passage of time. In our modern day society we can see the trappings of wealth that are associated with certain occupations. We can also see around us dire poverty and the undignifying effect of unemployment on both the individual, and communities at large.

Work and its many different occupations take up at least a third of our normal daily activities. The effect of work on man and the health conditions of man and their effect on work are well documented. It is vitally important, therefore, that within the nursing profession there is a practitioner who has the appropriate expertise to deal with work-related ill health and promote and champion the cause of prevention in the work place.

Today this status is owned by the occupational health nurse (OHN) who may find themselves working in industrial or commercial settings or within the National Health Service (NHS). This chapter then, using a historical perspective, looks at the role of the OHN – the micro aspects of that role and wishes to show how the micro has flourished into a macro evolution. This evolution has brought about great changes within the specialism of occupational health nursing, which with the passage of time has focused its attention on the more wider global issues that effect our environment. An old Buddhist teaching states that if you point your finger to the sky but only concentrate on the tip of the finger, you miss the beauty and the splendour of all that lies beyond. Occupational health nursing over recent years, underpinned by relevant and challenging educational courses, has been able to alter its focus and become a more interactive discipline capable of understanding needs, challenging the *status quo*, and researching to bring about new knowledge that will help the discipline to grow even stronger. This then is the blossoming evolution of the role of the OHN.

In the beginning

There is some debate as to who was the first actual OHN and one of the most popular theories lends itself to it being Phillipa Flowerday, who in 1878 was appointed as an industrial nurse with J.J. Colman in Norwich. Much of her work at that time was spent visiting the sick in their homes and so her role had almost a dual purpose to it, in so far as many of her activities boarded on what we would now regard as being the domain of district nursing as well as OHN activities.

To wonder about who was the first OHN is, of course, missing the point. What is important is that people had the foresight to create such posts for the benefit of employees. Even Florence Nightingale is attributed with having said that, 'Nursing is not only a service to the sick – it is a service to the well – we have to teach people how to live' (Radford, 1990). In other words she was already acknowledging that nursing in the main was reactive. It needed to be preventative and needed to promote well being through education and research.

Hippocrates, 400 years before Christ, described the symptoms of lead poisoning. He laid down many guidelines for his medical students in respect of questioning skills they should apply in helping them to reach a diagnosis. However, he failed to include a question related to occupation or how their patients earned a living. This is a legacy that still exists today within the medical profession. Many general practitioners (GPs) have little or no knowledge relating to occupational health and in fact this is an issue that the Trade Union Congress is raising, and requesting that doctors be better trained in relation to this discipline so that their members may, where appropriate, be more speedily diagnosed in the case of an occupational-health related condition.

Throughout history, many famous personalities have shown a considerable interest in the working practices of man. Agricola in Germany, Paracelsus in Austria and Ramazzini in Italy all contributed to the body of knowledge that was at the embryonic stage of occupational health. Bernadino Ramazzini (1633–1714) went one step further than Hippocrates of old and suggested in his treatise *De Morbio Artificium Diatribia* (Diseases of Tradesmen and Craftsmen) that a doctor should ask the occupation of the patient. This was a giant step forward, one which was not well received by his contemporaries but one which has stood the test of time and certainly one which is as much in vogue today as it was contentious in the days of Ramazzini.

With the hundred years of Industrial Revolution that followed between 1730 and 1830, a whole host of occupational conditions came to the fore. In the main, this was due to the fact that conditions were now being seen *en masse*. Workers were now working under the same roof, factories were being built and for the first time came the opportunity to be able to monitor and study the workforce. Previously, much industry was undertaken in cottages in rural outlying areas. What illnesses occurred went almost unnoticed; there was little opportunity to apply any basic criteria of incidence between them. The Industrial Revolution changed all that. This era saw the famous names of Percival Pott, Thomas Percival, Robert Peel and Charles Turner Thackrah, the latter regarded as the father of British occupational medicine, all working towards trying to provide and legislate for a better working environment. Their observations, and subsequent writings, helped to formulate the beginnings of a professional body of knowledge upon which occupational health today was originally based.

The reforms that were ratified in parliament in the nineteenth century leading to better hours of work for women and young people, better working conditions and a legislative framework to underpin the reforms was due in the main to enlightened employers and politicians such as Shaftesbury, Peel, Owen and Sadler. Legislation continued to spew out of parliament at a rate of knots throughout the nineteenth and twentieth centuries. The first Industrial Nursing Certificate was offered by the Royal College of Nursing in 1934. Following the deliberations of the Robens Committee between the period 1970 to 1972 their recommendations were eventually incorporated into the Health & Safety at Work Act 1974, perhaps the most important and far-reaching piece of legislation that we have yet seen within the disciplines of health and safety.

Today, with the European parliament issuing directives to all its member states, the OHN can be hard pressed to keep abreast with all that is happening within the field of health and safety. The Commission, the Parliament and the Council of Ministers are keen to make sure that we all as members of the European Union, even though we have different legal, institutional and cultural traditions, will with one voice endeavour to work together from a common position and will be seen as genuinely pioneering as our forefathers did before us, to build not just a better social country but a better social Europe.

The services offered

There is currently no mandate in the UK for occupational health nursing and, given that there is so much legislation available to employers today, there are still many companies who are unsure of the type of service that would suit them best. The development of occupational health services as stated in Harrington and Gill (1993) has in the main been through the willingness and voluntary provision of employers. As a consequence, occupational health nursing, as a service to industry and beyond, may have similarities with its counterparts in other nursing disciplines but still has no formalized identity.

OHNs can find themselves working in a wide variety of establishments offering a huge variety of services. The type of service offered may initially have been planned by the employer. The service may have been planned by a multiplicity of people from different backgrounds, all with an interest in the welfare of their employees and, of course, finally, the service may not have been planned at all.

Generally speaking there are three main types of service offered which roughly fall into the following categories.

TREATMENT-BASED SERVICE

By definition, this is a reactive type of service. It is responsible for dealing with accidents, trauma, etc. as and when the problems occur. The service is useful in that it provides a service that can deal with injuries in the work place in a professional manner without having to utilize external services. It enables employees to be treated at work so enabling to keep lost time due to injury to a minimum. It also allows specific expertise to be established in relation to dealing with common or frequently occurring injuries. The treatment service also encourages good rapport between the OHN and employee and often acts as a medium through which the OHN can learn more about the types of work activity that employees are undertaking. The service also creates an opportunity for issues of a wider nature, other than simply treatment, to be raised and dealt with on an informal basis. Sheila Danton (1984) would advocate that 'it is not realistic to dispense entirely with the treatment role of the occupational health nurse . . . some injury and illness is inevitable'.

PREVENTION-BASED SERVICE

Some sites have, however, left the treatment service behind in search of a more preventative type of service. Here the emphasis is on eradication of risk at source, trying to pre-empt problems arising and having an active awareness of potential hazards in the work place so that appropriate monitoring can be undertaken. In this type of environment one would expect to see a wide variety of screening services being made available to the workforce and the OHN having the appropriate competencies for not only undertaking such activities, but also being able to advise both employee and management on the way forward.

Mixture of prevention- and treatment-based services

From the author's own recent research, undertaken for this particular chapter, it would appear to be the more popular mode of service currently in the UK. Of the 34 OHNs who participated in the survey, 33 offered a service that provided for both treatment and prevention. Only one out of this particular sample offered a service that could only be described as purely preventative. The respondents saw both treatment and prevention working hand in hand and felt that they were natural partners in an ever changing occupational health environment. Treatment was considered to be an aspect of the role of the OHN even though in some companies the actual role of treating may be given over to first aiders.

Professional isolation

Professional isolation has for a long time been an excuse, and in some cases rightly so, for the non-advancement of Occupational Health Nursing Services (OHNS) working on their own have said that they feel isolated from both the mainstream of nursing and from within the specialism of occupational health. In the 1990s, and beyond, the aspect of isolation will cease to be a problem, if indeed it ever was. The main reason why isolation may have been a problem in the past was due to the fact that practitioners within the discipline were poorly equipped, professionally and academically, in dealing with their particular unique situations. The role of the OHN with its multivariate tasks and skills required is quite unique within a nursing orientation and its very uniqueness has to some extent caused it, in the past, to be considered almost 'outside' the realms of nursing and more akin and parallel with perhaps the disciplines of safety and hygiene. Of course, such observations were often made by those ill informed about occupational health and whose ignorance fuelled their opinions.

Education has done much to improve the professional profile of the OHN by providing appropriate courses such as diplomas of higher education in community health with discipline-specific awards that draw together all the many and varied disciplines working in the community. For once, the OHN has the opportunity to see themselves as having a much wider multidisciplinary function and very much a key figure in the primary health care team.

Research carried out by the author, has looked at a variety of aspects of the role of the OHN. Figure 11.1 indicates the number of nurses working

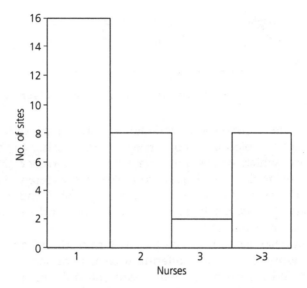

Figure 11.1 Number of nurses on site.

on sites that participated in a questionnaire research activity. The majority of sites had just one qualified OHN at their place of work. However, over 52 per cent of the sample had at least two nurses or more working on site. The aspect of professional isolation, working on one's own and the phenomenon of 'lack of identity', can arise when OHNs have little or no contact with their peer groups or strive to create better communications across disciplines which might include hygiene, safety, toxicology and other ancillary services utilized by an occupational health service.

One could, perhaps, anticipate that individuals working alone might not be as proactive as a group or dynamic team of OHNs working together. One might ask the question, just how professionally effective can nurses be when working in professional isolation; does it make them better nurses or is there a down side to such a scenario? To test this hypothesis the author created a correlation exercise based on data from the questionnaire in which numbers of nurses working on site were compared with types of service offered. Figure 11.2 indicates that, at least from this small sample, one respondent who is actually involved in purely prevention activities comes

NURSES	SERVICE			
	Total	TREAT	MIX	PREVENT
Total	34	0	33	1
ONE	16	0	15	1
TWO	8	0	8	0
THREE	2	0	2	0
>THREE	8	0	8	0

Figure 11.2 Correlation between number of nurses on site and type of service offered.

from the sample of nurses who work alone. In this instance it would appear that professional isolation is no barrier to progressing towards an avant garde service which concentrates on prevention rather than treatment. Clearly, one example is inadequate to make any sweeping generalizations but future studies might look at what is being offered and examine if there is a relationship between type of service offered and numbers of nurses working on a particular site.

Figure 11.2 also exemplifies the fact that from the sample there was no respondent who was actually offering a total treatment service. The vast majority offered a mixture of both treatment and prevention. Treatment, traditionally, has been seen as a large part of the role of the OHN. Today this is not often the case with OHNs wishing to broaden their skill base and create a more extended role within the framework of the specialism. Again

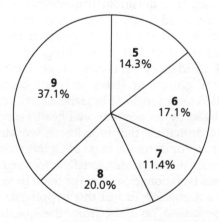

Figure 11.3 Percieved importance of treatment ranked on a scale containing nine elements. The respondents were occupational health nurses. Rank nine represents 'of least importance'.

this is borne out by the author's data as can be seen in Figure 11.3. Respondents were asked to rank various elements of their perceived role in order of importance, from a ranking scale containing nine elements. Treatment was listed as one of the elements. With a large majority the element of 'treatment' was considered to be of little importance by the sampled group. Thirty-seven per cent of the group actually ranked the element of treatment in ninth position (i.e. of least importance) as a characteristic of occupational health nursing. A further 20 per cent of the sampled group ranked the same element in eighth position. This gave a total of over 57 per cent of the group who attached little importance to treatment and yet almost 100 per cent of the group were involved in treatment processes to some extent. Might this lead one to believe that OHNs are not getting adequate job satisfaction from their current work activities?

The pie-chart also indicates that the highest ranking that 'treatment' received was fifth position (14.3% of the sample). This might go some way to explaining the recent advances made in the role of the first aider within occupational health (i.e. treatment activities are being taken away, with mutual agreement, from the OHN and given to first aiders). Theoretically, this should allow the OHN to concentrate more in proactive occupational health and preventative work. There is also a cost benefit in this transfer too. First aiders are cheaper to employ and if employers see 'treatment' as the only useful activity required by their workforce might they decide to disassociate themselves with the OHN?

Hopefully, the OHN within the work place is now creating a platform for itself in terms of its role and is educating both employers and employees into the many functions that fall into its remit, which to some extent are its sole preserve. This does not mean though that the OHN can rely on all employers to see its role in this way and become blasé or indifferent. The role has to be developed, promoted, sold and practised to an audience that can either be appreciative or not of the services rendered. Perhaps more so in occupational health nursing than in any other aspect of the profession has the OHN to be politically aware, managerially confident, capable of marketing, aware of client needs and competent in meeting them. The role should be such that employers in today's markets would find it difficult to manage their business enterprises without the facility of an occupational health service. They should see it as an integral part of their business plan just as much as they would attach importance to profit and loss on balance sheets and personnel and finance departments. They won't do this, however, if we have a dormant acquiescent service that doesn't really care and only pays lip service to the role.

In the real world, the OHN of today has to be equipped with the skills to negotiate against the many barriers that might be placed in its way. A recent study undertaken by the Health & Safety Executive (Dorward, 1993) looked at managers' perceptions of the role of the OHN. To some extent, the Dorward report validates the author's existing findings, albeit on a microscopic scale, that managers have a very poor reception of what OHNs are about. A review of the Dorward report in *The Newsletter* (1994: 11) issued by the Royal College of Nursing Society of Occupational Health Nursing, stated: 'lay managers see OHN's role as a treatment service for injury or illness at work. The study shows that both doctors and lay managers showed little interest in management courses for OHNs'.

Hopefully, the skills that the OHN is acquiring today are being laid down through a greater awareness of what is being made available to them through the medium of education. The theoretical input has a practical ability to be witnessed in the work place and the skills that are learnt can be used in the armourment required by today's OHN. As Garvey (1995) has stated, one of the main aims of education is to produce a critical practitioner who will develop a person-centred approach within the immediate environment of the practitioner and beyond into the wider community setting. So that the role is enhanced appropriately, five general objectives are given as an underpinning to practice, as follows.

1 TO GENERATE CRITICAL THOUGHT THAT WILL ENABLE STUDENTS TO BE REFLECTIVE OF THEIR OWN COMMUNITY PRACTICE

The word 'reflection' can conjure up many and varied ideas of thought processes and relaxation skills. True reflection has an element of action attached to it. As practitioners we need to learn to reflect, otherwise our work becomes aimless. As Palmer *et al.* (1994: 36) state: 'Reflection is a process of reviewing an experience of practice in order to describe, analyse, evaluate and so inform learning about practice. In contrast to the vision of quiet contemplation that the word used to create . . . there is an active element to reflection'.

2 TO DEVELOP A PERSON-CENTRED APPROACH WITH REGARD TO COMMUNITY HEALTH

The strategy here required by the OHN requires to view, along with other health care professionals, the client as the ultimate goal, attempting to provide the client with the type of service that he or she wants, not what we as practitioners think they want and having the ability to be able to step back from the issues and analyse them in conjunction with clients' requirements. Where a client is unable to make appropriate decisions or feels to be lacking in confidence, the OHN should be there to offer advice and assistance to promote informed decision making.

3 TO BROADEN THE KNOWLEDGE BASE BY THE UNDERSTANDING AND APPLICATION OF HEALTH FROM VARIOUS DISCIPLINES

OHNs should not view themselves in isolation. Though they have a very important part to play in the role of community health, they are part of a much wider team both within the work place setting, the primary health care setting and the wider community at large. There is a traditional Celtic quotation which is quoted in Crossley-Holland (1970) that states: 'It is better never to find the centre than to wander from the circle'. To some extent OHNs have to find the centre or try to solve all the solutions of community health on their own. They are a member of a team and should work together in creating a good team, a strong network and a large enough circle of expertise that can assist and help in contributing greater knowledge to both practitioners and clients. To do so requires a considerable amount of determination and vision on the part of the OHN, it may often mean abandoning short-term gains for long-term benefits.

4 TO GENERATE THE CAPACITY TO OFFER AND RECEIVE MENTOR-SHIP, SUPERVISION AND CRITICAL FRIENDSHIP

Interwoven into the life of any community health practitioner, comes the ability to be able to instruct others as well as to receive instruction, to give advice as well as to be advised, so that professional growth occurs. A blinkered view of our practice, our skills, our professional inter-relationships can only help to create the stereotype cobwebbed image of the OHN of yesteryear which some would still have the naivety to believe still exists. There is nothing wrong with criticism providing the critic who offers it does so in a constructive capacity, with the intention of generating positive growth from the situation. Criticism which is levied in a malicious manner, bent solely on destroying either the person, or the work that has been done, serves no purpose and falls outside the professional facade of nursing. Morris et al. (1988: 24) stated that 'Mentoring can be seen as a master craftsman/apprentice relationship in which the trained, skilled practitioner enables the learner to develop her skills, knowledge and attitudes. This could be described as professional nurturing and mentors seen as guiding lights'. Typical characteristics of a mentor have been described by Morris et al. as an 'envisioner', a 'standard prodder' and a 'challenger'. OHNs like all other members of the nursing profession have to be capable of breaking new ground, preparing for the future, and more importantly taking people along with them en route so that they receive support in the development of new ideas and practices and at the same time can support people in return when difficulties and problems occur.

The work of Daloz (1986) is often quoted for rendering an insight to the expected role of the mentor. He highlights three main facets of the role that of support, challenge and providing vision, very similar in many ways to those characteristics of Morris et al. Through giving support and providing challenging experiences, the OHN creates an atmosphere for others to be better able to understand. It is the element of understanding which is imperative to all that we do. People need to be cognizant and aware of what it is they are encountering and what significance such experiences have for them in their lives either as professional practitioners, employers or employees.

5 TO DEVELOP SKILLS NECESSARY TO ENABLE STUDENTS TO ENGAGE IN RESEARCH PROGRAMMES IN HEALTH-RELATED FIELDS

There is perhaps no other area within community health care that has exalted occupational health nursing to its current height than the field of research practice. Nurses in general and perhaps OHNs in particular have, at the risk of making a sweeping generalization, been inherently afraid of methods of enquiry and evaluation. Research methods have been wrapped in a jargon all of their own. Research was always something that somebody else did or was involved with. It was not considered to be the remit of the OHN. Today, we can make a positive statement that research is truly part and parcel of the skills that the OHN needs to function appropriately in a technological society. Areas of concern, problem issues and new information will all lend themselves to specific types of research methodology. If OHNs are not involved in the research pertaining to their own practice can they afford to wait for others to do it for them? If we call ourselves a profession shouldn't that profession be underpinned by a body of knowledge that has been created by its practitioners? Furthermore, research is a discipline which enables the user to formulate logical thought, analyse it and produce results. It is a discipline that we can all do well to practice. It requires a change of thought and a change of stance. Every time we embark on a research project we can never be sure of the outcome. We may have made various hypotheses but until the data are analysed we can never be sure that the results will confirm our original thoughts.

Neither should research be seen as something not related to everyday life. The process of research is undertaken by each and every one of us, day in and day out. Less formally we look for a specific item of furniture for the house, or a hi-fi system or even a new car. What do we do? Albeit, we might not go as far as designing a questionnaire or completing complicated statistical calculations such as T-testing, Kruskal–Wallis test variables or even Chi Square analysis, but we do involve ourselves with questioning, with interviews, observation and other forms of collecting data. Why? because we want to make an informed choice. We have to gather information about a product so that we can make a decision on whether that product is suitable or not. Some will be – others will be discarded. To a certain extent this is 'real world' research and examples of it abound every day of our lives. To be good at research requires nothing more than an interest in the topic concerned and the ability to be able to use a few tools to collect the information. Howard and Sharp (1983: 6) confirm this in their statement:

> Most people associate the word 'research' with activities which are substantially removed from day to day life and which are pursued by outstandingly gifted persons with an unusual level of commitment. There is of course a good deal of truth in this viewpoint, but we would argue that the pursuit is not restricted to this type of person and indeed

can prove to be a stimulating and satisfying experience for many people with a trained and enquiring mind.

It is important for the OHN to realize that in undertaking any research you start from your own focal point. The OHN is central to the research being undertaken, because the investigation that will ensue is important to them as a professional practitioner and they will interact with the process of investigation throughout the research exercise. As Kirby and McKenna (1989: 46) state: '... who you are has a central place in the research process because you bring your own thoughts, aspirations and feelings, and your own ethnicity, race, class, gender, sexual orientation, occupation, family background, schooling etc. to your research'.

Finally, research and the ability to be able to undertake enquiry is at times a complicated procedure. The OHN has to learn the appropriate skills, have an enquiring mind, be capable of asking the right sort of questions, be prepared to challenge in a structured way and have the power and ability to seek answers to problems in the work place environment. Without such skills, occupational health nursing will never be regarded as a professional discipline, thankfully more and more diplomate and bachelor degree students now have these capabilities and the future looks very good for occupational health in general and for occupational health nursing specifically. As Robson (1993: 4) reiterates: 'Entering into any kind of investigation involving other people is necessarily a complex and sensitive undertaking and to do this effectively you need to know what you are doing'.

Conceptual models for occupational health nursing

Nursing is said to be full of models, some of which are difficult to relate to practice while others are relevant and useful to the practitioner. Occupational health nursing until 1988 had not been blessed by any specific model pertinent to its own discipline. There were certainly many models abounding within the discipline of nursing but occupational health nursing was made to 'fit' the model rather than the other way round. A nursing model has to be systematically constructed and logically developed in an effort to make sense of what nurses do or should be doing. Basically, the key to understand a discipline is to understand its concepts and so conceptual frameworks are devised in an attempt to grasp ideas which help to form principles which may ultimately affect practice. Concepts were given a deal of thought at an international educational workshop in Hanasaari, Finland in September 1988. The outcome of this was the now renowned and famous Hanasaari conceptual model (Fig. 11.4) which has for some years helped to underpin occupational health nursing practice. Alston et al. (1988) in Finland are attributed with compiling the documentation relating to the Hanasaari model following the workshop meetings.

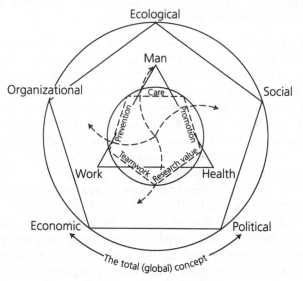

Figure 11.4 The Hanasaari model (after Alston *et al.* 1988).

There are three main concepts linked to the above model and briefly these are:

1 *The total environment concept.* This is the global concept of occupational health which is represented by the large outer circle in Fig. 11.4. Interwoven into the global concept come influences which, while general to society at large, can and do have direct and indirect influences on the health of us all and therefore influences on the practice of occupational health. These in the main are the areas of economics, politics, social, ecological and organizational factors. The OHN, today, cannot afford to be indifferent of these influences and how they will affect their practice. The OHN has to be aware, and education has to make that awareness a reality by providing the practitioners of today with the appropriate academic tools for the job.

2 *The man, work and health concept.* On the model (Fig. 11.4) this concept is represented by a triangle to indicate the close relationship between the three elements and how the three elements are bonded together within the total environment. Again various issues and aspects of politics and policies affecting social welfare can and do have an affect on the development and subsequent growth of an occupational health department. An organizational philosophy or culture may be seen to directly affect the strategy that an occupational health service has to follow. These influences can be exerted at times for totally the wrong reasons and the OHN risks being swept along with the tide if they are unprepared to take stock and negotiate sometimes what is best for occupational health and how the discipline will fit into the culture of the company, bringing with it rewards in terms of a more productive and a

more health-wise workforce. Occupational health cannot afford to be seen as an add-on function of a company's philosophy; it has to be seen as a driving force and integral part of that philosophy, to consider any other proposition is to court disaster.

3 *Occupational health interaction*. This is the key to the success of the Hanasaari model and indeed to nursing in general. The OHN has to be a person involved in proactive interaction. They must spearhead initiatives, not adopt a reactive stance, but be part and parcel of all aspects of health care being implemented for the good of the worker. Such a person becomes well known on site; such a person interacts well with colleagues; such a person is involved in the company, has an interest in the mission of the company and has vision to see how that overall picture incorporates occupational health. The model (Fig. 11.4) shows curving arrows to depict the element of flexibility and influence of the OHN. The arrows will widen and encompass larger areas on the model the more the OHN takes up the task of promoting their role. For the OHN who wishes to remain static, take a rigid stance and not be involved in any form of interaction the arrows on the model would encompass less space until eventually the arrows would cease to turn and disappear on the model as simply a dot. Various aspects of the role of the OHN were included on the original model, these included care, prevention, promotion, research/value and teamwork. This was by no means an inexhaustible list that was raised by the working party but these were skill areas that were identified as having some significance and priority.

A further model (Fig. 11.5), again specifically orientated towards occupational health, appeared in the occupational health literature in the early 1990s. Produced by Dr Wilkinson of the University of Arizona, it became known as the Wilkinson Windmill Model – (WWM) – a conceptual model of occupational health nursing. According to Wilkinson (1990: 73) 'such a model provides a tool for examining one's nursing practice'. The main purpose of the Windmill Model is to depict clearly and succinctly the inter-relationships among the various parts of the model and to explain the critical role of the OHN. In keeping with the underpinning philosophies that we have already seen attached to the Hanasaari model, the WWM uses a windmill to conceptualize how occupational health nursing helps convert managed labour into production. That is, the OHN tries to maintain the health of the workforce not only for the sake of the employees, but also for the organization; a healthy worker, as we have already postulated, is more likely to be a productive worker. For Wilkinson the model contains five major parts:

• *The core*. This represents the truly most important asset of a company the workers.
• *The hub*. This represents the OHN central to the model as in the Hanasaari conceptual model. Being at the centre enables the OHN to be creative and control the occupational health programmes in the work place. The

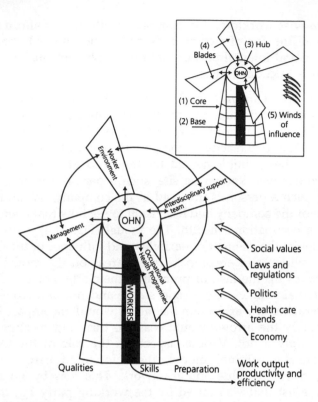

Figure 11.5 The Wilkinson Windmill model. Reprinted by permission of the American Association of Occupational Health Nurses, AAOHN Journal, Vol. 38, No. 2.

arrows around the hub indicate communication; that is, constant communication flowing in many and varied directions to particular groups.

- *The windwheel with four blades.* The blades represent: the working environment; interdisciplinary support team; occupational health programmes; and management. For Wilkinson, the blades of the windmill may be partially completed, be in tatters or may not be attached to the hub at all. Also the size of the blade will depend on just how well developed such things as the working environment, management and support teams are. If there are no occupational health programmes there will be no blade at all. The motion and turning of the blades represents the operation of the occupational health programme. If the blades turn the windmill will work, the fuller the blades the more wind the blades will catch in the form of the winds of influence.

- *The base.* On the model the base is constructed out of bricks. Each brick represents levels of professional training and skills of the OHN. The whole support structure of the windmill is dependent on the professional education that the OHN must receive in order to be able to be effective in the working environment. For Wilkinson the skills include: communication; collaboration; networking; diagnostics; administration; and the ability to meet self-care needs. The more the education needs of the OHN are being met, the more that pertinent qualifications are attained, the more bricks will be produced in the base and the higher the windmill will be elevated and will therefore catch even more of the winds of influence.

- *The winds of influence* are the driving force that drive the whole structure and with proper management the machine produces work in the form of output of products and/or services. Worker health and the health of the organization are seen in this model as two concepts being synonymous with each other.

In conclusion, Wilkinson (1990: 77) states: 'The OHN may function in varied roles while practising alone or as a staff member, a manager or corporate director, a consultant, a nurse practitioner, or a researcher'. The Wilkinson Windmill Model – with its core, hub, base, blades and winds – symbolically represents a conceptualization of nursing practice in an occupational health setting. It may be a useful framework for understanding the role of the OHN in many different work environments. It may prove valuable also as a research tool, for if an organization is not producing goods or services efficiently, the researcher can look carefully at the components of the system to evaluate its deficits.

Fairburn and McGettigan (1994a), both occupational health advisers, felt that both Hanasaari and the Wilkinson models did not provide an appropriate framework for problem solving as Henderson did for general nursing. How comforting it is that the enquiring mind of the OHN should now be publishing articles dealing with conceptual issues that directly affect practice – evidence, if it were needed, of the enquiring mind in action.

Fairburn and McGettigan (1994b) went some way towards developing and applying their own occupational health management model (adapted in Fig. 11.6). For them communication was still fundamental to the model as it had been with Hanasaari and the WWM. They stated that communication 'acts as a trigger point for the process. It may be direct or indirect communication . . . as in a face-to-face meeting or as a telephone conversation or written message . . . or even as non-verbal communication' (Fairburn and McGettigan, 1994b: 154). After the initial communication process the OHN moves into a process of exploration or evaluation of the problems or problem areas that have been realized in an attempt to formulate a resolution. Four key areas are highlighted on the model and include: organization, health, work and support. There are many similarities here to the previous two models but there is emphasis on realistic outcomes and good time management. Transactions are instigated by managing the outcomes of the exploratory phase and achievable goals are set which might require the support of the OHN or even managerial support of the worker within the work place. The model goes on to look at implementation or the action phase of the model. Here the activities that have been set in the goal-setting stage will be accomplished. The model at this point has a loop-back system to evaluate and assess if the goals have been achieved. If they haven't, additional communication has to be engaged and further

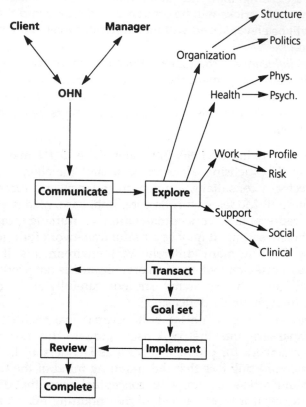

Figure 11.6 Fairburn and McGettigan's occupational health management model (After Fairburn, J. and McGettigan, J. 1994).

exploration of the problem or problems commenced. Finally, the process if completed, is recognized as such, and documented formally. An element of reflection on the whole process would be considered advantageous here and the positive learning that has arisen from the situation/s be extrapolated and internalized. In the words of Fairburn and McGettigan (1994b: 158), 'the aim of providing a system with sufficient flexibility to enable OHNs to deal consistently with problems has been achieved'. It is only with commitment from other OHNs and application in their own situations that this model can be truly tested.

Towards the macro . . .

The word 'environment' comes from the French *Les environs* meaning the neighbourhood; that which surrounds us, the surroundings. The word 'environment' for the OHN in days gone by was often a term used to describe the inside of the surgery, first aid room or clinic. OHNs were not encouraged to step beyond that environment. Their zone was clearly demarcated and to step beyond was to attract severe criticism from colleagues and management in the work place. Thankfully, those days should now have past and the word 'environment' has several meanings to the OHN. In its narrowest definition it can still mean the confines of the clinical setting and indeed attention has to be focused on this environment for all that is undertaken within it needs to be related and connected to the wider environment outside. The term 'environment' can also mean the actual work place of which the occupational health unit is just a part, albeit an integral and important part, of the whole commercial enterprise. However, the word 'environment' for the OHN must also mean 'beyond the factory wall'. The OHN of today has to focus on issues which go beyond their work place site. There may be issues within the immediate community that the OHN needs to know about, concerns from neighbours living near the site, causes for concern with the public at large, complaints that may damage the corporate image of a company, all of which to some lesser or greater extent fall within the province of the OHN role. The OHN, therefore, has to be concerned just as much about individuals within the work place setting as those that live beyond it. Their professional expertise and knowledge creates within them an expert practitioner who can advise appropriately giving due care and attention to both the health and welfare of people in general and the corporate image of their company.

The working environment can be bedecked with problems and poor standards such as extremes of temperature, poor lighting, poor ventilation, presence of dust, fumes, gases and noise. With such potential hazards in the work place pertinent legislation has tried to eradicate such problems by creating a legal framework against which such problem scenarios become the exception rather than the rule. Legislation such as the Health & Safety at Work Act 1974, COSHH Regulations 1988, the Environmental Protection Act 1990 and the Management of Health and Safety at Work regulations 1992, to mention but a few, have all helped to enshrine the employer's duty to provide a sound and healthy working environment both in relation to the actual organization of the environment and in the control of environmental stressors. Needless to say, environmental conditions have a direct effect on the way people behave at work, on the degree of risk of occupational disease and injury and on morale, management/worker relations, labour turnover and profitability. The OHN has to be focused and tuned in to all of these elements of everyday working life for they are all connected to their role by virtue of their unique position in the work place.

The OHN within their own environment may well have an important role to play in helping to control the environment along with other key members of the health and safety team. Advising on control strategies such as substitution, isolation, enclosure, exhaust ventilation, good housekeeping, reducing exposure time, appropriate training and the use of appropriate personal protective clothing and equipment, requires a competent and knowledgeable OHN.

The OHN is also involved in looking at much wider aspects of the work place environment that might at first not be considered to be threatening to health. While fumes and gasses might cause respiratory problems and working in noisy environments will cause deafness, it may be more difficult to assess the problems that might affect health when looking at office workers, who are employed in a potentially clean and warm environment. The OHN then has to be aware of ergonomic causes that might affect health. They may look at job movements, for example, typewriting which may cause repetitive strain injury if the work station is badly designed. Friction and pressure might cause bursitis or cellulitis. Indeed, the OHN should not find themselves, in the ideal world, responding in a reactive mode to such conditions, but should be involved in the initial design stages so that they can help to contribute and prevent ill health, in whatever guise it may appear, before it happens. Their multidisciplinary colleagues need to know their potential, need to know what they have to offer and what they can contribute to the overall grand scheme of events. They won't know, if the OHN is not prepared to tell them. As Garvey (1994: 53) has indicated in his work on sick building syndrome, such a condition: '. . . will benefit from a coordinated approach to the problem utilizing the expertise of many people beyond the traditional extended role of occupational health – but then again isn't that what the Hanasaari model for Occupational Health nursing is all about?'

Whether the OHN is treating a wound, counselling an employee, dealing with hazard and risk assessments, being involved in a multipartite discussion on the waste management and disposal of polychlorinated biphenyls, or commenting on the consultative document related to the Clean Air Act, the aim remains the same – prevention is the key. Their need to be able to communicate has already been seen and must not be underplayed. The OHN is the spokesperson for all in the work place and indeed beyond into any forum that is likely to have a tangible thrust into the realms of health and safety. Already there are several groups within Europe looking at ways and means of bringing together OHNs from all European states and beyond. The communication process is becoming global. OHNs are talking together, not just within the UK but across international boundaries; they are busy sharing and learning from one another, involved in collaborative research and documenting their progress as they move forward for the benefit of mankind at large. The old cartoon picture of the OHN sat knitting, with fag in mouth and cups of tea to hand is imagery from a bygone era. Wake up to the second millennium about to dawn; now is the time of a graduate profession, with sound research skills, a motivated professional nursing workforce that is hell bent on eradicating bad practice. Now is the time of the lap-top computer and the communication process of the Internet and the World Wide Web. The OHN has landed and arrived; their destiny is clear and precise. The world will be a better place for their skills and their mediation and they intend to utilize all that modern day technology can throw at them for the benefit of all their clients.

Global concerns, waste management, environmental protection and issues such as sick building syndrome may seem a long way removed from the days when Bernardino Ramazzini was formulating his ideas and opinions about workers' health. The evolution of the OHN has been at times a harsh and demanding one. It has created a position for itself within the primary health care team based on hard work, effort and determination to succeed. Perhaps more than any other nursing discipline, occupational health has earned the right to be considered equal to its peers and by its example will endeavour to lead nursing and occupational health into the twenty-first century.

References

Alston, R. *et al.* 1988: *The Hanasaari conceptual model for occupational health nursing.* Paper presented at the RCN OHN Forum, Scotland.

Crossley-Holland, K. 1970: *Celtic miscellany.* Middlesex: Penguin.

Daloz, L.A. 1986: *Effective teaching and mentoring: realizing the transformation power of adult learning experiences.* London: Jossey-Bass.

Danton, S. 1984: Prevention of injury and disease. In Harris, C.J. (ed.), *Occupational health nursing practice.* Bristol: John Wright.

Dorward, A.L. 1993: *Managers' perceptions of the role and continuing education needs of occupational health nurses.* Sheffield: HSE Books.

Fairburn, J. and McGettigan, J. 1994a: Development of an occupational health management model: part 1. *Occupational Health Journal* 46(4), 120–3.

Fairburn, J. and McGettigan, J. 1994b: Development of an occupational health management model: part 2. *Occupational Health Journal* 46(5), 154–8.

Garvey, J.P. 1994: Developing an integrated approach to SBS. *Occupational Health Journal* 46(2), 50–3.

Garvey, J.P. 1995: Delivering training and education in occupational health for nurses. In Pantry, S. (ed.), *Occupational health.* London: Chapman & Hall, 229–49.

Harrington, J.M. and Gill, F.S. 1993: *Occupational health.* Oxford: Blackwell Scientific.

Howard, K. and Sharp, J.A. 1983: *The management of a student research project.* Aldershot: Gower.

Kirby, S. and McKenna, K. 1989: *Experience, research, social change: methods from the margins.* Toronto: Garamond.

Morris, N., John, G. and Keen, T. 1988: Mentors learning the ropes. *Nursing Times* (November 16) 84(46), 24–7.

Palmer, A., Burns, S. and Bulman, C. 1994: *Reflective practice in nursing: the growth of the reflective practitioner.* Oxford: Blackwell Scientific.

Radford, J.M. 1990 (ed.) *Recent advances in nursing (occupational health nursing).* London: Churchill Livingstone.

Robson, C. 1993: *Real world research.* Oxford: Blackwell.

The Jerusalem Bible 1966: (Standard edition). London: Darton, Longman & Todd.

The Newsletter 1994: Winter issue, newsletter of the RCN Society of Occupational Health nursing, London, RCN.

Wilkinson, W.E. 1990: A conceptual model of occupational health nursing. *American Association of Occupational Health Nursing Journal* 38(2), 73–7.

12 Health visiting

Joanna Bateman

This chapter presents a comprehensive view of the health visitor. Following a brief history of the specialism, Joanna Bateman uses the present role to offer a useful exploration of the future of health visiting. Models of practice and the skills needed to be effective are described. A really useful addition is the frequent direction to further reading when issues are worthy of further exploration.

What is a health visitor?

Health visitors are all qualified nurses who have undergone a further course at a college or university, which is generally one year in length, and currently at either diploma or degree level. Alternatively, they may have completed an undergraduate degree programme from which they will have qualified as an RGN and health visitor at the same time.

As a result of the UKCC's recommendations in *Standards for Education and Practice Following Registration Report* (UKCC, 1994) the postregistration course will soon be only run at degree level.

Students from any branch of Project 2000 will be able to undertake the health visiting award, following a period of experience to consolidate the preregistration learning. It is envisaged that the course will take an academic year, which includes three months supervised practice. An important element of the course will be the common core modules which are undertaken with other professional branches, such as district nursing and occupational health.

There was previously a requirement that health visitors had midwifery qualifications or three months obstetric experience, but it is now felt that adequate experience is gained through RGN/Project 2000 training.

The history of health visiting

It is necessary to look at the history of health visiting as, unlike other specialist nursing branches, the first recruits were not qualified nurses. It was in 1858 that Florence Nightingale's *Notes on Nursing* drew attention to the social dimension of infant mortality, and she felt that household hygiene was a potential area for improvement.

The Ladies' Sanitary Reform Association of Manchester and Salford was formed and ladies visited the homes of the working class to teach hygiene, child care and feeding, taking pamphlets and tins of carbolic powder and soap. This work was voluntary until 1890 when Manchester Corporation paid the salaries of six health visitors.

In 1891, Florence Nightingale called for a special course to be established to train nurses in the field of public health. She wrote:

> . . . it is hardly necessary to contrast sick nursing with this . . . the needs of home health nursing require different but not lower qualifications . . . they require tact and judgement unlimited to prevent the work being regarded as interference and becoming unpopular . . . .She must create a new work and a new profession for women. (CETHV, 1977: 12)

It was in response to this that a training course was established in 1892, but it was not until 1909 that regulations regarding the qualifications of health visitors were stipulated, with them having to possess either a medical degree, midwifery certificate or nurse training. No generally recognized training was in existence until 1919 when a two-year course was recommended, with a shortened course for those with nursing experience or graduates. Following the 1915 Notification of Births Act, it was felt that health visitors needed midwifery training in order to effectively visit families following a birth.

It is important to understand that the role of the health visitor was initially to teach the lower-social class mothers in order to reduce the infant mortality figures: the role of the health visitor essentially '. . . combined the roles of inspector, social worker and teacher' (Symonds, 1991). The health visitor's role undermined the working classes and they and other professionals attributed poor child rearing practices to individual ignorance, not a response to appalling living conditions. Their interference was not surprisingly resented by the working class (Symonds, 1991).

In the 1930s, there was a rise in the number of health visitors and they joined with doctors to work in the speciality of social medicine. There was also a fall in infant and child deaths as a result of war-time rationing, welfare food introduction and medical advances. It was felt by many that the health visitor's work was over (CETHV, 1977).

However, in the 1946 NHS Act responsibility was laid on the local health authorities to make provision for visiting people in their home to give advice on care of young children, expectant and nursing mothers, and to prevent the spread of infection.

The Jameson Report (MoH, 1956) defined the role of the health visitor in terms of health education and social advice and suggested that while health visitors should maintain contact with families with children, they should also expand their role to become family visitors. Recommendations were made on entry requirements for health visiting and that a national syllabus and approved courses should be established (CETHV, 1977: 16).

The Council for the Education and Training of Health Visitors was formed, producing a syllabus of training and taking over responsibility for the examination and registration of health visitors. In 1977 they published the document *An Investigation into the Principles of Health Visiting* (CETHV, 1977) which defined the theory and principles behind health visiting.

Where are they based?

Most health visitors are now attached to general practitioners (GPs) and are based either in health centres, clinics or in the surgery premises. With large GP practices there may also be a geographical allocation of health visitors.

Following the NHS and Community Care Act (DoH, 1989a) GP fundholders have been given their own budgets and the powers to purchase a range of services including health visiting. They cannot directly employ the staff themselves, and may only purchase services from established NHS providers (HVA, 1994a).

What do they do?

It is often hard for other professionals to state what health visitors actually do, as in today's world of audit and measuring outcomes people look for hard quantifiable data, which are not always appropriate in health visiting. Indeed, it can take student health visitors several weeks to gain a true insight into the role, especially when they come from an acute background and are used to 'doing things for people'.

The definition of health visiting most widely accepted is that of the CETHV (1977: 8) which states that:

> ... the professional practice of health visiting consists of planned activities aimed at the promotion of health and prevention of ill-health. It thereby contributes substantially to individual and social well being, by focusing attention at various times on either an individual, a social group or a community. It has three unique functions:

1 identifying and fulfilling self-declared and recognised as well as unacknowledged and unrecognised health needs of individuals and social groups;

2 providing a generalist health agent service in an era of increasing specialisation in the health care available to individuals and communities;

3 monitoring simultaneously the health needs and demands of individuals and communities; contributing to the fulfilment of these needs; and facilitating appropriate care and service by other professional health care groups.

Underlying all the health visitor's work are the principles of health visiting. They were initially identified in 1977 and have been recently re-examined and found to be still relevant to health visiting in the 1990s (Twinn and Cowley, 1992). The four principles are:

- the search for health needs
- the stimulation of an awareness of health needs
- the influence of policies affecting health
- the facilitation of health enhancing activities (CETHV, 1977).

THE SEARCH FOR HEALTH NEEDS

This can be either on an individual or community level, and involves the health visitor empowering clients to identify their own health needs, or recognizing needs that the client may not be aware of. Here the health visitor is a facilitator and a resource for clients, having an up-to-date knowledge base about community health and epidemiology (Twinn and Cowley, 1992). An important element of this principle is community profiling which is discussed later.

THE STIMULATION OF AN AWARENESS OF HEALTH NEEDS

This involves empowering clients to be aware of their health needs and any available help. It is also important that those responsible for providing or commissioning services are aware of these needs, and also the public in general (Twinn and Cowley, 1992). This aspect of the health visitor's role has become more important recently with the increasing levels of poverty and the widening gap in health between the rich and the poor.

THE INFLUENCE ON POLICIES AFFECTING HEALTH

This can be at different levels, from local to national. Examples include campaigning for better nursery provision, well women's clinics, youth advice shops or against tobacco advertising.

THE FACILITATION OF HEALTH ENHANCING ACTIVITIES

Again, this can be at individual, family or community level. Examples include setting up a stress management clinic, local projects as a response to the health needs of the community, or the work of health visitors on the child development programme.

Time spent on various activities

The most recent research is the Audit Commission report (1994) which analysed health visitor time spent on various activities: 42 per cent of time was spent with young children including time spent on routine surveillance.

Twelve per cent of time was spent with adults, and 25 per cent on administration/clerical work.

Some health visitors are having to meet the requirements of trust policy which may state the number of visits to families with children of certain ages, or to GP fundholders who may specify certain visiting procedures. There is also the currently unresolved issue of the amount of time allocated to 'public health' in the contracts of health visitors attached to GP fundholders. This is discussed later.

Although traditionally the role of the health visitor has been concerned with the under fives, this is no longer their sole concern. Recent reports such as the *Health of the Nation* (DoH, 1992a) have given health visitors the opportunity and rationale to actively target other groups.

Community profiling

Health visitors must respond to the health needs of individuals and communities, and as such their role must be adaptable, responding to meet the needs of the community. One of the most important skills of the health visitor is that of health needs assessment, and this can be in the form of assessing the needs of a community, a family or an individual.

The importance of the health visitor in community profiling is widely documented (Twinn *et al.*, 1990; Blackburn, 1992a,b; DoH, 1993a; HVA, 1994a; RCN, 1994). Using skills in data collection and analysis, the health visitor should undertake a community profile regularly to identify the health needs of the defined population (this could be a GP practice or a defined community). It is useful to make the information collection a joint venture with residents and health professionals, as this not only utilizes the skills and knowledge of local people but can lead to an enhanced relationship between local residents and professionals (Blackburn, 1992a).

Community profiling can be seen as either having a top down approach, where the needs of the community are assessed by outsiders, or a bottom up approach, where the community is in charge of the process of profiling (Hawtin *et al.*, 1994). The ideal situation is a '. . . balance between the more objective, expert assistance from outside agencies and the enthusiastic, insider understanding of the community itself' (Hawtin *et al.*, 1994).

It is important that the information gained from the profile is shared as it is needed by purchasers. It can help raise the profile of the health visiting profession by ensuring that purchasers are aware that health visitors are assessing the health needs of the whole of the community and not just the 'under fives'. The sharing of the information with the primary health care team is paramount so that the team can work together to meet the local health gain targets (DoH, 1993a).

STRUCTURE OF THE PROFILE

There are many ways of structuring a profile such as using the community assessment wheel as described by Anderson and McFarlane (1988) or the format outlined by Luker and Orr (1992). A guide for the GP practice population profile is available from the RCN (1993a). Flexibility is essential as not all information will be relevant to every community and some will need expanding on more than others, according to need.

WHAT INFORMATION IS NECESSARY?

It is essential that the following data are included in a profile and are obtained at electoral ward level, or where possible, GP practice level.

Client group

(This can be a GP practice list or defined community.)

- age–sex structure
- social class
- unemployment rate
- ethnic minorities
- household structure
- levels of deprivation
- housing: type, condition, homelessness, overcrowding
- vulnerable families: those in B & B, travelling families
- prevalence of disability.

Environmental/social characteristics

- environmental characteristics, e.g. rural, industrial, etc.
- community support or isolation
- facilities, e.g. markets, shops, post office, etc.
- transport systems
- pollution levels
- water quality and fluoride levels
- crime rate, including domestic violence
- subjective data from residents regarding the area.

Health status

- mortality rates, concentrating on under 65s
- morbidity figures, e.g. asthma, diabetes.
- accident rates
- immunization uptake
- numbers on child protection register
- drug abuse/HIV/AIDS
- screening uptake for both adults and children
- clients' attitudes towards services provided.

Services provided

- health services – community and hospital
- liaison between community and hospital
- social services, e.g. day centres, nurseries
- liaison between health and social services
- educational provision
- leisure/recreation services
- voluntary/self-help groups

Where do you get the information from?

The OPCS census (OPCS, 1993) will provide much of the above data on social class, housing type, etc. and is available at ward level. This information can be obtained from the library or town hall. The last census data were collected in 1991 and are now a few years out of date. It is vital that the most recent sources of data are used: for example the unemployment figures are produced each quarter. All the statistics need comparing with the district, regional and national averages to establish a relative level of need.

Public health reports (and GP practice/Family Health Service Authority (FHSA) data) are a vital source of data on the health experiences of the community and it is necessary to obtain the following information:

- standardized mortality ratios (SMR) for the under 65s (preventable deaths);
- stillbirth, low birth weight and infant mortality rate;
- accident rates: it is necessary to obtain data on accident rates, which have been shown to be linked to social class (Child Accident Prevention Trust, 1991);
- morbidity rates: these are necessary for most illnesses, although are harder to obtain than mortality rates. It is essential to find out the estimated rates of depression or anxiety disorders in addition to the SMRs for suicide, especially as the suicide rates for men are increasing while women's are decreasing. Taking the SMRs at face value is misleading as women are twice as likely as men to become depressed or harm themselves (DoH, 1993b);
- immunization uptake (this will be available from each GP practice) and screening uptake for all ages;
- rate of dental decay;
- estimated rates of drug misuse;
- initiatives towards meeting the *Health of the Nation* (DoH, 1992a) targets.

Other primary health care team members can provide a different perspective on the needs of the community. Community pressure groups/voluntary groups/community health councils are all able to give an insight into the needs of the community, especially the Citizen's Advice Bureau, which deals with a wide range of client enquiries.

Local drugs teams can give you an idea as to the type of drugs being abused and the problems abusers and their families are facing. It is also necessary to be aware of the services they provide including needle exchange schemes, counselling, education programmes and support groups.

Local authorities will provide information on educational provision, child minders, day nurseries, day centres and other facilities for the elderly, recreational facilities, etc.

Some areas have several free local papers produced weekly which include what is happening socially and also meetings arranged by the community health council, community police or active voluntary groups.

It is necessary to obtain the resident's perspective of what it is like to live in the area (subjective data). For example, do women feel safe or are they frightened to go out to the evening clinics? What do they feel about the services provided and are they meeting their needs? This can be done formally through interviews or gathered informally by talking to shop workers and residents.

POVERTY PROFILING

While it is unfashionable to refer to social class, it must be recognized that most epidemiological data are broken down this way, and it is perhaps the easiest way of demonstrating the effect deprivation has on health. It is acknowledged that there are problems with the way social class is defined (with the male/head of household occupation being categorized) and the importance of not labelling is recognized.

In recent years there has been increasing recognition that the gap between the rich and the poor is getting wider in Britain, and there is no doubt that rates of poverty and social deprivation are rising (Blaxter, 1990; Blackburn, 1991). Health visitors are increasingly faced with families in hardship: it is estimated that there are 3.1 million children living in poverty in Britain (1988/89 figures) – a quarter of all children. Over recent years there have been changes to those in poverty: there has been a decline in the numbers of pensioners in the poorest 10 per cent and a rise in the proportion of families with children and single people (Oppenheim, 1993: 46).

All these changes have implications for the work of the health visitor who has traditionally been involved with families with children under five years. The rates of accidents, infant mortality, dental decay and sudden infant death syndrome (SIDS) have a strong social class relationship with higher rates from the lower social classes. It is, therefore, impossible for the health visitor to ignore the effects of deprivation on health.

This social class difference in health experience is seen right from birth to old age (Meredith Davies and Davies, 1993) and it is vital that any profile analyses the effect of deprivation on the health of all age groups. The process of poverty profiling is discussed by Blackburn (1992b).

WHAT DO YOU DO WITH THE INFORMATION?

It is essential to be analytical and look at whether the services provided are meeting the needs of the community; that is, what is being done about the identified health needs? For example, there may be a high rate of teenage pregnancies but are there facilities for teenagers to get contraceptive and health advice – youth shops, etc? What educational programmes are there in schools or youth clubs? Are they aware of the services provided? What facilities do they want?

There may well be good provision of services, but are they accessible to residents without a car? Can the unemployed afford to use them? What about the waiting list? Are there creches available for women with children? Are there services/facilities before or after work hours? Be critical and analytical about service provision.

Plan action

It is necessary to draw up a list of identified health needs and then to plan what action is required by or for the community.

Evaluation

The process of health need assessment needs to be undertaken annually and it is essential that any plans implemented are evaluated.

Models and assessing family health needs

The health visitor cycle (Robertson, 1991) is very similar to the nursing process and is an integral part of all visits. The basic activities being:

- assessing needs (this could be the family or community)
- planning action (in partnership with the client)
- implementing the plan
- evaluating.

This cycle then carries on to the next contact/visit and is a continuous process. There are a variety of ways to assess the needs of the family, one of these being the 'family health needs model' which outlines four areas of need: general environment, physical health, mental/emotional health and social aspects of health (Robertson, 1991). This is a basic tool which provides a useful framework for information to assist in assessment.

More comprehensive approaches can be found with the adaptation of many nursing models which provide both a philosophical and theoretical framework. Clark (1986) believes that not all nursing models are appropriate in health visiting as the focus needs to be on the family rather than the individual, the emphasis on needs rather than problems, and on long-term intervention aiming to maintain the health of the family rather than necessarily change it. Clark's (1986) model has been specifically written for health visiting, but has not been widely used in practice.

The Worcester models for health visiting have been devised from a variety of different models and outline a philosophy for health visiting, a conceptual framework and an assessment tool specifically designed for each of the three models: family care, child-watch (for children at risk) and caring (a model for the elderly) (Barker, *et al.*, 1991).

THE PREVENTION MODEL

This provides a philosophical structure for categorizing intervention, and has been adapted to include four foci for prevention by Downie *et al.* (1990) which are:

- 'Prevention of the onset or first manifestation of a disease process, or some other first occurrence, through risk reduction'. Examples of this include discouraging smoking, the adoption of safe sexual practices and promoting the use of safety equipment to reduce accidents.
- 'Prevention of the progression of a disease process or other unwanted state, through early detection when this favourably affects outcome'. The health visitor's work in surveillance fits into this category – hearing and developmental tests, cervical and breast screening and the use of the Edinburgh Postnatal Depression Scale.
- 'Prevention of avoidable complications of an irreversible, manifest disease or some other unwanted state'. This could include teaching to control blood sugar levels in diabetics with the aim of preventing complications such as vascular problems.
- 'Prevention of the recurrence of an illness or other unwanted phenomenon'. This may include the attempts to prevent a further heart attack, or counselling/support to prevent the recurrence of depression.

It is sometimes hard to fit health visiting actions specifically into one category as they often overlap, but this model of prevention can provide a useful framework through which to plan health education or promotion intervention, particularly on an individual or family level.

The process of assessment may take many visits as the needs of a family may be complex and ever changing. Whatever model is chosen to assess the needs of the client, it is important that it incorporates partnership with the client, and takes the social and environmental situation into account.

Communication skills

Perhaps the most important skills health visitors need to possess are good communication and counselling skills, as very little of their time is spent on 'hands-on care'. It is paramount that they are able to communicate effectively with all age groups and members of the public, as well as other members of the primary health care team. As there is no obligation by the public to use the health visiting service and health visitors have no right of access to the home, it is essential for health visitors to build up their relationship with families and communities to facilitate working in partnership with them.

An essential component of acute nursing is practical tasks, although with the increasing implementation of primary nursing there is less 'task orientation' than previously, but in many places 'doing something' still takes priority over talking to patients. Students who are observing the health visitor may, therefore, find the transition to listening and facilitation hard, and may feel frustrated that they are not solving the problems they are faced with in the community (Reed-Purvis and Dakin, 1994).

The art of listening and speaking is not simple, although '... to the untrained observer, who may lack insight into the health visitor's role, it can appear passive' (Brettell, 1994). Whilst the interaction may appear like a friendly conversation, the health visitor is constantly assessing the situation. Any advice given is not only in line with current research, Department of Health guidelines, local trust policy and UKCC standards, but at an appropriate level for the client and responsive to their needs, taking into account their personal and social situation.

A specific situation demonstrating the importance of listening, supporting and facilitating is postnatal counselling, which can improve psychological health. Reed-Purvis and Dakin (1993) feel this method to be beneficial as it can '... build women's sense of control over their lives and empower them to cope with, and often to change, the situations in which they find themselves'. Such approaches may not always be initially acceptable to clients who perhaps expect a more directive and authoritarian method, and an element of 'unlearning' may be required by both the client and health visitor to enable this approach to be utilized successfully (Reed-Purvis and Dakin, 1993).

One of the key components of counselling is self-awareness and it is essential that health visitors have insight into their background, upbringing, and life experiences which all affect, either consciously or unconsciously, the judgements and interpretations made in encounters with clients. You may notice that individual health visitors have different interests and approach clients with different priorities – for example, one may have a particular interest in postnatal depression, possibly because of personal experience, and is, therefore, keen not to let other women suffer. It is important to explore personal attitudes to subjects such as breast feeding, child abuse, drug addiction, poverty, bereavement and even conditions such as Myalgic encephalomyelitis (ME) and depression, as the professionals' attitudes towards these topics may have consequences for the client encounter. The skill of reflection is another important aspect of self-awareness in the health visitor.

Factors affecting the health visitor's role

Factors that influence the role of the health visitor include changes in the NHS, demographic and epidemiological factors and professional issues. Some of these are highlighted below. It is not possible to discuss all the issues here, but it is important to be aware of the effects of these factors and the changing nature of health visiting practice:

- rising numbers of families living in poverty
- increasing differences in health experience between the rich and the poor
- increasing numbers of elderly people
- needs of the ethnic minorities
- women's health and inequalities in treatment/attitudes
- needs of the homeless
- *Health of the Nation* (DoH, 1992a) targets
- changes in the NHS structure with GP fundholding, trust status and purchaser provider relationship
- skill mix
- the NHS and Community Care Act (DoH, 1989a)
- demands to meet GP or trust targets/visits
- public health role
- increased emphasis on clinical audit
- changes in nurse education
- community development work.

Aspects of the health visitor's role

For ease of reading the health visitor's role is outlined under the following headings: families with young children, needs of ethnic minorities, health visitor role with adults and the elderly. It is important to recognize that it is not easy to categorize health visitor's work as they often are involved with a variety of issues within one family unit.

FAMILIES WITH YOUNG CHILDREN

The role of the health visitor with families is outlined briefly here, focusing on preconceptual and antenatal care, postnatal role, postnatal depression, child development, special needs and child protection. The emphasis is on issues relating to children: the role with adults/parents is discussed later.

Preconceptual care

It is now widely accepted that the health of the parents prior to conception has long-term implications for the health of the baby. The diet is a major factor and the nutritional state of women in the early stages of pregnancy, before pregnancy is confirmed, is vital to the development of the foetus. Folic acid is recommended to reduce the rate of neural tube defects (DoH,

1992b). High levels of vitamin A may possibly cause birth defects (DoH, 1991a), and must be avoided. There is mixed research about anaemia in pregnancy: it is felt that if women have adequate iron stores prior to pregnancy they will not generally require supplementation as they naturally absorb more iron from the diet. Preconceptual screening is suggested by some. In addition to the above, the health of the foetus can be affected by smoking, alcohol, infections from toxoplasmosis, listeria and rubella.

'Foresight' is an association for the promotion of preconceptual care and it produces information for health professionals and clients, including a research-based quarterly newsletter and other publications.

Potential areas for targeting women about preconceptual care include schools, family planning clinics, GP surgery information boards, and through health visitor's contact with mothers who are considering having further children.

Antenatal care

The health visitor has a vital role in the antenatal period, both in terms of health education either in parentcraft groups or on a one-to-one basis, and this contact is useful for establishing a relationship with the client which is beneficial in the postnatal period.

A review of antenatal education shows a wide variety of health-visiting input to the antenatal client (Combes and Schonveld, 1992) and it has been suggested that health visitors have greater involvement in antenatal care, especially home visits. It is important not to ignore the social, emotional and psychological aspects of pregnancy, and to look at the needs of the women rather than concentrating on the baby (Braun and Schonveld, 1993).

Attendance at antenatal and postnatal groups is predominately by white, middle-class, educated women. Those who are young, single, working class or from an ethnic minority group are poor attenders (Combes and Schonveld, 1992). These groups are generally those who have the greatest need: they have poorer information, poor access to health services and a higher risk of ill health to both mother and baby, and need to be specifically targeted.

Ethnic minority groups have special needs both antenatally and postnatally and need targeting for improved antenatal care (Combes and Schonveld, 1992). There has been a recent increase in the number of leaflets produced in different languages and there are link workers employed in areas where there are large numbers of ethnic minority groups, although this service is by no means universal.

It is important that breastfeeding is promoted as the benefits are widely documented (DoH, 1989b) and the rates are currently low throughout Britain. Those more likely to breast feed are the higher social classes, those educated beyond 18 years, the over 25s, those having their first baby and living in the South East or London (White et al., 1992). It is felt that most mothers make up their minds on whether to breast or bottle feed long before the birth and are actually unlikely to change this decision (Oxby, 1994).

Efforts to increase the rate of breastfeeding would be appropriate preconceptually, and through education at schools with both sexes, as the attitudes of the partner has been found to be influential in the mother's decision. Whatever decision the parents make, it is vital that they are supported fully and not made to feel guilty if they have chosen not to breast feed.

Other areas which are relevant to discuss during pregnancy are:

- *Lifestyle*: smoking, diet, safe exercise levels, alcohol and drugs, avoiding infections, financial issues.
- *Physical changes*: both antenatally and postnatally, weight gain/loss, dental health, sexual health.
- *Postnatal issues*: feeding, minor ailments and immunization, emotional changes, coping with a new baby, parenting skills, support systems, preventing SIDS, equipment, home safety.

Health visitor role postnatally

The health visitor usually visits between 11 and 28 days postnatally, depending on authority/trust policy. Giving the family prior notice of the visit, either by a phone call or appointment letter, is good practice. Forms of identification must be carried by the health visitor and should be shown on first contact with a family. If there has been no contact antenatally then the role of the health visitor needs clarifying.

The following list gives an idea as to the range of topics that may be covered in the immediate postnatal period, but this is not conclusive and must be adapted to suit the needs of the client:

- *Mother*: feelings about the delivery and amount of control she had, experience in hospital, emotional health, attitudes towards infant feeding, physical condition, dietary intake, plans for postnatal check.
- *Baby*: feeding, sleeping (including position), general physical condition, weight gain, immunization schedule, environment (e.g. animals, smoking).
- *General*: partner's attitude, support systems available from family and community, sibling reaction, clinics and postnatal groups.

Postnatal depression

Postnatal depression is estimated to occur in approximately 10–27 per cent of women, although some studies have indicated a rate as high as 57 per cent when using a non-clinical definition of depression (McIntosh, 1993).

The Edinburgh Postnatal Depression Scale is a screening tool which has been shown to be sensitive and specific to postnatal depression, and also acceptable to mothers (Cox *et al.*, 1987). A training programme for health visitors in the use of the scale, in addition to non-directive counselling techniques and preventative strategies, was recently found to be effective, enabling health visitors to '. . . positively influence the emotional well-being of postnatal women' (Gerrard *et al.*, 1993). An input of eight hours counselling by health visitors can significantly improve recovery of postnatally depressed women (Holden *et al.*, 1989). Many areas now have postnatal depression support groups.

It is important to try to prevent the development of postnatal depression by supporting those considered to be at risk. Health visitors are in an ideal position to assess the family antenatally and postnatally, and it has been recommended that more input on the demands of motherhood and postnatal depression is included in antenatal education (Taylor, 1989).

Two useful texts on the psychological care of families in the period around childbirth are Niven (1992) and Raphael-Leff (1991).

Sudden infant death syndrome

Whilst the rate of sudden infant deaths has reduced dramatically in recent years there are still 0.78 deaths per 1000 live births attributed to SIDS, which accounted for 531 deaths in England and Wales in 1992 (FSID, 1994). This rate varies across the country with the North Western regional health authority having the highest rate in 1992, and there being a strong relationship with social class: the rate in social class V is over twice that in the professional, managerial and skilled classes (FSID, 1994).

It is important that health visitors are not complacent about the reduction in the rate of SIDS and continue to advise on sleeping position, smoking, temperature and signs of illness as recommended in the Department of Health publication *The Sleeping Position of Infants and Cot Death* (DoH, 1993c).

CONI (care of the next infant) is a support system for subsequent children where families have suffered a previous cot death. Parents get extra support and advice in a structured way, which involves weekly home visits by the health visitor. Parents are taught resuscitation skills and have access to an apnoea monitor if required (Baumer and McLindon,1994).

How often are families with young children seen?

This very much depends on the needs of the family and other factors such as local policy, services available such as postnatal groups, and the type of area. The Audit Commission (1994) recommends that following an initial contact all visits should be based on assessed needs and against agreed priorities, in order that resources are available for where needs are clearly defined. The report encourages health visitors to '... move away from historical patterns of universal service delivery to a more focused approach' (p. 23). This approach has been adopted by some areas, where health visitors form a contract with clients outlining agreed contact patterns.

It is unlikely that one visit is adequate to assess the complex needs of the family and most health visitors see clients either in clinic or at the home on further occasions. Some trusts outline the numbers of visits health visitors have to make to families at certain ages.

In most cases, the health visitor will see clients either at baby clinic, or when they have immunizations, in addition to home visits. The current immunization schedule is: two, three and four months for diphtheria, tetanus, pertussis, polio and haemophilus influenza type B (HIB), and 13 months for measles, mumps and rubella. The preschool booster is given at four years (DoH, 1992c).

Nutrition issues

Health visitors are expected to be a source of advice about a range of nutritional issues including infant feeding, and must provide research-based advice about breast and bottle feeding, weaning, allergies and intolerance, and dental decay.

With the high level of mothers who give up breastfeeding in the first few weeks it is necessary to look at what support breastfeeding mothers receive in the community, and to ensure that the advice given is in line with the RCM (1991) guidelines. Health visitors can work together with the National Childbirth Trust, who provide excellent support to mothers in terms of breastfeeding advisors and social support, and also loan out electric breast pumps, etc. A number of joint initiatives are now running between midwives, health visitors and voluntary agencies to ensure that the breastfeeding mother gets adequate support. One such scheme is outlined by Stokoe (1994).

There has been recent concern about the prevalence of iron deficiency anaemia among Asian infants and toddlers in particular, with one study in Nottingham finding 39 per cent of Asian children anaemic (Marder *et al.*, 1990). The effects of anaemia in children are well documented and can affect growth, resistance to infection, behaviour and cause diminished mental performance, and there is current debate as to whether the psychomotor delay related to iron deficiency can be fully reversed by iron therapy. A recent study has suggested that giving iron supplements to non-iron-deficient children can impair growth (Idjradinata *et al.*, 1994), and it is recommended that parents are educated about dietary sources of iron and vitamin C, to aid adsorption.

Child development

As much of the health visitor's time is spent with families with young children, they need to be knowledgeable about child development and growth, and must be able to assess children of all ages and refer to appropriate agencies. A useful outline of development is found in Sheridan (1992).

The Hall Report (1992) recommends that there is a core programme for child health promotion, with the emphasis on health rather than disease, and supporting the concept of partnership with and empowerment of parents and carers. The aims of this are first that all children should have the opportunity to realize their full potential in terms of good health, well being and development, and second that remediable disorders are identified and acted upon as early as possible (Hall, 1992).

The following programme has been recommended (Hall, 1992):

- Neonatal examination: by hospital doctor
- First 2 weeks: physical check by GP

- 6–8 weeks: by doctor
- 6–9 months: HV: hearing, hips and testicular descent
- 18–24 months: HV at home
- 36–54 months
- 5 years: school entrant medical.

There is now debate as to the effectiveness of the hearing tests which have traditionally been carried out by health visitors at about 7–8 months. Some areas have stopped using the tests routinely but are using them selectively for children who they are concerned about (Mott and Emond, 1994).

Health visitors also need to be aware about child behaviour and what is 'normal' for a particular age. They are a vital source of advice to parents about child behaviour issues such as discipline, temper tantrums, eating and sleeping problems, and toilet training. There is currently much debate on smacking and whether this form of physical punishment is acceptable. The Health Visitors Association (HVA) is affiliated to EPOCH (End Physical Punishment of Children) and produces a useful document on the issues surrounding punishment (HVA/EPOCH, 1991).

Special needs

On most health visitors' caseloads there will be some children with special needs, and there are specialist health visitors who work predominately with such families on child development teams. However, generic health visitors still have an essential role in supporting these families. One survey found that 40 per cent of parents were the first to identify their child had a problem, but many felt that health professionals did not take their concerns seriously (Audit Commission, 1994). A Spastics Society Report makes recommendations aiming to prevent the unnecessary distress caused by: '. . . clumsy handling of diagnosis and disclosure of disability' (Leonard, 1994). Parents want clear and honest information and to be treated with respect and understanding.

The 1989 Children Act and the 1993 Education Act both state that parents must be treated as partners, and that voluntary and statutory agencies must also work together more. The Children Act (DoH, 1991b) lays clear duty on the local authority to identify the numbers of children in need, provide information about the services provided and give children '. . . the chance to lead lives which are as normal as possible'.

Health visitors have an essential role in maintaining a holistic view of the family and it is important to consider the impact of the child's condition on the parents and siblings, as discussed by Gath (1985, 1990). It is necessary for the health visitor to be aware of local services, both voluntary and statutory, and to refer and liaise as appropriate. National organizations/ charities often produce excellent publications and are a vital source of support for families.

Accident prevention

The health visitor has a clear role in the prevention of accidents in children and suggested intervention for different age groups has been outlined by the Department of Health (DoH, 1993d) in the *Key Area Handbook*. It is important to have an understanding of the epidemiology of accidents: there is a very strong social class gradient, with as many as five times more children dying in house fires from social class IV and V than from I and II (CAPT, 1991). Different types of accidents are more likely to occur at certain ages.

While certain health visitor action may be in terms of education regarding safety and safety equipment, there is also a role for assessing other issues, such as poor housing, inadequate play facilities, and the way poverty affects families' choices regarding safety issues. Health visitors have initiated a variety of schemes, including safety equipment loan schemes, roadshows and parent support groups.

Child protection

In recent years the number of children registered on child protection registers in categories of physical injury, neglect, emotional and sexual abuse has risen, although the removal of the category 'grave concern' has meant the total number registered has fallen. There were a total of 32 500 children on the register in 1993 (DoH, 1994).

The health visitor has a key role in child protection 'to observe, assess, record and refer. It is not her responsibility to diagnose, nor to investigate child abuse' (HVA, 1994b). Health visitors are supported by child protection advisors, who are health visitors with additional training and experience in the management of child abuse. In addition, there are local policy and procedure guides which clearly outline the steps to be followed should child abuse be suspected. At a child protection conference a 'child protection plan' is formulated to ensure that the needs of the child are being met: this outlines the professionals' and the parents' role and is co-ordinated by a key worker.

It is necessary for health visitors to have understanding of the following:

- variables associated with abusive behaviour
- screening for child abuse, and whether this is both practical and ethical (Barker, 1990)
- preventive services/strategies
- signs of the different types of abuse
- local policy/procedure for assessment/referral
- support systems for parents and children locally and nationally
- child protection procedures under the Children Act 1989
- parenting skills: how these can be improved.

For further reading on child abuse see Corby (1993) or HVA (1994b).

NEEDS OF ETHNIC MINORITIES

It must be recognized that Britain is a multicultural society and in most areas there will be a variety of minority groups. Regardless of the make up of the local population, the services provided must be responsive to their needs.

It is essential that health visitors have an understanding of different health experiences of ethnic minority groups and also know and respect their cultural beliefs, religion, diet and attitudes to health. While there are inequalities in health status, there is also much evidence to suggest that other factors such as poor housing, unemployment, lower income, poor educational experience and racial discrimination all affect the health needs of these groups (HVA, 1989).

A summary of the major differences in health experiences is outlined below:

- Lower uptake of health services during pregnancy and reduced access to written information due to communication barriers (Combes and Schonveld, 1992).
- Higher stillbirth, neonatal and postneonatal mortality rates, especially if the mother was born in Pakistan (Parsons et al., 1993).
- Sickle cell disease affects approximately 1 in 200 Afro-Caribbeans but is not routinely screened for.
- Higher prevalence of iron deficiency anaemia among Asian infants and toddlers, with one study in Nottingham finding 39 per cent of Asian children anaemic (Marder et al., 1990).
- Increased susceptibility of vitamin D deficiency, rickets and osteomalacia (HVA, 1989).
- Higher rates of coronary heart disease among Asian men and women, despite lower rates of smoking and other risk factors (Coronary Prevention Group, 1986).
- Higher levels of diagnosed mental illness, especially schizophrenia, and different types of treatment once in hospital (Sashidharan and Francis, 1993).
- Higher suicide rates among young Asian women (DoH, 1993b).
- Higher rates of diabetes mellitus among Asians.
- Higher rate of disability among Afro-Caribbean people than whites, but slightly lower in Asians (Pickin and St Leger, 1993).

Rather than taking a medical view of the differences in health status in ethnic minority groups, it is necessary to look at their access to health services, and whether the services provided are meeting their needs (e.g., do meals on wheels cater for the different dietary patterns of the ethnic groups?).

It has been noted that when services have been specifically developed for ethnic minority groups with link workers, they have been predominately for the maternity and child health services. No initiatives involving health visitors and the black elderly have been documented (Pharoah and

Redmond, 1991). Some research has suggested that information regarding the services in the community is not available to the black elderly: 58 per cent of Asians had not heard of meals on wheels compared with none of white elderly surveyed (Atkin *et al.*, 1989). For further reading regarding the experiences of black elderly, Blakemore and Boneham (1994) is excellent.

HEALTH VISITOR ROLE WITH ADULTS

It is not possible to discuss all aspects of adult's health here but possible areas for health visitor intervention are highlighted.

Women's health (see Chapter 4)

As most of the health visitor's contact is with women, they are ideally positioned to become involved in women's health issues and to raise women's awareness about their health and social needs. It is necessary to be aware of the different health experiences of women: they are more likely to be given a psychological diagnosis than men, and less likely to have investigations for certain conditions such as coronary heart disease. Issues commonly discussed by health visitors include:

- cervical screening
- breast awareness
- contraception
- Premenstrual tension (PMT)
- menopause
- lifestyle factors
- adaption to various changes in role, e.g. motherhood and carer.

Osteoporosis is potentially preventable but attracts little attention, despite the devastating personal effects on sufferers in terms of hip and other fractures. The financial cost of femoral fractures and associated expenses by health and social services is estimated to be in excess of £500 million a year (Wallace, 1987). Health visitors are ideally situated to target young women to increase awareness of osteoporosis before bone mass starts to reduce at 35–40 years.

Health visitors are likely to visit women affected by domestic violence. The size of the problem is unknown, but every year in England over 30 000 women and children seek refuge to escape violence. Many women have suffered abuse for many years before seeking help, and are reluctant to take action. Health visitors must be aware of the possible signs of physical or emotional abuse, and have the necessary communication skills to discuss the issue. Specialist agencies such as Women's Aid provide emergency accommodation, support, advice and information.

Many health visitors have responded to the needs of women by setting up a well women's clinic, where women are holistically assessed, rather than the traditional medical approach of breast and cervical screening. A useful resource for such groups has been produced by the Health Education

Authority (1993), and includes activities covering a range of issues for different client groups.

The health visitor's role extends beyond providing resources or advice, and involves empowering women to demand better treatment, services and information from health professionals. The inequalities in health between the sexes is widely researched: what is needed is action to redress the imbalance.

MEN'S HEALTH

Health visitors should also be targeting men's health issues as part of their role with families and communities. Males have a consistently higher mortality rate for all ages from foetal mortality onwards, and lower life expectancy (DoH, 1993b). Particular areas relevant to health visitors are:

- testicular cancer/examination
- prostate problems and cancer
- stress and mental health issues
- coronary heart disease
- lifestyle factors.

There has been a recent rise in the incidence of testicular cancer, with the risk doubling in the past 20 years. It predominately affects men between 19 and 44 years, with about 1420 new cases each year. Despite the disease being easily treated if caught early by examination, very few men regularly check their testicles. This is an important issue for health visitors to discuss when visiting families.

Recent surveys have highlighted the low levels of exercise by both men and women in England, with only 19 per cent of men in the 45–54 age group meeting their age appropriate activity levels (Allied Dunbar/HEA, 1992). This is of concern in view of the high risk of coronary heart disease for this group. Exercise has been shown to not only reduce the risk of heart disease by lowering blood pressure and cholesterol, but to be beneficial in reducing depression, strokes, osteoporosis, testicular tumours and obesity.

Some health visitors have set up groups for men and women to attend following a myocardial infarction, which involves practical advice to reduce the risk of a further heart attack, exercise programmes and support for both the individual and their partner. Such schemes are often run in conjunction with physiotherapists.

Well men's clinics have been established in some areas, although they are generally not as well attended as women's groups. One way to target men is in the workplace as recommended in the *Health of the Nation* (DoH, 1992a).

ELDERLY (SEE CHAPTER 8)

There are rising numbers of the elderly in the UK and forecasts predict the rise in the over 85 year age group will continue. The demographic changes will affect the work of all health professionals, in addition to the carers of the elderly which are predominately women (Hamner and Statham, 1988).

Some areas have specialist health visitors who work solely with the elderly and in others the amount of involvement the health visitor has with the elderly varies, depending on factors such as trust policy and the demands of GP fundholders.

Screening the over 75s is now required annually as part of the GP contract (DoH, 1989a). There is current debate as to the most appropriate professional to undertake the screening and the content of the assessment which varies from practice to practice (Richards, 1993a,b). It is important for health professionals to be aware of their attitudes towards the elderly and ageing, as research has suggested that many do not see the importance of health education and promotion with the elderly and, instead, see the aging process as a time of '... deterioration, increasing dependency and a high likelihood of disability' (Pursey and Luker, 1993). The value of professionals with such attitudes visiting the elderly must surely be doubtful.

As a result of the community care White Paper *Caring for People* (DoH, 1989a), social services have a lead role in assessing the social care needs of elderly people. Health visitors frequently undertake joint assessments with social services, and are involved in planning the package of care to meet the identified needs. Health visitors can be involved in the following:

- health needs assessment, including mental health needs (see RCN, 1993b)
- supporting both the elderly and their carers
- bereavement counselling
- health promotion advice and activities such as 'Look after Your Heart'
- referral to specialist agencies
- providing information about community services, voluntary and statutory.

The health visitor's role with the elderly is discussed fully by McClymont *et al.* (1991).

Future of health visiting

There is current uncertainly about the future direction of health visiting but the UKCC (1994) recommend the specialism is named 'public health nursing specialist – health visiting'. This clearly indicates the importance of public health work which has been highlighted in other reports such as *New World, New Opportunities* (DoH, 1993a) and a *Vision for the Future* (DoH, 1993e). It is not yet clear what the effect on the health visiting service will be with increasing attachment to GP fundholders. Public health is an integral part of the health visitor's role (HVA, 1993); however, some health visitor contracts specify a certain amount of time to be allocated to 'public health'. Many areas are now employing health visitors as community development workers, particulary in deprived areas.

Skill mix is another contentious issue (see Chapter 7). There are many advantages to skill mix when correctly implemented, as it will free health visitors to work on projects which require their complex skills, rather than the 'routine' work which could be delegated. At present, skill mix is not that widespread in health visiting: a bottom up approach is preferable where health visitors themselves decide which activities they would like nursery nurses or health visitor (HV) assistants to undertake, rather than having decisions forced on them by management. The distinction between skill mix and grade mix is important (HVA, 1994a).

Nurse prescribing could affect the future of health visiting practice if it is implemented. At present there is a pilot scheme with health visitors prescribing from a Nurse Prescribers' Formulary, following an additional training course.

The future of health visiting lies in its marketing. This is basically an exercise in communicating with purchasers, other health professionals and client groups to ensure they understand the role and functions of the health visitor. In order for health visiting to move forwards, it is important that past misconceptions about the role are squashed and that all concerned, including health visitors themselves, understand the potential for health visitors and the exciting future ahead.

References

Ahmad, W.I.U. 1993: *Race and health in contemporary Britain.* Buckingham: Open University Press.
Allied Dunbar/Health Education Authority (HEA) 1992: *National fitness survey.* HEA/Sports Council.
Anderson E. and McFarlane J.K. 1988: *Community as Client.* Philadelphia: Lippincott.
Atkin, K., Cameron, E., Badger, F. and Evers 1989: Asian elders' knowledge and future use of community social and health services. *New Community* 15(3), 439–5.
Audit Commission 1994: *Seen but not heard: coordinating community child health and social services for children in need.* London: HMSO.
Barker, C., McCurry, M., Yates, J. and Parry, E. 1991: *Health Visiting: the Worcester Models.* Worcester and District Health Authority.
Barker, W. 1990: Practical and ethical doubts about screening for child abuse. *Health Visitor* 63(1), 14–17.
Baumer, D. and McLindon, H. 1994: Support after a cot death: the CONI Programme in action. *Professional Care of Mother and Child* 4(5), 131–3.
Blackburn, C. 1991: *Poverty and health.* Buckingham: Open University Press.
Blackburn, C. 1992a: *Improving health and welfare work with families in poverty.* Buckingham: Open University Press.
Blackburn, C. 1992b: *Poverty profiling.* London: HVA.
Blakemore, K. and Boneham, M. 1994: *Age, race and ethnicity.* Buckingham: Open University Press.
Blaxter, M. 1990: *Health and lifestyles.* London: Tavistock/Routledge.
Braun, D. and Schonveld, A. 1993: *Approaching parenthood: a resource for parent education.* London: Health Education Authority.
Brettell, K. 1994: Doing through speech: the health visitor's skill. *Health Visitor* 67(10), 344–6.
Child Accident Prevention Trust 1991: *Preventing Accidents to children: a training resource for health visitors.* London: CAPT.

Clark, J. 1986: A model for health visiting. In Kershaw, B. and Salvage, J. (eds), *Models for nursing*. London: John Wiley, 97–109

Combes, G. and Schonveld, A. 1992: *Life will never be the same*. London: Health Education Authority.

Corby, B. 1993: *Child abuse: towards a knowledge base*. Buckingham: Open University Press.

Coronary Prevention Group 1986: *Coronary heart disease and Asians in Britain*. London: Coronary Prevention Group.

Council for the Education and Training of Health Visitors (CETHV) 1977: *An investigation into the principles of Health Visiting*. London: CETHV.

Cox, J.L., Holden, J.J. and Sagovsky, R. 1987: detection of postnatal depression. *British Journal of Psychiatry* **150**, 782–6.

Department of Health (DoH) 1989a: *Caring for people: community care for people in the next decade and beyond*. London: HMSO.

Department of Health (DoH) 1989b: *Present day practice in infant feeding*. London: HMSO.

Department of Health (DoH) 1991a: *Dietary reference values for food energy and nutrients for the United Kingdom* (Report no 41). London: HMSO.

Department of Health (DoH) 1991b: *Working together under the Children Act 1989*. London: HMSO.

Department of Health (DoH) 1992a: *The health of the nation: a strategy for health in England*. London: HMSO.

Department of Health (DoH) 1992b: *Folic acid and the prevention of neural tube defects*. London: DoH.

Department of Health (DoH) 1992c: *Immunisation against infectious disease*. London: HMSO.

Department of Health (DoH) 1993a: *New world, new opportunities*. London: NHSME.

Department of Health (DoH) 1993b: *On the state of public health 1992*. London: HMSO.

Department of Health (DoH) 1993c: *The sleeping position of infants and cot death*. London: HMSO.

Department of Health (DoH) 1993d: *The health of the nation: key area handbook: accidents*. London: DoH.

Department of Health (DoH) 1993e: *Vision for the future*. London: NHSME.

Department of Health (DoH) 1994: *Children and young people on child protection registers*. London: HMSO.

Downie, R.S., Fyfe, C. and Tannahill, A. 1990: *Health promotion models and values*. Oxford: Oxford Medical Publications.

Foundation for the Study of Infant Deaths (FSID) 1994: *Factfile 1: cot death – facts, figures and definitions*. London:FSID.

Gath, A. 1985: Parental reactions to loss and disappointment: the diagnosis of Down's syndrome. *Developmental medicine and child neurology* **27**, 392–400.

Gath, A. 1990: Siblings of mentally retarded children. *Midwife, Health Visitor and Community Nurse* **26**(4): 116–18.

Gerrard, J., Holden, J.M., Elliot, S.A., McKenzie, P. and Cox, J.L. 1993: A trainer's perspective of an innovative programme teaching health visitors about the detection, treatment and prevention of postnatal depression. *Journal of Advanced Nursing* **18**, 1825–32.

Hall, D.M.B. 1992: *Health for all children*, 2nd edn. Oxford: Oxford University Press.

Hamner, J. and Statham, D. 1988: *Women and social work*. London: BASW/Macmillan..

Hawtin, M., Hughes, G. and Percy–Smith, J. 1994: *Community Profiling: auditing social needs*. Buckingham: Open University Press..

Health Education Authority 1993: *Every woman's health*. London: HEA.

Health Visitors Association (HVA) 1989: *Entitled to be healthy: heath visiting and school nursing in a multi–racial society*. London: HVA.

Health Visitors Association (HVA)/EPOCH 1991: *Positively no smacking*. London: HVA.

Health Visitors Association (HVA) 1993: *Health visiting and public health* (position statement). London: HVA.

Health Visitors Association (HVA) 1994a: *Action for health*. London: HVA.

Health Visitors Association (HVA) 1994b: *Protecting the child*. London: HVA.

Holden, J.A., Sagovsky, R.S. and Cox, J.L. 1989: Counselling in a general practice setting: a controlled trial of health visitor intervention on postnatal depression. *BMJ* 298, 233–6.

Idjradinata P., Watkins, W.E. and Pollitt, E. 1994: Adverse effects of iron supplementation on weight gain of iron-replete young children. *The Lancet* 343, 1252–4.

Leonard, A. 1994: *Right from the start: looking at diagnosis and disclosure*. London: The Spastics Society.

Luker, K. and Orr, J. 1992: *Health visiting: towards community health nursing*. Oxford: Blackwell Scientific.

McClymont, M., Thomas, S. and Denham, M.J. 1991: *Health visiting and elderly people*. London: Churchill Livingstone.

McIntosh, J. 1993: Postpartum depression: women's help–seeking behaviour and perceptions of cause. *Journal of Advanced Nursing* 18, 178–84.

Marder, E., Nicoll, A., Polnay, L., and Shulman, C. 1990: Discovering anaemia at child health clinics. *Archives of Disease in Childhood* 65, 892–4.

Meredith Davies, B. and Davies, T. 1993: *Community health, preventive medicine and social services*, 6th edn. London: Baillière Tindall.

Ministry of Health (MoH) 1956: *An enquiry into health visiting* (Jameson Report). London: HMSO.

Mott, A. and Emond, A. 1994: What is the role of distraction tests of hearing? *Archives of Disease in Childhood* 70, 10–13.

Niven, C.A. 1992: *Psychological care for families before, during and after birth*. London: Butterworth Heinemann.

Office of Population Censuses and Surveys (OPCS) 1993: *General household survey 1991*. London: HMSO.

Oppenheim, C. 1993: *Poverty: the facts*. London: CPAG.

Oxby, H. 1994: When do women decide? *Health Visitor* 67(5), 61.

Parsons, L., Macfarlane, A. and Golding, J. 1993: Pregnancy, birth and maternity care. In Ahmad, W.I.U. (ed.), *Race and health in contemporary Britain*. Buckingham: Open University Press, 51–75.

Pharoah, C. and Redmond, E. 1991: Care for ethnic elders. *The Health Service Journal* **16 May**.

Pickin, C. and St Leger, S. 1993: *Assessing health needs using the life cycle framework*. Buckingham: Open University Press.

Pursey, A.C. and Luker, K. 1993: Assessment of older people at home – a missed opportunity? In Wilson-Barnett, J. and Macleod Clark, J. (ed.), *Research in health promotion and nursing*. London: Macmillan, 132–9.

Raphael-Leff, J. 1991: *Psychological process of childbearing*. London: Chapman and Hall.

Reed-Purvis, S. and Dakin, S. 1993: Listening: an undervalued health visiting skill. *Health Visitor* 66(10), 367–9.

Richards, D. 1993a: Screening the over 75s. *British Journal of Nursing* 2(16), 827–32.

Richards, D. 1993b: Screening the over 75s: 2. *British Journal of Nursing* 2(17), 879–83.

Robertson, C. 1991: *Health visiting in practice*. London: Churchill Livingstone.

Royal College of Midwives (RCM) 1991: *Successful breastfeeding*, 2nd edn. London: RCM.

Royal College of Nursing (RCN) 1993a: *The GP practice population profile*. London: RCN.

Royal College of Nursing (RCN) 1993b: *Guidelines for assessing mental health needs in old age*. London: RCN.

Royal College of Nursing (RCN) 1994: *Into the 90s: a discussion document on the future of health visiting practice*. London: RCN.

Sashidharan, S.P. and Francis, E. 1993: Epidemiology, ethnicity and schizophrenia. In Ahmad, W.I.U. (ed.), *'Race' and health in contemporary Britain*. Buckingham: Open University Press, 96–113.

Sheridan, M.D. 1992: *From birth to five: children's developmental progress*. Windsor: Nfer-Nelson.

Stokoe, B. 1994: Failure breeds success. *Health Visitor* **67**(5), 170.

Symonds, A. 1991: Angels and interfering busybodies: the social construction of two occupations. *Society of Health and Illness* **13**(2), 251–63.

Taylor, E. 1989: Postnatal depression: what can a health visitor do? *Journal of Advanced Nursing* **14**, 877–86.

Twinn, S. and Cowley 1992: *The principles of health visiting: a re-examination*. London: HVA/UKSC.

Twinn, S., Dauncey, J. and Carnell, J. 1990: *The process of health profiling*. London: HVA.

UKCC 1994: *Standards for education and practice following registration* report. London: UKCC.

Wallace, W.A. 1987: The scale and financial implications of osteoporosis. In RCN 1993: Nursing update: established osteoporosis: a time for action. Learning unit 35. *Nursing Standard* **7**(33).

White, A., Freeth, S. and O'Brien. 1992: *Infant feeding: 1990*. London: OPCS/HMSO.

PART FOUR

And that special flavour . . .

13 Learning disability

Peggy Cooke

Peggy Cooke offers a thought-provoking chapter whilst examining this specialism which is becoming increasingly marginalized. Provision for people with learning disabilities has been consistantly eroded over the years. It could be argued that 'normalization' has been used in both health care and education to disguise the structured neglect of this group. At the time of writing, this specialist branch of nursing is very much under threat and looks in danger of failing to survive. It would be a tragedy if this specialism were to disappear since it attracts nurses with a genuine interest in the lives of this disadvantaged group. Great strides have been made in the care of people with learning disabilities because there has been a specialist branch; without it a part of nursing could return to the 'unenlightened' age.

Introduction

The impact of community care policy on people with a learning disability and their carers has been great. The effects of relocation and closure plans of long-stay residential settings and day care settings have not always been positive for people with a learning disability, their families and service providers. Rationing of services has impacted upon both residential and day care provision with the effects being felt mainly by people with learning disabilities who live in the family home being cared for by informal carers. The introduction of the principle of normalization (more recently described as social role valorization) as a foundation for providing effective services has further exacerbated the problems that rationing introduced and has provided problems of its own due in part to service providers mis-interpreting its meaning. These problems have resulted in limited and often poor services for people with a learning disability and their carers. Whilst we have seen reductions in the service provision these effects can only be minimized if two things occur. First, community learning disability nurses and other service providers need to supply a more effective service for people with a learning disability and their carers than has occurred in the past. Second, if the philosophy of care is to be based on the principle of normalization, its ideals must be accepted by the community as a whole rather than just a select few professionals.

Terminology

Within this chapter the term 'learning disability' is used as a descriptor of the client group under consideration. It is the present terminology used and as Thompson and Mathias (1992) note 'in 1991 the Minister of Health announced that, in England, the term learning disability would be used instead of mental handicap by the Department of Health'. Rose (1993) points out that: 'this was widely accepted as a significant step forward; even though the term "learning difficulties" which the people who have to carry the label say they would prefer was not chosen'.

The problem with the terminology used by professionals is that the jargon means very little to the lay person. What is a learning disability? How can we define this concept? One of the difficulties of truly defining the phrase learning disabilities is that the term is too broad. To the lay person, learning disability could be almost anything. Anyone can have a learning disability, from the person who cannot understand statistics to the person who cannot read, to the person with such additional labels as Down's syndrome or cerebral palsy. However, if you ask a nurse or other professional who works in the area of learning disabilities, the question: 'What is learning disability?' you would expect a clear answer. In reality, the answer is unlikely to be clear but the indication will be that the nurse or other professional intuitively knows that a person with a learning disability has a learning disability and therefore if the individual is referred to the team for a service then the person will be accepted by that team. But that gets us no further in explaining learning disability. We can consider the previous terminology used: mental handicap or learning difficulty. These terms may provide better descriptors of the people we are considering but as Ashton and Ward (1992) point out 'there is no universal definition of mental handicap'. Frazer and Green (1991) provide a useful explanation, indicating that learning disability is 'a condition of lifelong intellectual impairment and accompanying disabilities in social functioning. It is not simply a clinical diagnosis: it is a social process of changing expectations, labelling, and families coming to some understanding of what handicap (or learning disability) means'.

Labelling

Whilst there is a need for a label (if only as a means of planning future services) some would argue that the labelling process is damaging to the individual. The label becomes stigmatizing so devaluing the individual and as a result organizations start to look for less stigmatizing labels to refer to the client group under consideration. The people do not go away, the client group does not change and in many respects the service does not change – the only thing that does change with monotonous regularity (at least four times in the last 20 years) is the label. The devaluing process cannot be changed purely by altering the label.

Some may argue that categorizing people is inappropriate but it is an essential part of the structured society in which we live. It allows us to make appropriate policies and provide services for those varied groups in society. Tuckett (1976) indicates that Parsons, when discussing the label 'patient', identifies that labelling individuals as patients 'is not socially valued' and can reduce an individual's status either temporarily or permanently. Wolfensberger and Thomas (1994) indicate that 'people who are societally devalued . . typically get cast and kept in social roles that are not valued'. People with learning disabilities have been labelled for many centuries. This categorization effectively provides labels by which others can codify individuals. This labelling may have negative aspects but on the positive side it provides parents with a reason and understanding of the disability their child experiences and it allows services to be set up to meet the needs of people who are deemed to have the label learning disability.

Wolfensberger is often recognized as the person who made service providers aware of the devalued lives people with learning disabilities were living in long-stay institutions; 'he made a quantum leap in the way service workers could understand the lives of people with disabilities in terms of them being a "devalued" group' (Brown and Smith, 1992). The issue of relocation of people with learning disabilities from hospitals to community settings was taken up by him and his supporters in order to provide people with a learning disability a more valued lifestyle. Unfortunately, recognizing that a group of people is devalued does not remove the devalued status from that group – relocation does not provide a more valued lifestyle, a more fundamental shift in the attitudes of society is needed. This change cannot occur overnight and indeed if this shift in attitude is to occur it may take many decades. That attitudinal shift may be helped if people within society have contact with, and knowledge of, the devalued groups within society.

Relocation

The move of that relatively small number of people with a learning disability from long-stay hospitals to the community setting has been heralded as a good move – a positive step forward for people with a learning disability. However, 'whilst radicals within and beyond the movement' [of normalization] 'were using the ideology to work towards the closure of large inhumane institutions, the government was using community care to limit spending on the elderly and handicapped' (Brown and Smith, 1992). The combined efforts of policy and these supporters of the principle of normalization have effectively reduced the facilities (both buildings and people) available to people with a learning disability and their carers. Whilst the aim may have been to close inhumane institutions, the result is inadequate provision for many and no service for some.

The process of resettlement from the old-style institutions to community settings is well underway. This move to care for all people with learning disabilities in a community setting is valuable provided it ensures a bet-ter quality of life for the individual. Whilst recognizing that hospital care was not ideal and indeed was often extremely poor, we have the prob-lem of throwing the baby out with the bath water. The problems of insti-tutional care cannot be swept under the carpet but the resulting changes have occurred in the belief that all institutional care was poor. It appears that good care in institutions has been ignored rather than maintaining or replicating it in the community setting. By getting rid of everything from the past in order to start anew we have a situation where some community care is excellent but other care is equally as poor if not poor-er than that previous institutional care. We have seen the closure of those hospital and hostel environments (poor and good) but have maintained many of the (good and poor) staff from those institutions and replaced others with untrained and poorly paid care assistants. The enquiries of the late 1970s and early 1980s highlighting poor care and practice, in places like Ely Hospital Cardiff, was one of the factors that resulted in the closure of long-stay hospitals. Whilst these closures have reduced the numbers of people being cared for in one setting, they have also reduced the opportunity of identifying and challenging poor practice where it exists in small community homes. The practice of encouraging people with learning disabilities to live either alone or with one or two other people results in minimally staffed homes where only one member of staff is on duty at one time. The effect of dispersal of these many people with a learning disability has in many cases hidden the problem of lack of ser-vices and as a result has lost what little voice was available to fight for better services. More importantly, monitoring of quality practice and the opportunity to share that good practice has been reduced whilst the oppor-tunity for poor practice to develop and go unnoticed has increased.

Community care

The idea of community care is not new but one that has been considered by policy makers for almost a century. Parker (1990) notes that: 'the 1904–08 Royal Commission on the Care of the Feeble Minded . . . did . . . advocate guardianship and supervision "in the community" where appropriate'. Much of the support for community care has been based on the issue of cost, with benefit to the individual being a secondary gain. Recognition that institutional care is an expensive option has long been identified and the idea of identifying cheaper options has been welcomed. The discussions surrounding community care policy have highlighted the importance of improving care for the vulnerable in our society, however, progress has been slow. When discussing community care for people with a learning disability the focus is often the move from hospital care back into the community but for the majority of the population, who have always lived in the community, it means care at home.

Ashton and Ward (1992) indicate that: 'community care has no precise definition'. This lack of clarity is evident as people's perceptions of community care are varied. DoH (1989) indicate that 'community care means providing the services and support which people who are affected by problems of . . . mental handicap . . . need to be able to live as independent as possible in their own homes, or in homely settings within the community'. Whiting, cited in Benson (1987), highlights 'the burden of care has been shifted from the trained professional to the untrained and isolated – the family'. Wilkin (1979) argues that 'community care does not mean care by the community, nor does it mean care by the family, it means maternal care with varying but generally low levels of support from others'. Whilst this quote may be seen to be dated, particularly as the role of male carers is being acknowledged, the reality is that little has changed.

Whilst it is evident that most care for people with a learning disability has always been provided within the home it is also apparent that the paid support available in the community is being reduced. The availability of day care and respite care is reducing and support staff is rationed. The need to make savings on the health and social services budget seems to be paramount. If paid support is reducing and informal carers are to continue to care there is a need to mobilize the local communities to support these informal carers and the individuals with a learning disability.

Family care

For those being resettled back into the community, residential support in group homes is assured but for those people with a learning disability living with carers the options are limited. Ham (1992) suggests 'that there will be an increase in self care and care in the home . . . stimulated by . . . the shift from residential to domiciliary support for those needing long-term care'. The reality is that the closures of institutions has resulted in a dearth of both short- and long-term day and residential care facilities for those people still living within the family home. As a result care in the family home will, in the future, be the only option available for many people with a learning disability regardless of the quality of care available in that setting. As Parker (1990) points out:

> official policy statements have increasingly argued that not only is the state unable to bear the cost of . . . institutional care, it also cannot afford to provide a comprehensive network of health and welfare services to support the many . . . who live outside formal institutions.

Horne (1989), when discussing the introduction of the 1990 NHS and Community Care Act, indicates that 'the Government is clearly banking on increased effort, resources and commitment from the families and friends of . . . disabled people . . .'. It is, however, unclear if there are the human resources and commitment available to provide this increase in unpaid care.

An additional problem for people with learning disabilities is that, whilst they have family to support them, their bank of friends is likely to be small and to consist mainly of other people with learning disabilities. This is due to the segregated lifestyle that many people with a learning disability have had imposed upon them from the early years of their lives.

Normalization

The philosophy of care used by many community teams and services for people with learning disabilities is said to be based on the principle of normalization or social role valorization. Evidence of its wide service base is described by Rose (1993) who argues that today normalization is 'a guiding principle standing for a whole new ideology of human management' and provides 'a set of service principles that govern many services throughout health services, local authority services and the voluntary sector'. That principle of normalization is said by Wolfensberger (1977), cited in Tyne (1981) to be 'the utilisation of culturally valued means in order to establish and/or maintain personal behaviours, experiences, and characteristics that are culturally normative or valued'.

Tyne (1981) identifies Wolfensberger's five accomplishments which are essential for a valued lifestyle: dignity and respect, community presence, community participation, choice and competence. To these five accomplishments were later added 'expression of individuality and the experience of continuity in one's life' (Frazer and Green, 1991). Those service providers with a philosophy based on the principle of normalization attempt to ensure that provision for people with learning disabilities is based on these beliefs.

The terminology used by exponents of the principle of normalization has been misinterpreted and misapplied by many in the past and, as Jackson (1988) points out, the result is confusion over Wolfensberger's meaning of the principle of normalization. As a result of this Wolfensberger himself advocates the use of social role valorization instead of normalization. Rose (1993) indicates that 'it may seem strange that something can simultaneously be widely misunderstood and yet extremely influential'. Garety (1990) highlights that 'its influence is controversial', it is 'a principle, which has been presented in many different ways and with different shades of emphasis by its many proponents'. It is evident that problems exist with, not only the interpretation of the principle of normalization but also the implementation of its principle.

The reasons for the use of normalization as a guiding principle for service provision are at times unclear. The problem appears to be that many service providers and policy makers have needed something to cling on to in the wake of the disquiet about both residential and day care service provision for people with a learning disability. As Garety (1990) points out 'the term "normalisation" is to be found liberally scattered through current policy documents' like 'the House of Commons Social Services Committee Report on Community Care (1985)'. Policy makers and community teams seem to have accepted that a change in philosophy was needed and the way forward was through the principle of normalization without acknowledging that this can only be implemented effectively if the commitment, training and finances are available and society's attitudes can be changed. Instead, what we have seen in many services is a half-hearted attempt to implement the principle of normalization resulting in mediocre or poor service provision. Indeed, in many situations services are no better, if not worse, than those provided in the old institutions. What has happened is that normalization has been accepted as the way forward without sufficient acknowledgement of its implications or recognition by service providers that in a world of rationed services the reality is that we place the burden of implementation not on service providers but on the people with learning disabilities themselves and their informal carers.

The belief that people with learning disabilities should live in the community like anyone else – living in ordinary houses in ordinary streets, having ordinary jobs and leisure opportunities – has to be supported. Whilst it may be possible to achieve presence in the community, Wolfensberger's other accomplishments, described above, are more difficult to achieve. Effective application of the other accomplishments relies not only on the individual, carers and service providers but also on the many people in society that the individual will come into contact with on a day-to-day basis.

Ryan and Thomas (1993) consider the argument of equal rights for people with learning disabilities and question how in a society where 'material, psychological and cultural inequalities are overlooked' we are to ensure equality. As Tadd (1994) indicates 'we live in a divided society in which class, ethnic and religious ghettos abound'. The reality is that we cannot achieve equality for the many minority groups in society including those with a learning disability. In this society we are unlikely to achieve equality and total integration but what we may be able to achieve is ordinariness. A principle of ordinariness, however, may include poor-quality housing, inadequate or inappropriate diet and clothing, little money and no job; these experiences may be culturatively normative but far from the culturally valued lifestyle espoused by Wolfensberger and many service providers. In reality, this principle of ordinariness provides a worse quality of life for some people with a learning disability than the old-style residential care that so many people fought to remove.

Ryan and Thomas (1993) point out that 'normalisation can mean much greater pressure on mentally handicapped people to adjust to prevailing customs and standards'. Tadd (1994) indicates that 'people with learning difficulties are rarely given the choice of deciding whether they want to adopt the social and cultural norms of the community in which they live'. He goes on to indicate that 'undoubtedly they will stand more chance of acceptance if they conform as much as possible to public perceptions of what constitutes "normal" standards of behaviour'. Unfortunately, the reality of life is that we all have to conform to the customs and standards of the society in which we live and if we choose not to do so then we have to accept the penalties of not conforming which may include exclusion from that society. If people with a learning disability are to be accepted into their community, then they also must accept the pressure of adjusting to the existing standards and customs.

What are coming to the fore are the varied problems that exist with using the principle of normalization as a service philosophy. Whilst the problems may be many, the two major ones, which are affecting the implementation of the principle of normalization, are a lack of training and a lack of finance to ensure effective implementation.

Finance

Ryan and Thomas (1993) indicate that the issue of financial cost for introducing services based on the principle of normalization has often been dodged by many reforming groups. The present climate of care further heightens the problems of funding services based on this principle. Small group homes have been the focus of community care replacing the hospitals and hostel care of the past. This type of care is not, however, a cheap option. Spreading the client group out into many homes has resulted in the need for many staff to support these people with learning disabilities in these homes. Equally, finding day and leisure services using the principle of normalization as a basis for provision may be more costly (at least initially if not long term). At the moment money continues to go into bricks and mortar rather than people, and changes in this outdated system of care will take many years. Finances are limited and indeed are becoming more scarce. The result is that authorities can no longer afford to employ well-qualified and consequently well-paid individuals.

The reality is that rationing of health and social care has always occurred; today it has become more explicit. The result of this rationing seems to be that many service providers have either put their heads in the sand and carried on as before or become angry that management has allowed this to happen. The need is to relook at service provision for people with a learning disability and to identify ways of improving the provision for as many people as possible. There is a need to balance quality with quantity and whilst service providers may sometimes have to accept that if more money were available better services could be found, that has to be balanced with both the needs of clients and carers.

This issue of funding significantly affects informal carers. Glendinning (1986) highlights that 'community care may look cheap because it involves less public expenditure; but it imposes substantial financial costs on individual members of the community'. The introduction of the NHS and Community Care Act 1990 has not seen a reduction in this financial burden and indeed its implementation may further disadvantage those people with a learning disability living at home with informal carers. The decision that 'clients and their carers will face an increase in means testing before resources are allocated' (Horne, 1989) will place further pressures on informal carers.

In theory, resources and finances are indirectly available for the service user or a group of service users to have a choice of service; however, in reality users do not have ownership of that service. As a result of this, the service providers maintain a powerful role whilst the service users continue to retain the position of weakness. Recent changes in policy have done very little to alter this position. Unless there is a system where money goes to the individual to buy the service that they need we will never satisfy all client needs.

The use of brokerage, described by Brandon (1988) as a system that 'links the person, the funding body and community resources', could have helped to address the issue of funding for individuals' needs and may have encouraged choice for the individual and transferred some of the power from providers to the client in need of the service. Salisbury *et al.*, cited in Brandon and Towe (1989), indicate that service brokerage is based in part 'on the traditional, if overlooked, principle that the proper role of human service professionals is that of "adjunct" or "auxiliary" to the individual who seeks to arrive at informed decisions while pursuing appropriate goods and services'. The opportunity to move service providers to their proper place as assistants in ensuring appropriate care be identified for people with a learning disability could have occurred with the introduction of case management but was not recognized and as a result the continuation of provider power remains. The move to see the individual with a learning disability as the central person when considering the funding of care has been overlooked for too long and is still to be addressed.

Training

The issue of continued training of service providers is important, particularly with the large increase in unqualified people working in services for people with a learning disability. Many community teams, on setting up a service based on the philosophy of normalization, provided some training for their team members. Unfortunately, that training seems to go little further than the qualified community team members, so we have a small, elite, group who have the appropriate normalization/social role valorization training. They have a clear understanding of the principle of normalization but many others working with people with a learning disability, such as volunteers and care assistants, have inadequate or no training. Equally, it is rare to see informal carers and people with learning disabilities themselves being offered an awareness of this philosophy of care. Additionally, training is in the main offered when the service considers its operational philosophy. Many people who join the service at a later date are offered nothing or only a diluted form of training (i.e. cheaper and shorter in length). In many situations it is this lack of training which results in misinterpretation of normalization theory which can, and has, led to poor service and at times neglect. Jackson (1988) highlights that 'a significant proportion of front line staff working in facilities for children and adults with mental handicaps are young, or inexperienced, or untrained'. He goes on to point out that 'the lack of adequate training is at the heart of the problem'. The use of the principle of normalization as a foundation for the setting up of community-based services, in particular homes, has exacerbated this problem as it means that many more people are using this as a basis for their work with little understanding of how best to provide a service using this principle. This problem is further heightened as in many situations the turn over of unqualified staff is high.

If effective service provision based on the principle of normalization is to be provided then a bottom up approach to training must be provided rather than the top down approach that presently exists. But that training must go further; it must encompass work with the community as a whole if we are to see effective integration of people with a learning disability.

Integration

A fundamental problem with introducing the principle of normalization is the segregationist policies within which people with learning disabilities have to live. The problem starts with the label that is attached at or soon after birth and reinforced with the introduction of specialist services. This is closely followed by education policy which, whilst seeming to support integration with the 1981, 1988 and 1993 Education Acts, in most cases makes access to ordinary education difficult to implement. The exclusion from local services at an early age adds to the problems of integration as it makes the later reintroduction of people with learning disabilities to ordinary services extremely difficult. Whilst policy makers and supporters of the principle of normalization are advocating integration into ordinary community-based services the reality is that there are too many specialist buildings that need filling and too many paid people with vested interests who want to see those specialist buildings maintained. Whilst Brandon argued in 1987 that 'both day services and accommodation projects are at last discovering what users need and want and moving towards more individualised services' the problem still remains that the majority of service users are having to use those outdated day and residential services that exist. Large amounts of money continue to go into this provision in the form of maintenance and also to pay the large numbers of personnel employed as carers and managers of such services. Idealists could argue that units do not exist to employ people, but that the people should be employed to meet the needs of individuals as cost effectively as possible whilst maintaining a quality provision. Whilst one may agree with this, it would appear that the reality is that service users' wants or needs for both day care and residential accommodation will not be met whilst old-style facilities still exist. The majority of financial resources will continue to be placed in a few buildings resulting in limited choice for the service user.

Some could argue that there are sufficient generic services in the community for people to use, but the reality is that whilst services exist the support mechanisms to facilitate the integration of the person with a learning disability into the service has disappeared. Indeed, Tadd (1994) argues against the 'ethically dubious ways of pursuing the goal of integration' highlighting that it is unfortunately the case that 'much of the responsibility for attaining successful integration is being placed on the clients rather than upon society'. If the onus is to be placed on clients and carers, they must decide if integrated activities are what they require. We may find that integration is a professional ideal rather than something that clients and carers are aiming for.

Consumerism

We have recently seen the introduction of consumerism used in the provision of health care. Trnobranski (1994) highlights that 'the current socio-political philosophy in the United Kingdom promotes the belief that consumers of health care should exercise choice and express opinions about the care they receive'. Many of the policy documents of recent years, including the Griffiths Report, White Paper, and National Health Service and Community Care Act, make reference to consumerism (Walker, 1993). Trnobranski (1994) emphasizes the White Paper 'Working for Patients' 1989 indicating it 'explicitly promotes patient choice and asserts that the planning and delivery of health services should be aimed at meeting people's expressed needs'.

Lewis (1991) highlights that the spread of consumerism to the public sector 'is increasingly focusing on providing a high quality, valued service where good managers know their customers and their needs and preferences'. Monach and Spriggs (1994) point out that 'user involvement is no longer simply a good thing: users' organisations demand it, legislation requires it and much has been written about it'. The discussion of people with a learning disability having a say in the care they receive has been ongoing for many years (Brandon, 1987). The move to provide quality services which have a focus on the needs of the user can only be to the advantage of those people with learning disabilities that use services. The consumerist emphasis is one where choice is applauded, and if we accept that people with a learning disability are to be offered choices, then it is only natural that they be offered the choice of service they receive. The issue of finding out what service users want and need is a valid aim. However, the consumer needs to be provided with the knowledge to make effective contributions to that process, in fact the empowerment of the individual is an imperative if consumer choice is to be a reality.

In this society, it is the norm for individuals to expect some choice in the things that they do, that they think and that they buy. Even those most basic of choices that are made on a day-to-day basis are, however, usually limited – it is rare to be offered a free choice, owing to the unavailability of goods, time, finances or resources. Most people are usually trusted to make appropriate choices from a limited range and also to live with or learn from any mistaken choices. Each opportunity to make choice provides the service user with some ownership of what is done and some satisfaction in having been a party to the decision making. The value of choice in one's life cannot be overemphasized and the idea of encouraging people with a learning disability to make choices in their lives should be supported. However small or however limited that choice may appear to the service provider is immaterial as long as the service user values and benefits from the choice making. Williamson (1992) points out that 'those choices retain in reality, and in symbol, power and control over some aspects of life, as well as expressing and defining the self'.

Choice of service, however, whilst applauded rarely exists. With limited provision available and lack of experience of having choices, the person with a learning disability is left with little say in what service they receive. Of equal significance is the fact that whilst some people want a say in the service that they get, others may not be in a position to give a clear idea of what they want or may want others to make the choice for them. As Walker (1993) indicates 'in the field of social care many people are mentally disabled, frail and vulnerable; they are not in a position to "shop around" for services but have to accept what is offered'. Brown and Smith (1992) point out that 'describing service users as consumers evades the immense vulnerability and dependence on services of the people themselves'. Certainly, the person with a learning disability may have learned to be grateful for what they receive, particularly if that person has at some time been in institutional care of one form or another and may not previously have had the opportunity to evaluate critically the service they receive or to make choices about those services. Monach and Spriggs (1994) also highlight the problems that people with a learning disability have in making representation. They highlight that few ever use the complaints procedure for fear of adverse consequences and 'the possible damage to their relationships with carers'. If people with learning disabilities are to be allowed to make choices, then they must be able to challenge service providers without fear of retribution. As many people with a learning disability have accepted without question the services that are offered/ provided to them in the past, they are unlikely to rock the boat at this stage. Others may still have an attitude that the provider knows best. Whilst this situation remains, it is unlikely that we will see service users having fair and just choices of services.

The issue of encouraging people with learning disabilities to make choices raises the issue of informed choice. An essential element when offering choice is that of ensuring that people have the knowledge to make wise choices. It is not worth asking someone who has lived in an institution for many years to choose in which town they would like to live. Knowledge of the environment, the inhabitants, the facilities and the support mechanisms is essential as are such things as the feel of the place. These individuals may not be in a position to make informed choices owing mainly to lack of experience in the area of choice. As Brandon (1987) points out 'many consumers have been treated in a child like way and lived for years in segregated settings with choices being made for them'. Therefore the introduction of choice making must be done gradually, and as Ryan and Thomas (1993) indicate, if we offer 'a greater degree of choice . . . we have to ensure that these experiences are not overwhelmingly negative'. However, we must take into consideration Brandon's (1987) point that 'in our enthusiasm we often fail to examine consumer's capacity for meaningful choice'. If we are to provide choices, then we must ensure the independent support mechanisms are in place to secure well-considered choices. This support mechanism will ensure that people with learning disabilities are not only given the opportunity to make choices but are also able to learn about the consequences of their decisions. Brandon (1987) highlights the need for individuals to take on the responsibilities for the decisions they make indicating that 'choice is a complex concept – we learn to make better choices through making mistakes'.

Lewis (1991) indicates that consumerism 'has attempted to redress the balance of power between producers and purchasers of goods and services'. The reality is that service providers cannot give everyone what they choose. Equally, we have to accept that choices in the real world are painful and 'the best choice available is really the least worst' (Brandon, 1987). Lawson (1993) supports the view that 'we should offer people choices, along with a clear explanation of the consequences of decisions. We should negotiate to produce an outcome which is acceptable to all and we should intervene where necessary to protect the vulnerable from exploitation and abuse'. Lawson (1993) clearly paints a picture of 'we' the professionals offering what 'we' perceive as the choices to 'them' the service users. Brandon (1987) is more honest suggesting 'we haven't the money, resources or detachment to make good choices'. The unfortunate point is that people with learning disabilities or their carers are not the purchasers but the recipients of the product that the purchasers choose to buy. Indeed the introduction of the purchaser/provider split has sharpened a situation that has always existed – the purse-holding authority, in this case local authority, health authority/trust, GP or government, decides if there is the money to provide a service and if there is not then the needs of an individual will not be met. The consumer does not have purchasing power, therefore the power clearly remains with the provider.

Power

Whilst it can be seen that there is a move to consumer participation and choice, this involvement is still very limited and users still lack the power to make significant changes to the service that they receive. Consumerism is a fashionable term in learning disability services yet this consumerist model, whilst a little more open than the paternalistic model, still leaves the power with the service providers. It is not in the interests of service providers to encourage change as their power over people with learning disabilities and maintaining the *status quo* allows their survival. As Brandon and Towe (1989) indicate 'traditional approaches are not structured to respond adequately to the needs of people with disabilities and their families. They are inherently autocratic and bureaucratic'. Brandon and Towe (1989) further criticize service provision indicating that 'the system of the key worker does not indicate individualised funding but "sophisticated paternalism" '.

If we consider those people who live independently with minimal support from workers within a community team, these people are often those who have in the past been resettled either from hospital care or from social services hostel care. They have often been managed, and still are, by carers who hold the power and have the final say in the care received. The move to care in the community and living in one's own home should have allowed a change in the person's life with them managing their own life and holding the power. In many cases this is not so. The individual with a learning disability may live independently and be responsible for their own lives for most of the time but when a member of the community team appears that person may become subservient, recognizing the power and authority of the person.

Griffiths (1988) highlighted that community care services should be geared to the needs of the individual and carer and that local authorities should assess the community care needs of the locality, set local priorities and service objectives and develop local plans in consultation with health authorities. He emphasized that local authorities should also identify and assess individual's needs, taking account of personal preferences. They should arrange delivery of packages of care to individuals using the system of care management; clearly, an indication of a move of power towards the person with a learning disability. However, Means and Harrison (1988), cited in Hawker and Ritchie (1988) indicate that 'it is suggested that the Griffiths proposals might offer greater choice (to individuals) but that professional staff retain their key powers'. As Hawker and Ritchie point out 'the (Griffiths) white paper does not in itself create greater consumer choice and power'.

Communicare (1993) when discussing mental health services points out that 'for most of us' [service users] 'there are no real alternatives and no choice at the moment'. The editorial goes on: 'what is proving difficult is to get action on what users say, even when extensive consultation takes place'.

The aim must be for the development of a user-led service if we are to develop a service that meets the needs of the service users rather than one that maintains the role of the service providers. The idea of letting go of power and allowing users to retake responsibility for their own lives is difficult for some people to accept but is increasingly being challenged by user groups and within standard setting and quality documents.

The emphasis must be on service-user participation in the making of choices. However, we must accept that there will be provider unease regarding the shift in power and loss of control. This, however, is no reason for that shift not taking place, provided that the service user gains the necessary support to make choices that are right for them and at the same time ensuring that the service provider is not put into a risky position due to the consequences of that user's choice. With an effective, independent, advocacy system in place to support individuals with a learning disability, the power and control of service providers can be minimized whilst allowing people with learning disabilities to make choices regarding the decisions that affect their lives.

Informal carers

Twigg et al. (1990) point out that 'over the last decade, the subject of informal care has increasingly been in the forefront of policy'. The reasons for this may be many, but the main one seems to be the increasing costs involved in supporting sick or disabled people (Twigg et al., 1990). But of major importance is the political climate in which we live, where public services are being privatized and public expenditure is being reduced (Finch and Groves, 1983), and for the individual, or family group, responsibility of paying for one's own is seen to be paramount. Parker (1990) focuses on this change from formal carer to informal carer indicating that 'now, rather than services being provided to support informal carers, informal carers have increasingly been viewed as a substitute for formally organised services'. Twigg and Atkin (1994) indicate that whilst carers are visible in the policy debate, policy itself 'remains undeveloped and seldom goes beyond bland statements of the importance of supporting carers'.

Government health and social policy still focus attention on family care due to concerns that if services are substituted for informal care it 'will encourage people to do less for their dependants' (Twigg, 1989). She goes on to discuss the emphasis of the New Right 'on family obligation and the need not to undermine this by incentive systems that "encourage people" to substitute welfare provision for their own activities'. This point of encouraging family obligation and unpaid help is supported in an unlikely quarter. The normalization principle espouses valuing of individuals, particularly those people with disabilities, but whilst valuing people with disabilities and supporting the use of unpaid help one may be devaluing the informal carer.

Whilst a small number of people are being cared for in a range of residential settings the majority are being cared for by informal unpaid carers, usually the family. These families get very little support from the service providers. The recent move, defended by those supporters of normalization, to close devaluing residential and day care services has left carers with less support and less services. Brown and Smith (1992), in their discussion of normalization, point out that 'Wolfensberger explicitly values unpaid help over paid help', the idea being that this unpaid help is more socially valued than paid help and possibly less stigmatizing. This idea of valuing unpaid care is challenged by Brown and Smith (1992) who highlight 'women who work outside the home constitute a class of wage earners whilst women who do the same task, but in the domestic sphere, have terms and conditions reminiscent of servants in bygone households'. It appears contradictory that whilst advocating the need to provide a valued lifestyle for one group in society (i.e. people with a learning disability) we are devaluing another group: their carers.

The costs of caring for a person with a learning disability has long been recognized (Bayley, 1973; Wilkin, 1979; Ayer and Alaszewski, 1984). Challis and Davies (1986) indicate that the major costs are in terms of 'stress, strains and social limitations'. Seale (1990) highlights the social isolation of carers which can produce 'feelings of resentment and guilt'. He indicates the high percentage of carers who had their lives severely restricted as they did less visiting, went on less holidays, gave up entertaining at home and did less work. Whiting, cited in Benson (1987), discussed figures provided by the Association of Carers and highlights the severe problems faced by carers with two out of three in poor physical health, half are at serious risk of becoming mentally ill, 70 per cent have become physically injured as a result of caring – many with back problems from lifting, and 83 per cent receive no assistance from any other person, professional or relative or friend. Challis and Davies (1986) also highlight the high proportion of carers suffering from mental distress. It is of concern that carers are not getting the necessary support to keep these negative factors of caring to a minimum.

It is evident that carers do need the help of professionals in looking after the person with a learning disability. The reality is that community learning disability nurses are still unclear about their role with carers, particularly if the needs of the carers are at odds with the needs of the person with a learning disability. There is a need to recognize the importance of the carer's role and accept that without these unpaid carers the quality of life for most people with a learning disability would be significantly worse. If professionals are not in a position to provide a better quality of care they should at least help the informal carers to continue to care. The important thing is that any help provided should be flexible enough to meet the needs of both the person with a learning disability and the carer, so improving the quality of life for both. It is, however, essential that carers get the support that they need if the deleterious effects of caring are to be minimized.

Community nursing service provision

Many community nurses for people with learning disabilities have highlighted that their philosophy of care is one of normalization but the reality is that the care they provide is paternalistic with providers of services maintaining the power. This may be because they have not had the appropriate training regarding the normalization principle or have not accepted the philosophy of normalization. This paternalistic attitude is particularly evident in the doctor/patient relationship but equally if one considers the plethora of service providers one can identify the powerful role that they hold as gatekeepers to the services available. This power base is an effective way of service providers maintaining the *status quo* and excluding or minimizing the role of people with a learning disability from the important decisions in their lives. Brandon and Towe (1989) point out that 'the professional journals run endless articles about involving consumers of services in management, planning and the running of projects. But does the participation movement really amount to anything – or is it simply the new paternalism?'.

Much has been written on the role of the community team for people with a learning disability (Community Mental Handicap Nurses Association, 1985; Royal College of Nursing, 1985; 1992). It is sufficient to indicate that different community teams have different roles and functions but the main focus is the support of people with a learning disability in the community. Services have been provided in most areas for between 15 and 20 years, so we can see the service is still young and finding its feet. This service, however, does not have the advantages of time that health visitors have had to develop their role. If this developmental stage goes on much longer there will be no specialist community nursing service for people with a learning disability. The problem that this group of community nurses has is that they have a wide role which they are unable to explain clearly and as a result have difficulty in justifying their existence, a problem compounded by the service philosophy of normalization. Indeed, if taken to its natural conclusion, the principle of normalization advocates the use of ordinary services which could be provided by other community-based nurses such as paediatric community nurses or district nurses or indeed health visitors.

Community learning disability nurses have spent too long worrying about whether or not they will continue to have a job (next year, at the next election, to see themselves to retirement age). Unfortunately they forget that the important consideration is whether the person with a learning disability will get a service (next year, at the next election, etc.). It is time community learning disability nurses were concerned about the client group they work with and whether people with a learning disability and their carers will miss their service if they do not have a job.

The reality is that there are many people with learning disabilities living in the community who are in need of a service, whether that be developmental, health promotional or behavioural, that is, not presently being provided by generic services. Equally, there are carers in the community who need a service if they are to continue to provide quality care for the person with a learning disability. But equally real is that the demise of community learning disability nurses will occur unless they learn to speak out for their client group and ensure they provide the sort of service that clients and carers need. The time of going in to a family and putting extra pressure on them by getting them to do the assessments and the interventions and maybe evaluations, is past. The wasted time spent in ineffective meetings and office discussions is gone. So has the time of referring difficult work on to anyone else who will do it. The grim reality is that if community nurses do not go out there and do the work that is there waiting for them someone else will. At the moment they have the skills to work with people with learning disabilities who have problems or needs and the expertise to resolve those problems/needs. They must not only do this, but be seen to do this work.

The future of learning disability nursing

The recent concern regarding the future role of community learning disability nurses has resulted in uncertainty and a lack of direction. The future of learning disability nurses has been in question for many years (e.g. Chudley, 1987). That uncertainty came to a head in 1993 with the consensus conference (DoH, 1993) recommending a range of options for the future care of people with learning disabilities which may or may not include learning disability nurses. The effect of that conference seems to have been three-fold. For some it has heightened the disillusionment in the profession (Brown, 1993); for others it has encouraged a fighting stance with arguments for the continuation of that role (Cox, 1993; Kay, 1993; Balkizas, 1994), whilst for others it has highlighted the need to consider development of the role so allowing a more secure future (Jukes, 1994).

For community nurses the uncertainty has increased as a result of the implementation of the NHS and Community Care Act 1990. Its introduction saw social services taking the lead role for people with learning disabilities and again nurses were fighting for survival (McMillan, 1991). However, as Turnbull (1993) suggests, with adaptability and flexibility to meet local client needs, the future is more promising.

Whilst GP fundholding is another threat, particularly as from 1993 GPs have been in a position to purchase community nursing services (Crail, 1992), nurses are again rising to the challenge by making fundholders aware of their skills and contributions in the care of people with learning disabilities. This acknowledgement of the ongoing community learning disability nurse role is further supported by recent reports (DoH, 1995; Kay et al., 1995).

The future of community learning disability nursing is in the hands of the nurses themselves. They must clearly identify the needs of the individuals with a learning disability and their carers. They must be prepared to market their skills and ensure they can meet the needs of the market. They must provide quality provision and be able to clearly show purchasers what they have provided, why it was good in terms of value for money and long-term health gain. Gone are the days when nurses can say we can only offer this in a particular way. If they want to survive and continue to provide a quality provision for their client group, they must learn to play the market.

Conclusion

Whilst agreeing that it was important to recognize that people with a learning disability were being devalued, in part, as a result of the system but also as a result of people's perceptions of learning disability, and there was a need to change that devalued status, it is questionable whether this has been achieved. Indeed it can be argued that it is impossible to provide care for people with a learning disability in the community or indeed in an institution based on the principle of normalization because of the overwhelming external factors that disallow the individual carer or professional service provider to work effectively in this way. We are still living with a service history that has provided segregated buildings and specialist people to work in those buildings. We must accept that for many people with learning disabilities along with the principles of normalization come services that, whilst more culturally normative, may provide less support and opportunities for the individual. Recognition of the problems of devaluation of people with a learning disability by an elite few professionals will not improve the lives of those people. The reality is that a few people with ideals will not make a significant impact on people's lives. If the principle of normalization or social role valorization is to be successful in improving the lives of minority groups, then it must be taken up by all in society.

The future care of people with a learning disability seems to be clearly placed in the hands of informal carers. Policies of segregation are still in existence and the will to change these policies at national and local levels is weak due to the fear of change. As the *status quo* remains, service providers must make the best of the existing facilities and their own skills in order to improve the lives of individuals within the various community settings.

References

Ashton, G. and Ward, A. 1992: *Mental handicap and the law*. London: Sweet & Maxwell.
Ayer, S. and Alaszewski, A. 1984: *Community care and the mentally handicapped: services for mothers and their mentally handicapped children*. London: Croom Helm.

Balkizas, D. 1994: *Status quo. Nursing Standard* 8(40), 44–5.

Bayley, M. 1973: *Mental handicap and community care.* London: Croom Helm.

Benson, S. 1987: Caring for the carers. *Community Care* **664**, 25–7.

Brandon, D. 1987: When free choice becomes a tyranny. *Community Living* 1(4), 3.

Brandon, D. 1988: Brokerage gives consumers power. *Community Living* 2(2), 17.

Brandon, D. and Towe, N. 1989: *Free to choose: an introduction to service brokerage.* London: Good Impressions Publications.

Brown, H. and Smith, H. 1992: Assertion, not assimilation – a feminist perspective on the normalisation principle. In Brown, H. and Smith, H. (eds), *Normalisation: a reader for the nineties.* London: Routledge, 149–71.

Brown, J. 1993: Consensus or confusion? *Nursing Times* 89(22), 67.

Challis, D. and Davies, B. 1986: *Case management in community care.* Aldershot: Gower.

Chudley, P. 1987: We wont be missed until we're gone. *Nursing Times* **March 18**, 19–20.

Communicare 1993: Editorial. *Communicare* 1, 2.

Community Mental Handicap Nurses' Association 1985: *Community mental handicap nursing and management: roles and functions.* Bolton: Community Mental Handicap Nursing Association.

Cox, Y. 1993: Tailor-made for the job. *Nursing Times* 89(22), 66.

Crail, M. 1992: Managing in the community: new money. *Health Service Journal* **10 Dec**, 33–6.

Department of Health (DoH) 1989: *Caring for people: community care, the next decade and beyond.* London: HMSO.

Department of Health (DoH) 1993: *Opportunities for change: a new direction for nursing for people with learning disabilities.* London: DoH.

Department of Health (DoH) 1995: *Learning disability: meeting needs through targeting skills.* London: DoH.

Finch, J. and Groves, D. 1983: *A labour of love: women, work and caring.* London: Routledge & Kegan Paul.

Frazer, B. and Green, A. 1991: Changing perspectives on mental handicap. In Frazer, B., MacGillivray, R. and Green, A. (eds), *Hallas' caring for people with mental handicaps.* Oxford: Butterworth Heinemann, 1–7.

Garety, P. 1990: Housing. In Lavender, A. and Holloway, F. (eds), *Community care in practice: services for the continuing care client.* Chichester: Wiley, 143–60.

Glendinning, C. 1986: The costs of caring. *Community Outlook* **September**, 11–14.

Griffiths, Sir R. 1988: *Community care: agenda for action.* London: HMSO.

Ham, C. 1992: *Health policy in Britain: the politics and organisation of the National Health Service*, 3rd edn. London: Macmillan.

Hawker, C. and Ritchie, P. 1988: *Contracting for community care: strategies for progress* (Project Paper No 84). London: Kings Fund.

Horne, E. 1989: Who cares in the community? *The Professional Nurse* 4(12), 577.

House of Commons, Social Services Committee 1985: *Community care with special reference to adult mentally ill and mentally handicapped people.* Second Report from the Social Services Committee. London: HMSO.

Jackson, R. 1988: Perils of 'pseudo-normali ation'. *Mental Handicap* **16**, 148–50.

Jukes, M. 1994: Development of the community nurse in learning disability: 1. *British Journal of Nursing.* 3(15), 779–83.

Kay, B. 1993: Keeping it in the family? *Nursing Times* 89(22), 64–5.

Kay, B., Rose, S. and Turnbull, J. 1995: *Continuing the commitment: the report of the Learning Disability Nursing Project.* London: DoH.

Lawson, B. 1993: The quiet revolution. *Primary Health Care* 3(5), 25.

Lewis, A. 1991: Public participation in decision making. In Ramon, S. (ed.), *Beyond community care.* London: Macmillan, 137–61.

McMillan, I. 1991: Split provision. *Nursing Times* 87(28), 18.

Manthorpe, J. 1994: The family and informal care. In Malin, N. (ed.), *Implementing community care.* Buckingham: Open University Press, 97–121.

Monach, J. and Spriggs, L. 1994: The consumer role. In Malin, N. (ed.), *Implementing community care*. Buckingham: Open University Press, 138–53.

Parker, G. 1990: *With due care and attention: a review of research on informal care*. London: Family Policy Studies Centre.

Rose, S. 1993: Social policy: a perspective on service developments and inter-agency working. In Brigden, P. and Todd, M. (ed.), *Concepts in community care for people with a learning difficulty*. Basingstoke: Macmillan, 5–28.

Royal College of Nursing. 1985: *The role and function of the domiciliary nurse in mental handicap*. London: Royal College of Nursing.

Royal College of Nursing. 1992: *The role and function of the domiciliary nurse in mental handicap*. London: Royal College of Nursing.

Ryan, J. and Thomas, F. 1993: Concepts of normalisation. In: Bornat, J., Pereira, C., Pilgrim, D. and Williams, F. (eds), *Community Care: A Reader*. London. Macmillan, 242–6.

Seale, C. 1990: Caring for people who die: the experience of family and friends. *Ageing and Society* 10(4), 413–28.

Tadd, V. 1994: Learning to accept. *Nursing Standard* 9(5), 42.

Thompson, T. and Mathias, P. 1992: New approaches to competence: examples from nursing and social work. In Thompson, T. and Mathias, P. (eds), *Standards and mental handicap: keys to competence*. London: Baillière Tindall, 3–15.

Trnobranski, P. 1994: Nurse–patient negotiation: assumption or reality. *Journal of Advanced Nursing* 19, 733–7.

Tuckett, D. (ed.), 1976: *An introduction to medical sociology*. London: Tavistock.

Turnbull, J. 1993: Diverse options. *Nursing Times*. 89(22), 62–3.

Twigg, J. 1989: Models of carers: how do social care agencies conceptualise their relationship with informal carers? *Journal of Social Policy* 18(1), 53–66.

Twigg, J. and Atkin, K. 1994: *Carers perceived: policy and practice in informal care*. Buckingham: Open University Press.

Twigg, J., Atkin, K. and Perring, C. 1990: *Carers and services: a review of research*. London: HMSO.

Tyne, A. 1981: *The principle of normalisation: a foundation for effective services*. London: CMH.

Walker, A. 1993: Community care policy: from consensus to conflict. In: Bornat, J., Pereira, C., Pilgrim, D. and Williams, F. (eds), *Community care: a reader*. London. Macmillan, 204–26.

Williamson, C. 1992: *Whose standards? Consumer and professional standards in health care*. Buckingham: Open University Press.

Wilkin, D. 1979: *Caring for the mentally handicapped child*. London: Croom Helm.

Wolfensberger, W. and Thomas, S. 1994: An analysis of the client role from a social role valorization perspective. SRV-VRS: *The International Social Role Valorization Journal* 1(1), 3–8.

14 Mental health

Len Bowers

On the day that I was editing this chapter there was a news report that NHS executives were to be given three months to improve psychiatric community care, following bad reports (24.8.95). There was no mention, from the government source, of extra funding or resources. Against this backdrop I found Len Bowers' chapter all the more poignant since he highlights some of the current dilemmas facing community psychiatric nurses (CPNs). Without the knowledge of what was to come, Len has offered a view of the changing and expanding role that CPNs face.

The beginnings of community psychiatric nursing in the UK are inextricably linked to the development of a community care policy within psychiatry. Declining numbers of inpatient beds resulting in the more recent phenomenon of psychiatric hospital closure has meant that the locus of psychiatric care has moved from the institution to the community. However, the sufferers of mental illness still required practical care, a service traditionally provided by nurses. Thus, nurses moved with their patients into the new arena of community psychiatric care.

Key sources for information about the history of community psychiatric nursing are: Hunter (1974), Parnell (1978) and Peat and Watt (1984). These sources relate how the first 'outpatient nurses' were created at Warlingham Park Hospital, Surrey in 1954. A similar service was started at Moorhaven Hospital, Devon in 1957. Lena Peat (the first community psychiatric nurse (CPN) in the UK) relates that the outpatient services by nurses were the idea of a consultant psychiatrist (Dr Rees) who was also the driving force behind their establishment. The duties of these prototype CPNs were to run day care facilities and to visit and care for discharged psychiatric patients in their own homes. The Surrey service, and many subsequent ones, started with home visiting and follow-up by ward-based nurses who had cared for the patient during admission. This became more and more difficult due to rostering problems, the nurses involved being unable to meet the dual commitment to cover and manage an inpatient ward at the same time as trying to deliver flexible support to the mentally ill living in the community. Full time CPN posts were, therefore, created. The process is described by Parnell's (1978) respondants. Prior to the inception of these services the only route for psychiatric nurses to work in the community was for them to become mental health social workers, a situation reflected in the fact that 10 per cent of mental health social workers in Lancashire in 1953–5 had previously been trained as psychiatric nurses (Jones, 1972: 302).

Early CPNs were known under a number of different titles, for example outpatient nurses, psychiatric community nurses, aftercare nurses, domiciliary nurses, and members of the extra mural service. It was not until the 1970s that the term community psychiatric nurse emerged as the most popular. The links these early CPNs had with the wards is emphasized by some of the terminology they used, referring to their caseload as their 'ward' and their discussions with the medical staff as 'ward rounds'. In these early days no courses existed for postbasic training of CPNs and some sought and gained places on district nursing courses as an alternative. Indeed, there is some evidence that in this period district nurses themselves may have been seeking to expand their role to cover the community care of the mentally ill (Gunn, 1969).

However, from these humble beginnings in Surrey and Devon, a new psychiatric nursing specialism has developed which is now nationwide in scope. Hunter (1974) refers to an unpublished Royal College of Nursing investigation in 1966 which charted the steady growth in community psychiatric nursing services. By that time 42 psychiatric hospitals were using 225 nursing staff on community work. By 1980, 1667 CPNs were in employment (CPNA, 1981). Five years later this was up by nearly two thirds to 2758 (CPNA, 1985), and the most recent information (White, 1990) shows that there are now very nearly 5000 practicing, full-time CPNs in the UK.

The typical CPN team of an NHS trust will now usually consist of several groups. The most central and long-established CPNs will be termed 'generic' or 'acute' and work with all the mentally ill between the ages of 16 and 65 years. Their base office might be either in a local health centre, or in the hospital. A second group is likely to be those CPNs offering a specialist service to the elderly mentally ill. A third group may be those CPNs involved in resettling and relocating long-term patients who are being moved out of the older psychiatric hospitals into the community. In addition, it is possible that a health authority may have specialist CPNs operating in the fields of drug abuse, alcoholism and child psychiatry. All such CPNs are usually, but not always, part of a unified management structure.

With the expansion of community services in recent years, the inception of new forms of working, policy and organizational changes, it is not always clear which psychiatric nurses should be considered CPNs and which not. In some parts of the NHS the title is restricted to those at a certain grade, in others the title expands to cover those working in a range of day and residential care settings. Management structure and team organization also vary quite widely from place to place. As a consequence, when one tries to talk about CPNs in general, much ambiguity exists. In addition, the survey figures quoted above should be taken only as rough estimates of the numbers of psychiatric nurses actually working all or part of the time in settings outside the traditional psychiatric hospital or unit.

mental health problems, the CPN will make a comprehensive psycho-social assessment incorporating not just the symptoms of the illness and its treatment, but also the patient's social/leisure needs, emotional support needs, self-care abilities, housekeeping, accommodation needs, employment/vocation, physical health, the financial situation of the patient, the needs of carers, and again the risk to self and others.

PSYCHOTHERAPY

In common with the whole of psychiatry, CPNs hotly dispute with each other precisely which psychotherapeutic approaches are correct to use or effective in practice. Nevertheless, psychotherapy is widely applied by CPNs. Most common are various types of counselling, such as Egan's problem-solving approach, or Rogers' client-centred therapy. Behavioural aproaches are also widely used, particularly systematic desensitization and various anxiety management techniques. More recent additions to the CPN repertoire are family educational approaches in schizophrenia, cognitive behavioural techniques, and methods of working with adult survivors of childhood abuse.

CASE MANAGEMENT

This incorporates two types of activity. The first can roughly be called keyworking. For many patients and their carers, the CPN will be the main point of contact with the psychiatric services, and therefore the person who co-ordinates packages of care which may involve services from different parts of the organization. The second could be called systematic case management and is the use of the nursing process in structuring care. CPNs make assessments, draw up written care plans involving their own and other professionals' interventions, and they periodically review and evaluate that care package.

PHYSICAL TREATMENT

CPNs administer medication, educate patients on its costs and benefits, provide expert advice and monitor side effects. In order to do all this they work closely with prescribers, GPs and consultant psychiatrists, in order to provide the best and most efficacious treatment.

RISK MANAGEMENT

Risk of harm to the patient and to others is assessed and continually monitored. Risk management strategies may involve all of the four preceding activities, but may also involve increasing contact frequency or even arranging for an admission to hospital. Although CPNs have no statutory responsibilities with regard to compulsory detention, they may instigate such an event by mobilizing those who have, should the necessity arise. Follow-up on discharge is also a significant part of the CPN role, in particular for those patients who tend to be non-compliant with treatment plans. CPNs are likely to have a significant role in the administration of supervision registers and community supervision orders, as these are introduced.

Current issues for CPNs

Without a doubt the most acute dilemma for CPNs at present is the relative distribution of their services between the seriously mentally ill and primary health care referrals. It has become apparent that community care for the seriously mentally ill has been far from perfect in many areas. This may be partly the responsibility of CPNs, but not wholly so. Other professional groupings have also struggled with the changes in role necessitated by community care. It must not be forgotten that the policy of community care is relatively new, and that it has taken some time for its problems to emerge and for new management strategies to be devised. However, now that the essential components of good case management and community care for the seriously mentally ill are known (Bowers, 1994a,b,c), CPN services are left in a dilemma. On the one hand government policy and much public criticism is pushing them towards committing all their resources towards prioritizing those with serious illnesses. On the other hand, the introduction of GP fundholding creates organizational pressures towards the prioritizing of GP-referred patients. As always, resources are so tight that the needs of either group cannot be satisfied. Even in those areas where more resources have been secured, it is no easy matter to determine priorities. Prioritization on the grounds of diagnosis is possible, but incorporates many well and stable sufferers of psychosis and in any case does not help determine the most needy among those suffering a mood disorder. Prioritization on the grounds of recent admission penalizes those who are quietly neglected at home or who are managed at great cost at home by relatives. In this area there are no easy distinctions to be made.

The inception of GP fundholding presents another and different challenge to CPNs. There were initial worries that GPs would employ their own counsellors, and that referrals to CPNs would dry up. This does not appear to have been the case. Although some counsellors have been employed by GPs, they do not seem to have had an impact upon the rate of referrals to CPNs at all. However, in order to secure contracts from fundholding GPs, many CPN teams are altering their organizational structure to match up CPNs to GP practices, and altering CPN working methods to match rigid contractual formulations such as 'one assessment followed by six one-hour intervention sessions'. Whether this is working to the benefit of patients or not is unknown, and urgently requires monitoring, as does the use of non-professionally trained or organizationally integrated counsellors in GP surgeries.

The nature, status and content of training courses for CPNs has been a matter for argument and debate among CPNs for many years. Only 38 per cent of CPNs have completed the CPN course, mainly due to logistical and funding difficulties. In the early 1980s there was some unsuccessful agitation for the course to be made mandatory and thereby brought into line with health visitor training. Debate then passed to the issue of whether and to what degree the CPN course should consist of a period of practical skills training or academic instruction. This critique of CPN courses led to curriculum changes and increased emphasis on skills training in many courses (Bowers and Crossling, 1994). Over the late 1980s and early 1990s, numbers of students on CPN courses fell into a gradual decline which has only recently been reversed. The current debate over CPN training now seems to be shifting to discussion on exactly which skills CPNs should be trained in. The creation of new and efficacious intervention techniques for the long-term mentally ill, known generally as psycho-social interventions, has been coupled with discussions about prioritizing the care of this group of patients in order to argue that these should be the sole skills taught to CPNs. This of course ignores not only the fact that psycho-social interventions are only one part of wider case management for such clients, but also that CPNs are involved in the care of many clients for whom such skills are irrelevant. Further changes to CPN education are already imminent due to Community PREP (the new guidelines on post-registration education and practice issued by the UKCC , 1994). How the profession will respond to degree level education is yet to be seen.

Conclusion

Community psychiatric nursing is one of the youngest community professions in nursing and a completely new development for psychiatric nursing. From its small beginnings 40 years ago it has expanded to become a significant presence and contributor to psychiatric care in every part of the UK. Along with psychiatry itself, it has undergone many changes and will continue to do so. It would seem that neither psychiatry nor community psychiatric nursing has achieved any level of stability in recent years. However, change represents the opportunity for improvement in services to the patients with whom CPNs work and to whom CPNs devote their professional careers. As such, the work of CPNs remains both exciting and challenging.

References

Altschul, A. 1973: A multidisciplinary approach to psychiatric nursing. *Nursing Times* 69(15), 508–11.
Barker, C. 1977: A community psychiatric service. *Nursing Times* 73(28), 1075–9.

Beard, P.G. 1980: Community psychiatric nursing – a challenging role. *Nursing Focus* **1**(8), 306–7.

Bowers, L. 1994a: Towards a definition of community care. *Mental Health Nursing* **14**(3), 14–16.

Bowers, L. 1994b: Organisation and management of community care. *Mental Health Nursing* **14**(4), 8–11.

Bowers, L. 1994c: Quality of community care. *Mental Health Nursing* **14**(5), 12–13.

Bowers, L. and Crossling, P. 1994: Skills training in community psychiatric nurse education. *Mental Health Nursing* **14**(2), 13–17.

Caplan, G. 1964: *Principles of Preventive Psychiatry*. London: Tavistock.

Carr, P., Butterworth, C.A. and Hodges, B.E. 1980: *Community Psychiatric Nursing*. Edinburgh: Churchill Livingstone.

Corser, C. and Ryce, S. 1977: Community mental health care: a model based on the primary health care system. *British Medical Journal* **2** 936–8.

CPNA 1981: *The CPNA national survey*. Bristol: CPNA.

CPNA 1985: *The 1985 CPNA national survey update*. Bristol: CPNA.

Greene, J. 1968: The psychiatric nurse in the community. *International Journal of Nursing Studies* **5**, 175–83.

Griffith, J. 1978: Community psychiatric nursing. *Community Outlook* Nov, 357–8.

Gunn, M. 1969: District nursing and the mentally ill. *Nursing Times* **65**(16), 497.

Haque, G. 1973: Psychosocial nursing in the community. *Nursing Times* **69**(2), 51–3.

Henderson, J., Levin, B. and Cheyne, E. 1973: Role of a psychiatric nurse in a domiciliary treatment service: the treatment team and the clinical operation of the service. *Nursing Times* **69**(41), 1334–6.

Hunter, P. 1960: The changing function of professional staff in the mental hospital. In *Association of Psychiatric Social Worker Ventures in Professional Cooperation*. London: APSW.

Hunter, P. 1974: Community psychiatric nursing in Britain: an historical review. *International Journal of Nursing Studies* **11**, 223–33.

Jones K. 1972: *A History of the Mental Health Services*. London: Routledge and Kegan Paul.

Kirkpatrick, W.J.A. 1967: The in–out nurse – some thoughts on the role of psychiatric nursing in the community and preparations required. *International Journal of Nursing Studies* **4**, 225–31.

Leopoldt, H. 1973: Psychiatric community nursing. *Health and Social Service Journal* **83**(4324), 489–90.

Leopoldt, H., Hopkins, H. and Overall, R. 1974: A critical review of experimental nurse attachment scheme in Oxford. *Practice Team* **39**, 2–6.

Leopoldt, H. and Hurn, R. 1973: Towards integration. *Nursing Mirror* **136**(22), 38–42.

Leopoldt, H., Robinson, J.R. and Corea, S. 1975: Hospital based community psychiatric nursing in psychogeriatric care. *Nursing Mirror* **141**(25), 54–6.

Macdonald, D.J. 1972: Psychiatric nursing in the community. *Nursing Times* **68**(3), 80–3.

Macleod, W.G. 1970a: Domiciliary psychiatric nursing observed, 1. *Nursing Times* **Occasional Paper**, 185–8.

Macleod, W.G. 1970b: Domiciliary psychiatric nursing observed, 2. *Nursing Times* **Occasional Paper** 189–91.

Mangan, S.P. and Griffith, J.H. 1982: Community Psychiatric Services in Britain: the need for policy and planning. *International Journal of Nursing Studies* **19**(3), 157–66.

May, A.R. 1965: The psychiatric nurse in the community. *Nursing Mirror* **120**(3156), 409–10.

May, A.R. and Moore S. 1963: The mental nurse in the community. *Lancet* **i**, 213–14.

Moore, S. 1961: A psychiatric out-patient nursing service. *Mental Health Bulletin* **Summer**.

Parnell, J.W. 1978: *Community psychiatric nursing: a descriptive study.* London: Queens Nursing Institute.

Peat, L. and Watt, G. 1984: The passing of an era. *Community Psychiatric Nursing Journal* 4(2), 12–16.

Pollock, L. 1989: *Community psychiatric nursing: myth and reality.* Lancaster: Scutari.

Pullen, I. and Gilbert, M.A. 1979: When crisis hits the home. *Nursing Mirror* 149(14), 30–2.

Robertson, H. and Scott, D.J. 1985: Community psychiatric nursing: a survey of patients and problems. *Journal of the Royal College of General Practitioners* 35, 130–2.

Rodger, W. 1973: Community psychiatric nursing in the health centre: a Devon development. *The Practitioner* 210, 799–802.

Royal College of General Practitioners 1981: *Prevention of psychiatric disorders in general practice.* London: RCGP.

Royal College of Psychiatrists, Social and Community Psychiatry Section Working Party. 1980: Community psychiatric nursing: a discussion document. *Bulletin of the Royal College of Psychiatrists* 4(8), 114–18.

Ryce, S. 1978: Psychiatric nursing from a health centre. *Nursing Mirror* 147(7), 35–6.

Sharpe, G. 1975: Role of the community psychiatric nurse. *Nursing Mirror* 161(2), 39–41.

Shaw, A. 1977: CPN attachment in a group practice. *Nursing Times* 73(12), Suppl. The Health Centre ix–xvi.

Sladden, S. 1979: *Psychiatric nursing in the community – a study of a working situation.* Edinburgh: Edinburgh University Monographs.

Spy, T. 1980: Point of view. The CPN as a counsellor. *Community Psychiatric Nursing Association Journal* 1(4), 2–3.

Stewart, M., Kerr, S. and Dunlop, W. 1974: Psychiatric nurse in the community. *Nursing Mirror* 139(1), 84.

Stobie, E. and Hopkins, D. 1972: Crisis intervention, 1: a community psychiatric nurse in a rural area. *Nursing Times* 68(43), Occasional Paper, 162–5.

UKCC 1994: *The future of professional practice – the Council's standards for education and practice following registration.* London: United Kingdom Central Council for Nursing, Midwifery and Health Visiting.

Warren, J. 1971: Long acting phenothiazine injections given by psychiatric nurses in the community. *Nursing Times* 67(36), Occasional Paper 141–3.

Weeks, K. and Greene, J. 1966: Psychiatric nurses in the community. *Nursing Times* 62(8), 257–8.

White, E. 1990: *Community psychiatric nursing: the 1990 national survey.* Bradford: CPNA publications.

Wooff, K., Goldberg, D.P. and Fryers, T. 1986: Patients in receipt of community psychiatric nursing care in Salford 1976–82. *Psychological Medicine* 16(2), 407–14.

15 Substance abuse

I. Smith, T. Carnworth, N. Prinjha, and
M. Smith

This chapter visits the specialism of managing substance abuse. The authors, because of space, can only skim the surface but still manage to produce an informative and thought-provoking narrative. Smith et al. place addiction in context, highlighting the many other things (such as sport) that people abuse. Their argument can be alarming and many readers may leave this chapter recognizing their own addictions. The notion of a rising tide in addiction to hard drugs (a popular media theme) is debunked and we are reassured that the majority of drug use is experimental and recreational rather than dependency.

The second half of the chapter focuses on dependency and discusses some of the intervention strategies that have been useful with regard to the four categories of dependent user the authors describe. This is by no means a pessimistic viewpoint and the authors conclude that the '... once an addict, always an addict' notion is a myth when one considers the empirical data. Quite rightly, they argue that this area is no longer the preserve of the specialist; the recognition of substance misuse, they argue, should be a standard part of the skills required for community practice.

Introduction

The primary purpose of this chapter is to enable community health workers to feel more confident when confronted by individuals with drug-related problems. It is our belief that drug use, even of a problematic kind, is no more difficult or mysterious than many other health issues which appear on the community practitioner's agenda.

Towards this end we offer a preliminary guide to drugs and drug usage and an estimate of prevalence in the population; an indication of the different kinds of harms which can accompany certain substances and patterns of use; the policies and treatment philosophies which underpin work with drug users; the kinds of community services available to individuals seeking help in this area; the range and types of intervention on offer and the kinds of outcome we can expect from these. In relation to the latter topics, we will restrict our discussion to dependent users of heroin and other opiates as these form the bulk of individuals presenting to treatment services.

We would like to emphasize, if only for limitations of space, that this does not pretend to be a comprehensive or definitive account of the field.

If you wish to specialize in this area, there is no substitute for wide reading, training and education and, of course, clinical experience. We do want to say, however, that specialism aside 'Everyone can be a drug worker'.

Our justification for this claim lies in the fact that problems of dependency and 'addiction' are not confined to intravenous heroin users or smokers of rock-cocaine ('crack'). Millions of people struggle with cravings for nicotine; with a desire for excessive consumption of food or alcohol; with the effects of large amounts of caffeine in daily beverages; and often with combinations of all these addictions. Many others are afflicted with a compulsive appetite for gambling or other forms of risk-taking and sensation seeking.

Many of you who are reading this chapter will have experience of the inappropriate, excessive and even harmful use of some of the substances mentioned, or of overindulgence in food, sugar or salt, shopping, repetitive habits such as nail biting, gum chewing, the habitual pursuit of sports such as skiing, rock-climbing or even running and aerobics or the purchase of scratch cards and lottery tickets. You might have had an overattachment to electronic games in your youth. Some of you may be self-confessed 'workaholics'.

For socio-cultural reasons, habits centring on the use of illicit psychoactive substances seem to attract the bulk of critical and moralistic attention, perhaps because they are thought to be more dangerous than other dependencies. We would challenge this belief. Overeating, excessive sexuality, anorexia nervosa and gambling, can be as compulsive and harmful as intravenous heroin use or freebasing cocaine. Moreover, they can be as difficult to treat. Excessive training and participation in marathon running can cause illness.

A pharmacologist might argue that what distinguishes the compulsive use of substances from other forms of behaviour is that drug-based compulsions are characterized by *tolerance*. This means that the organism requires ever greater amounts of the substance to produce the same physiological response. Yet it would seem that we can discern a similar process at work in other habits. Stepney (1981: 233), from the perspective of psychology argues that:

> For the confirmed gambler, the amount of stake or risk involved must be increased to produce the same thrill of uncertainty or euphoria of winning. A similar phenomenon is observed in certain aspects of delinquency, in which those involved seem to find themselves on a gradient of escalating damage and violence, whilst those who derive their excitement from challenging authority may progress from the home to the school to the police in their search to find a sufficiently arousing source of confrontation. The development of tolerance is in fact a very general feature of the family of habits. For the confirmed athlete no speed is fast enough, for the stamp collector no specimen rare enough, for the anorexic no weight low enough, for the businessman no bank balance large enough.

We would also challenge what sociologists call 'the retreatist theory', the argument that we can distinguish between drug use and other habits in terms of its function as an escape attempt from everyday life. There are many habits which may in the beginning serve as a temporary retreat or escape strategy from the stresses of everyday life but end in a more permanent retreat from reality (Cohen and Taylor, 1976).

It is our view that there is no clear way to distinguish an 'excessive appetite' (Orford, 1985) for licit substances or behaviours from an overattachment to illicit psychoactive substances, except through referral to their criminal status.

All of you, either at a personal level or, at least, through the behaviour of a relative, partner or friend, have experience of appetitive disorders. Millions of us have to deal with our own and others' excessive appetites. The majority of us resolve these problems by ourselves or they are resolved for us by the passage of time and increasing age. Few of us are averse to giving advice or help when we see people suffering these difficulties.

What is it then that makes us feel powerless when confronted with someone using heroin or cocaine? Why do we feel confident enough to deal with our children's youthful experimentation with alcohol or tobacco yet contact specialized treatment services because we find our 14-year-old experimenting with cannabis? We suggest that what distinguishes one response from another is a lack of understanding, and a belief that addiction and dependency pertain only to illicit substances. We believe that 'addicts' are different. When thinking about drugs, we rely on fictions, misinformation, stereotypes and media myths.

Rather than perceiving drug users through stereotypes such as 'junkie' or 'druggie', rather than seeing them as 'hopeless addicts' and believing myths such as 'one hit and you're hooked' and 'cannabis leads inevitably to heroin', we should think about our own dependencies, our own and others' experiences with psychoactive substances and our own failures and successes with our own appetites and attachments. We should think about the fact that we live in a society in which the belief that physical, psychological and even social problems are amenable to chemical solutions is almost universal. And, as health care professionals, we should remember that we already have skills which could enable us to deal with many of the people who present with drug problems, if only we could see beyond the myths and value judgements which cloud our view. Drugtakers, problematic or otherwise, are not 'them': they are 'us'.

What drugs?

It is an almost impossible task to list the different substances which our species has chewed, swallowed, sniffed, smoked, drunk, injected and ingested in a variety of other ways for the purpose of altering consciousness. Listing and describing the full range of substances used in our society would take up the rest of this chapter. We will confine ourselves here to listing those drugs the community practitioner is most likely to encounter (see ISDD (1994a,b) for a full discussion).

The classification of drugs is an arbitrary exercise. Most systems allot substances to categories on the basis of their effects. This approach is flawed, because the effects a person experiences from a particular substance will depend as much on his or her psychological characteristics and on the social context in which the substance is consumed as on the pharmacological properties of the drug in question (see Gossop 1993: ch. 2, for an extended discussion of this point). Nevertheless, a system of classification based on effects allows us to get a first idea of the major substances and their functions. Broadly speaking, drugs can be allotted to the following groups:

- *Drugs that depress the nervous system* – alcohol, barbiturates, benzodiazepines, the solvents, etc.
- *Drugs that stimulate the nervous system* – amphetamines, cocaine, caffeine, etc.
- *Drugs that reduce pain* – opium, heroin, morphine, pethidine, methadone, codeine, etc.
- *Drugs that alter perception* – LSD (lysergic acid diethylamide), cannabis, MDMA (ecstasy), magic mushrooms (psilocybin), etc.

Kinds of drug use

It is important to recognize and, particularly in the assessment of drug use, to be clear about the different kinds of drug use that exist. Drug use takes many different forms. It can be:

- *Experimental* – this kind of use is typical of adolescent or pre-adolescent patterns of use. It often arises out of a combination of individual curiosity, availability of a given substance or substances and favourable peer attitudes. Tobacco, alcohol and cannabis presently typify pre-adolescent drug experimentation. Among older adolescents we might find LSD, ecstasy and even cocaine and heroin being used in this fashion. Experimental use can embrace one or two substances or possibly a whole range of drugs. Its major feature is its short duration.
- *Recreational* – this term (often seen as condoning drug use by moralists of various persuasions) refers to drug use which is designed to enhance the enjoyment of leisure or particular leisure activities. An example is provided by ecstasy in the dance scene. Use is regular but controlled. Alcohol use is recreational for most drinkers.
- *Dependent or compulsive* – here drug use has become central to an individual's life. All else – work, leisure, family obligations, non-drug social relationships – have become secondary. The contemporary phrase '24/7' as in 'He's 24/7 him' (24 hours a day, seven days a week) when applied to a drug user sums up this pattern particularly well. It is around this kind of compulsive use that terms like *physical* and *psychological*

dependence come into play. Physical dependence is usually defined in terms of the presence of a physical withdrawal syndrome of the kind we see in compulsive daily opiate users (diarrhoea, cramps, muscular pains, vomiting, sleeplessness) or compulsive daily drinkers or a proportion of daily benzodiazepine users. Psychological dependence is said to involve an overwhelming desire or craving to continue using the substance either for the psychological pleasure it affords or to avoid the psychological distress caused by its withdrawal (as is often seen with cocaine and the amphetamines, for example). Compulsive heroin, barbiturate, alcohol and benzodiazepine use can create both psychological and physical dependence.

In addition to the different patterns of use we also need to consider the different types of methods (modes of administration) in which drugs can be used. These include *injecting*, intravenously, intramuscularly or under the skin, *orally*, by swallowing, *sniffing* and, of course, by *smoking*.

Drugs and social acceptability

Drugs differ in their social acceptability. Some substances such as alcohol, tobacco and caffeine are legal in the UK and their use is generally accepted or tolerated. Other substances, heroin for example, are legal in certain circumstances, as when a doctor uses heroin for the relief of terminal pain, but are illegal in others, as when an individual self-administers for the sake of pleasure. Furthermore, the social acceptability and legality of substances differs between cultures (cf. alcohol in some Islamic societies) and over time (cf. opium and cannabis in nineteenth century Britain – see Berridge and Edwards (1981) for the historical background to drug use in this country). To remind us that acceptability and legitimacy are matters of social definition and not the necessary result of inherent dangers, consider Table 15.1 (see over).

Prevalence of illicit drug use

The term 'prevalence' simply refers to the proportion of a population which uses illicit drugs. Various problems exist when we try to assess the prevalence of illicit substance use in the UK. First, and most obvious, is the fact that, because these behaviours are against the law, they are generally concealed. A second complicating factor is the widespread regional and local variations in patterns of drug use in the UK. What holds true in Manchester will not necessarily hold true for Leeds. Prevalence and incidence in one health district may not be mirrored in an adjacent area. Thus, the results of prevalence studies in one area may not be generalizable beyond that specific locality. Third, enormous variations can occur in illicit drug use over relatively short periods of time.

Table 15.1 Number of drug-related deaths in England and Wales

Cocaine	6
Heroin	40
LSD	2
MDMA (ecstasy)	?0
Methadone	101
Amphetamine	10
Cannabis	0
Solvents	68
Alcohol	25 000
Tobacco	111 000

Figures for drug-related deaths taken from 1992 or 1993 Home Office figures – deaths registered as suicides or undetermined are not included. Alcohol and tobacco figures taken from OPCS and Department of Health.

If we wish to find out how many people use illicit drugs in the UK, then we have to rely on bits and pieces of information from a wide variety of sources, both official statistics and surveys. Fortunately, the task of assembling these varied and disparate pieces of information has been done by the Institute for the Study of Drug Dependence (ISDD), which publishes an annual assessment of the extent of Britain's drug problem (ISDD, 1994). But again, let us stress the provisional nature of these data. We are dealing with 'guesstimates' in relation to the overall picture.

The most widely used illicit drug in Britain is cannabis. From surveys, the ISDD calculate that some 2.5 million people take the drug, mainly by smoking but occasionally by eating. If we look at the official criminal statistics we find cannabis featuring in 80–90 per cent of all drug convictions and seizures, involving over 40 000 offenders a year since 1990.

Second in popularity to cannabis is amphetamine. Between 1989 and 1992 police seizures of amphetamine tripled. In 1993, 11 of the 18 illegal 'drug laboratories' discovered in this country were devoted solely to the production of the drug. Indeed, much of the amphetamine consumed in this country is in the form of heavily adulterated amphetamine sulphate powder illegally manufactured in the UK itself. Customs seizures of £75 million of the drug in 1993 have been attributed to the fact that domestic producers have simply been unable to cope with the increased demand for the drug. This demand is linked to the rise of 'dance culture'. Amphetamine sulphate can be sniffed, swallowed or injected and in parts of the country where injecting is frequent, amphetamine is thought to rival heroin as a preferred drug of injection.

LSD, the drug of the 1960s hippies, has recently enjoyed a revival, thanks to the mass youth culture associated with the rave scene. Surveys of the UK population as a whole give us an estimate of 3 per cent of the population

prescription, counselling, advice and support, whereas the voluntary sector generally offers counselling, advice, support and, often, alternative therapies such as acupuncture or aromatherapy. There is widespread geographical variation in the provision of community treatment and advice services and considerable variation in the range of interventions on offer. The current Effectiveness Review commissioned by the Department of Health (Polkinghorne, 1995) is expected to correct some of these anomalies, and to recommend plugging some of the more obvious gaps in services.

Typically, dependent opiate users present to services when the costs of their drug use have begun to exceed any benefits they might have perceived at the start of their drug-using career. They may be experiencing family or relationship difficulties; they may be involved in the machinery of the criminal justice system; their habit may have reached such proportions that they are no longer able to sustain it physically or financially; or they may be experiencing medical consequences of their drug use (e.g. septicaemia, hepatitis, HIV, cocaine or amphetamine psychosis, recurrent depression, etc.). It is usually some combination of external and internal forces which propels them forward to seek treatment.

There are a variety of interventions available to treat dependent opiate users, each appropriate for different circumstances. The most easily available treatment in the UK is gradual opiate withdrawal, although this may well change in the light of the new three-year National Drugs Strategy and the Effectiveness Review. This reduction programme involves the prescription of the substitute opiate drug methadone, almost always in oral form (Methadone Mixture DTF 1 mg/1 ml), generally over a period of weeks and often months. The idea behind this programme is that dependence will often be cured by a gradual reduction in opiate dosage (eventually to zero), usually accompanied by some form of support and counselling. High drop-out rates from such programmes, coupled with equally high relapse rates after treatment, have induced a certain pessimism regarding this approach among many practitioners, who have consequently come to favour longer and higher dose regimes. This view is supported by much evidence from the USA and elsewhere (see Ball and Ross, 1991; Ward et al., 1992).

Alternatively, or if a user's problems are particularly severe, what is called 'maintenance' substitute prescribing may be offered. 'Maintenance' involves prescribing oral methadone for the long term, possibly over many years. In this treatment, the immediate and intermediate goals are not abstinence-related: what is sought is stability in the individual's use of drugs and in their personal and social life, as well as the removal of the need for drug-related crime. No controlled study of methadone maintenance has been conducted in Britain for 20 years. As part of the Government Task Force on Drugs' review of treatment effectiveness, a National Treatment Outcomes Review study is currently under way at the time of writing. As we have already noted, outcome research elsewhere supports the contention that oral methadone maintenance programmes can achieve considerable reductions in illicit drug use, criminality and frequency of injecting particularly where high doses (around 80 mg or more daily) are prescribed. They have also been shown to reduce user mortality.

It is also possible to prescribe injectable drugs. These may include heroin, when a doctor is licensed by the Home Office. This policy was part of what was known as 'the British System': this system came into operation shortly after World War I and remained in place until the late 1960s. The prescribing of injectable heroin has steadily declined over the years, in spite of some vocal advocates. Today, only a small proportion of Britain's notified addicts receive supplies of the drug but the controversy for and against its prescription continues. A limiting factor for those who support heroin maintenance ('like for like' prescribing) is the fact that, with the exception of one study at University College London in the 1970s, which compared injectable heroin with oral methadone, there has been no published examination of this treatment approach. Currently, there is a large-scale trial going on in Switzerland and we await the results with interest. In the present climate, however, it is difficult to see the readoption of heroin prescribing on any large-scale in this country.

THE INJECTOR

Services for injectors, whether dependent or non-dependent drug users, centre around the provision of needle and syringe exchange schemes. This is achieved through the provision of dedicated needle exchanges (ranging from hospital-based services through to mobile facilities such as that provided by the voluntary organization Manchester Action on Street Health) or through community pharmacy-based schemes. The aim of such schemes is to reduce the sharing of injecting equipment and the harm arising from continued injecting, by promoting safer injecting practices through the provision of clean needles and syringes, and by encouraging the safe disposal of blood-borne diseases such as HIV/AIDS or hepatitis B and C. Exchange schemes increasingly provide citric acid: this is used as a substitute for acidifying agents, which are used to increase the solubility of heroin powder. Normal acidifiers such as vinegar and lemon juice are often associated with infections such as candidiasis. Evaluation of syringe exchange schemes reveals evidence of good effectiveness (Donoghoe et al., 1992) and the low prevalence of HIV among injecting drug users in England and Wales is a tribute to their utility. (Scotland has only recently adopted syringe exchange schemes on a wide scale.)

THE USER IN WITHDRAWAL

As we have already noted, the interruption of a regular supply of a dependence-producing drug leads to a withdrawal syndrome. Amongst the opiates, heroin produces the shortest syndrome (the earliest symptoms appear within 6–12 hours after the last dose, peak at two to three days and subside within seven to ten days) and methadone the longest (withdrawal from methadone may need two days to become apparent, and the symptoms may take up to six to seven weeks to decline). Unlike barbiturate and alcohol withdrawal, opiate withdrawal is not life threatening, but care is required in its management. Management can be undertaken as an inpatient, or within the community through home detoxification. This can be achieved through a variety of methods. In the inpatient setting, methods of detoxification range from rapid detoxification (around 48 hours) employing naltrexone (an opiate antagonist), benzodiazepines (for sedation) and clonidine or lofexidine (antihypertensive drugs which also relieve opiate withdrawal symptoms), to a methadone withdrawal regime over a period of two to three weeks.

There is no good evidence available concerning the effectiveness of rapid withdrawal techniques. Effectiveness studies of inpatient detoxification over a two-to-three week period, show that three quarters of opiate addicts voluntarily comply with treatment through to the completion of withdrawal. However, there is a high drop-out rate in the following two weeks when withdrawal distress can remain high. Relapse rates in the first few weeks after treatment also remain high. Currently, there are few data concerning home detoxification, although our own service is currently evaluating a pilot scheme. Initial results are promising and community management is potentially much more cost effective than inpatient treatment.

THE ADDICT IN RECOVERY

Community services for ex-opiate users in recovery are minimal. Drug treatment agencies often have a problem in finding suitable premises. Providing rehabilitation services on the same site as services to current users may be unwelcome to those in recovery, who may not wish to meet former drug-using associates and for whom the premises themselves may well act not only as a reminder of their previous careers but actually serve as a facilitating cue for relapse. Certainly, after-care groups when run by such agencies have rarely functioned particularly well, in terms of uptake or longevity.

Self-help groups, most notably Narcotics Anonymous (NA – a 12 step programme based directly on the fellowship of Alcoholics Anonymous) have been much more successful in keeping groups together over time. To date, outcome research on 12 Step self-help groups is conspicuous by its absence and the effectiveness of NA and Cocaine Anonymous is confirmed only by anecdote.

As regards residential rehabilitation services, the picture is somewhat more rosy. Despite pessimistic predictions at the time that community care funding was introduced, the structure of residential care for addicts in recovery remains intact. Such projects are run almost entirely by non-statutory agencies and range from therapeutic communities based on hierarchical structures (e.g. Phoenix House) through to relatively un-structured programmes (City Roads) to various forms of Christian-based houses. Programmes can last from as long as 15–18 months to 3–6 months.

The variety of available houses and programmes allows referrers to match clients quite closely to rehabilitation regimes.

The development of community care funding has led providers of residential care to engage in evaluation of outcomes but hard evidence has yet to appear. Residential rehabilitation is one of the areas of investigation for the DoH Effectiveness Review.

Dependency, treatment and outcome

There has been a tendency, particularly within the medical profession, towards 'therapeutic pessimism' with regard to the treatment of opiate dependency. Opiate addiction has been seen, to use the medical cliché, as 'a chronic relapsing condition' with a poor prognosis. But is this pessimism justified? There are a number of issues here but because of limitations of space we have to confine ourselves to making the most important points in summary form.

- Longitudinal studies both here and in America do not lend support to the conclusion 'once an addict always an addict'. Lee Robins' (1993) painstaking epidemiological work with heroin-addicted US soldiers returning from the war in Vietnam found that in Vietnam 43 per cent of the sample used opiates. On return to America, however, at 12 months follow-up only 10 per cent had used opiates and only a small minority were doing so on a daily basis. Stimson and Oppenheimer (1982) conducted a long-term follow-up study of addicts attending London drug dependency units (DDUs) and found 40 per cent of their sample drug-free at 10-year follow-up. There is, it appears, a general, long-term trend towards abstinence among heroin users consistent with the 'maturing out' hypothesis advanced over 30 years ago by Charles Winick (1962).
- Pessimism about the outcome of heroin addicts in treatment rests on a particular view of the goal of treatment, namely that it should be directed towards abstinence. However, as we saw in the discussion on maintenance prescribing, good outcomes in terms of reduction of illicit drug use and drug-related criminality can be gained from long-term prescribing. The reduction of both individual and community harms features prominently here. Two recent studies in the US applied rigorous cost–benefit analysis techniques to the question of the benefits of treatment. The first conducted for the State of California concluded that every dollar spent by the state on drug and alcohol treatment saved the taxpayer $7, largely through reduced crime (NOPCR, 1994). A Rand Corporation study of cocaine use revealed that treatment was seven times more effective in reducing cocaine consumption than the most effective law enforcement measures and cut the cost to society through crime and lost productivity (Rydell and Everingham, 1994).

- We also have to be clear about how far treatment is the important factor in effecting recovery. In the last few years there has been a development of interest in processes of 'natural recovery' in the addictions. Many people give up addictions without any recourse to formal treatment (it has been estimated, for example, that up to 95 per cent of ex-smokers gave up smoking without formal interventions). George Vaillant (1983) describes similar findings in problem drinkers, and Biernacki (1986) in heroin addicts. These 'natural pathways' out of opiate dependency include pressure from peers or partners, negative experience with peers, increased awareness of the stigma of addiction, a geographical move, disappearance of a supplier/dealer and positive experiences such as the discovery of religion. Such findings also support the concept of 'maturing out' of heroin addiction and remind us that what happens in formal treatment is only a small part of the wide range of influences that can influence the outcome of addiction. We have to be aware of the limitations of treatment. As Griffiths Edwards (1989) puts it, 'Treatment is more accurately conceived as being at best a timely nudge or whisper in a life-long course'.

Philosophy and aims of community drug services

From the 1980s until the publication this year of the government's new three-year strategy on drugs *Tackling Drugs Together* (Interdepartmental Group, 1995), drug services have taken their aims from the various recommendations of the Advisory Council on the Misuse of Drugs.

The establishment of community services for drug users in the form of community drug teams derives directly from the Advisory Council on the Misuse of Drugs 1982 report (ACMD, 1982) as does the concept, which implicitly informs our work, of 'the problem drug user':

> any person who experiences social, psychological, physical or legal problems related to intoxication and/or regular excessive consumption and/or dependence as a consequence of his (*sic*) own use of drugs or other chemical substances . . .' (p. 35).

Its 1984 report on prevention first drew attention to the need to develop service responses which reduced the harm that develops from continuing drug use, as well as more orthodox primary prevention approaches. Its 1989 report, following the Public Health Laboratory's report of HIV prevalence among injecting drug users three years before, stated that the prevention of AIDS was more important than the prevention of injecting drug use (ACMD, 1989). These reports laid the foundation for the development of what has become known as *harm reduction*. Harm reduction has informed policies such as maintenance prescribing, syringe exchange schemes, publications such as the 'Peanut Pete' leaflets and the harm reduction comic 'Smack In The Eye' produced by the Lifeline organization. Alongside these developments we have seen a focus on the health care needs of drug users, the provision of 'well drug-users' clinics and an emphasis on the treatment of injecting drug users in primary health care settings.

The most recent statement of aims is that provided by central government in the previously mentioned White Paper. *Tackling Drugs Together* focuses attention on three areas: crime, public health and young people. Community drug services have a role in all these three areas and the government sees its strategy as being delivered through multi-agency partnerships. In relation to health issues, and in particular the goal of treatment, the government has stated that the goal of treatment must be abstinence and that harm reduction strategies can only be seen as intermediate measures along the road to that goal. Harm reduction, it states, must be seen as a means to an end, not as an end in itself.

This re-emphasis on abstinence, and the consequent devaluation of harm reduction, have alarmed many workers in the drugs field who fear a new moral backlash against drug users. Our own feeling is that this is a thoroughly pragmatic document and that the focus on abstinence has no sinister connotations. Discussions of abstinence must take account of the factors mentioned above in the section on outcome. Harm reduction will always remain a principle in the treatment of drug users. Anyone involved in treating drug users, however opposed to harm reduction as an end, will at some time apply it in their own practice. We will have to wait until the end of the three-year period for evaluation of this new strategy which, it must be said, has not been backed by the release of major new resources.

Conclusion

Over the last 10 years, the frequency of illicit drug use has increased dramatically. Drug treatment can no longer be the preserve of the specialist. GPs have long become accustomed to taking a major role in the treatment of alcohol dependence: in some parts of the country they are also realizing that the recognition and treatment of drug misuse should also be a standard feature of community medical care. We believe that primary health care teams should play a key role in drug services, and that the interest and support of local GPs is at present a good indicator of the success of local community drug services. In our service, and in a few other districts such as Edinburgh, and the Wirral, much effort has been put into the education and support of GPs and their teams. We have demonstrated the benefits of treating drug users in primary care rather than at specialist facilities: where proper support is provided to GPs, medical care is better, stigma is reduced and users are more contented.

We believe that 'harm reduction' will remain the main goal of drug services, and will in time be more widely accepted as a sensible strategy by primary care teams and other treatment providers. Much more research is needed, in order to identify ways in which drug use can become safer: this must focus both on better ways of helping users achieve abstinence, but also on safer ways of continuing to use drugs. The available knowledge concerning cocaine and LSD is minimal compared with that accumulated concerning legal drugs, such as nicotine and alcohol.

Increased knowledge derived from research on illegal drugs will also bring the requirement for increased skills on the part of those working with drug users. None the less, we believe that most community practitioners already have the skills to deal with many problems presented by users. It is the job of community drug teams, and other specialist services, to provide support and training to help these skills develop, while at the same time remaining available to handle the more complicated problems. Our own research shows that younger practitioners already feel more confident in dealing with drug users. We would predict over the next few years a gradual integration of addiction treatments into mainstream services.

References

Advisory Council on the Misuse of Drugs (ACMD) 1982: *treatment and rehabilitation*. London: HMSO.

Advisory Council on the Misuse of Drugs (ACMD) 1984: *AIDS and drug misuse Part I*. London: HMSO.

Advisory Council on the Misuse of Drugs (ACMD) 1989: *AIDS and drug misuse Part II*. London: HMSO.

Ball, J.C. and Ross, A. 1991: *The effectiveness of methadone maintenance treatment: patients, programs, services and outcome*. New York: Springer.

Berridge, V. and Edwards, G. 1981: *Opium and the people: opiate use in nineteenth century England*. London: Allen Lane.

Biernacki, P. 1986: *Pathways from heroin addiction*. Philadelphia: Temple.

Cohen, S. and Taylor, L. 1976: *Psychological survival: the theory and practice of resistance to everyday life*. Harmondsworth, Middlesex: Penguin Books.

Donoghoe, M.C., Stimson, G.V. and Dolan, K.A. 1992: *Syringe exchange in England: an overview*. London: Tufnell Press.

Edwards, G. 1989: As the years go rolling by. Drinking problems in the time dimension. *British Journal of Psychiatry* 154, 18–26.

Farrell, M. 1991: Physical complications of drug use. In Ilana Belle Glass (ed.), *Handbook of addiction behaviour*. London: Routledge, 120.

Gossop, M. 1993: *Living with drugs*, 2nd edn. Aldershot: Wildwood House.

Institute for the Study of Drug Dependence (ISDD) 1994a: *Drug abuse briefing: a guide to the effects of drugs and to the social and legal facts about their non-medical use in Britain*. London: ISDD.

Institute for the Study of Drug Dependence (ISDD) 1994b: *Drug misuse in Britain*. London: ISDD.

Interdepartmental Group 1995: *Tackling drugs together*. London: HMSO.

National Opinion Research Centre (NOPCR) 1994: *Evaluating recovery services: the California drug and alcohol treatment assessment*. Fairfax VA: Lewin-VHI Library.

Orford, J. 1985: *Excessive appetites: a psychological view of addictions*. Chichester: John Wiley.

Polkinghorne, J. 1995: The Department of Health's task force to review services for drug misusers. *Druglink* 10, 5.

Robins, L. 1993: Vietnam veterans' rapid recovery from heroin addiction: a fluke or normal expectations? *Addiction* 88, 8.

Rydell, C.P. and Everingham, S. 1994: *Controlling cocaine: supply versus demand programs*. Santa Monica: Rand Corporation.

Stepney, R. 1981: Habits and addictions. *Bulletin of the British Psychological Society* **34**, 233–5.

Stimson, G. and Oppenheimer, E. 1982: *Heroin addiction: treatment and control in Britain*. London: Tavistock.

Strang, J. 1993: *Drug abuse*. Epidemiologically based needs assessment reviews: Management Executive of the National Health Service. Leeds: Quarry House.

Vaillant, G. 1983: *The natural history of alcoholism: causes, patterns, and paths to recovery*. Cambridge: Harvard University Press.

Ward, J., Mattick, R. and Hall, W. 1992: *Key issues in methadone maintenance treatment*. New South Wales: New South Wales University Press.

Winick, C. 1962: Maturing out of narcotic addiction. *Bulletin of Narcotics* **14**, 1.

PART FIVE

Bake for several hours

16 Asking the questions

Christopher Wibberley

The person best placed to effectively research practice is the practitioner. Most practitioners are engaged in research without recognizing the same; they observe and interview, develop case studies and measure efficacy. Often they are reluctant to publicize their observations because they hold the belief that research belongs to another world; that is, academia. Christopher Wibberley discusses the arena of practitioner research prior to offering a very useful, step-by-step guide to developing research questions. He does not offer advice in methodology – there are many excellent texts available that do this – but focuses on the most important phase: getting started.

Introduction

Community health practitioners, along with other professional groups, are being encouraged to be 'research-minded'; not only in keeping up to date, but also in becoming actively involved in carrying out research (DoH, 1990, 1991, 1993). When confronted with the prospect of having to carry out research, novice researchers often concentrate most on the question of how they are going to collect the data (and later on how these data might be analysed) – the mechanics of the research process. The more conceptual element of the research process – identifying, developing and contextualizing the problem and questions to be addressed in the first place, is usually assumed to be of less importance.

However, if research is to be fruitful, then the way in which research problems and research questions are identified and developed must receive adequate attention. Research effort is often wasted because this initial step is given too little consideration. Such consideration should also ensure that design issues are addressed as a whole, as opposed to being split into data collection and data analysis issues.

Unfortunately, the issue of identifying and outlining research problems and research questions is often given scant, if any, consideration in research methodology texts. One result of this is that people will allow topics, or sometimes approaches, to drive their intended research in a direction which is not always most appropriate.

In the film of Steinbeck's *Cannery Row*, there is a scene where the 'Doc' decides to do some research. He says to another character 'Mac':

Hell every year, you know, I go up to the Congress of Marine Biologists in San Francisco and every year I have to listen to a bunch of god damn guys reading papers on all the dandy stuff they know. Well hell this year they're going to sit through a paper of my own for a change. I know these animals as well as anybody . . . I ought to be able to find out something about them that's worth knowing. I think I'll call my paper 'Symptoms in some Cephalopoda approximating apoplexy'.

A voice over then notes that:

The Doc plunged into his octopus studies with all the professional dedication he could muster. He prodded, injected various chemicals into their water, and generally did everything he could to get the little buggers to react. Unfortunately the conclusions to be drawn from all this were slow in coming. But Doc knew he was on to something, even if he couldn't figure out what it was.

Obviously, research undertaken by practitioners should have a sounder base than the Doc's. Some texts suggest that research should be based on the researcher's personal interests; but, obviously, this alone – as evidenced by the Doc's research – is not enough. Another possible starting point is other investigators' theories and research. However, problems presenting to practitioners that require research are, in the words of Schon (1987): '. . . often messy, indeterminate situations'. Published research may give some peripheral insight to the problem – but the reason why the practitioner needs to undertake the research is that published research does not help solve the actual problem that they are presented with.

In the case of practitioner research, previously published research should not dictate the form of the stated research problem and research questions asked but aid the development of the research design, once the problem(s) and questions are clearly identified. Previous experience and learning will probably shape the way a person looks at the problem facing them; but they should try to avoid tunnel vision in terms of being blinkered by the findings of previous studies that they either know or find, in the process of their study.

Practitioners may also be affected by the confines of their occupational/ professional practice – as Schon (1987) notes: 'When a practitioner sets a problem he (sic) chooses and names the things he will notice'. Schon (1987) continues by detailing the differing ways that nutritionists, agronomists, epidemiologists, demographers, engineers and economists may view the issue of malnourishment among children in developing countries – adding that other influencing factors may include the individual's interests and political and economic beliefs. A similar discussion of both food shortages and energy problems is provided by Pacey (1983) who observes the negative aspects of this problem – that experts: '. . . learn to examine specialized aspects of problems with a concentrated attention that blinds them to other issues', whilst Schon (1987) considers that:

Those who hold conflicting frames pay attention to different facts and make different sense of the facts they notice [so that] It is not by technical problem solving that we convert problematic situations to well formed problems; rather, it is through naming and framing that technical problem solving becomes possible.

In other words, for individual practitioners, problems become soluble through the research process by 'framing' them in certain ways – certain questions arising out of the problem being given more attention than others. Practitioners should be aware of this framing process as they work through the stages of problem identification and the conversion of this problem into questions which can be appropriately addressed through research. Such awareness can then be communicated to others, with assumptions being made by the practitioner being articulated and justified.

So given the above: how do you identify a research problem? What makes a good research problem? How do you go about converting the problem into research questions which will then allow you to design a programme of research to carry out? This chapter now considers these questions from an individual perspective.

The process of generating a good research problem and moving it on

You may already have some ideas about your research problem – but make sure that it is a problem to be solved, not just a general topic area that you're interested in. If you have some ideas, keep a note of them. If you don't, you need to start ruminating over what problems there are in your work that warrant a systematic approach to their study, in the form of research. Keep a pen handy, ideas may crop up at the strangest times and may be forgotten if they're not committed to paper. Talk your ideas over with colleagues and then see if they are generally recognized as 'good' research problems.

Ensure that the problem is stated in a form which represents the problem as it presents to you as the practitioner – thus it should be grounded in your experience and perhaps those of colleagues. Additionally the problem should be stated clearly and concisely in a form easily understandable by colleagues working in the same 'field' (and probably by others) with little or no further explanation. This task, of setting the problem, can be difficult and time consuming – it is best undertaken with the help of others (both those with and without direct experience of the 'field'; outsider and insider perspectives can be equally illuminating).

A good problem should result in the potential to generate a range of questions – although only some of these may be researchable. Once you have a firm idea of your research problem, you can start generating a list of research questions. The first stage in this process is to generate a list of 'first thoughts' – aiming for quantity and breadth and not worrying about wording or how important the question may appear to be. Again, other people can be helpful in brainstorming these ideas. Having scribbled down all the 'first thoughts' you can start prioritizing and focusing down on specific questions, and fine tuning them into research questions.

As you begin, and continue, to focus and fine tune your research question(s), existing literature should be explored. The specific detail of the intended research should be related to themes generated from the literature. Searching and reviewing of literature should be broad based in nature as any, let alone the best, 'research base' may not be immediately obvious for all research problems. It is, however, important that the problem should define the research base and not vice versa – and it may not always be the research base that you expected. Additionally, the base may be related to different and diverse fields of work and academic disciplines. Some interesting research may well cross disciplinary boundaries; although perhaps for the novice researcher it might be simpler merely to note cross-disciplinary issues within which to contextualize a particularly focused approach.

The literature search and review should also result in some certainty that the problem is *sufficiently* new. The identification of a 'gap in the literature', tied in with the short-list of research question(s) should result in the development of aims which are considered to be of sufficient significance or importance with respect to the development of knowledge of relevance to your own practice. The aims should state clearly what it is you are aiming to find out. Such aims may then be translated into a relatively general statement of intent, proposition or series of propositions or into a more specific hypothesis.

It is important to note at this point that the research questions and aims of the study should not be written in tablets of stone. The research process, in reality, is often far less tidy than depicted through the medium of research reports; and the study will probably evolve and develop with time as fresh ideas emerge.

Finally, once the ideas have been tied down questions have to be asked about the 'doability' of the research with respect to time frames, budgets, access to and availability of data or data sources, and the methodological skills of the practitioner and/or other researchers.

At this stage, assuming a decision has been made as to the value and 'doability' of the research, a research proposal should be developed. This should include:

1 A background to the proposed study both in terms of the identification of the problem and the existing literature relating to the problem.

2 Clearly stated aims which identify what it is you are trying to find out.

3 A plan of enquiry including an indication of the proposed methodology, and a justification for this methodological approach which relates to the aims of the study (this may include setting objectives).

4 Discussion of any ethical issues arising from the proposed research approach.

The exact nature of the research proposal should, however, be considered with respect to any institutional requirements that you, as the practitioner researcher, may have to comply with.

The following worksheets may help you work through the process of identifying a research problem and appropriate research questions, so that you can then move onto refining these ideas in the form of a research design – finally writing a proposal in whatever standardized form is required. It should also be noted that practical and political factors may affect the research design adopted. Often the ideal design has to be traded down if you are actually going to carry out the research.

IDEAS FOR RESEARCH I: identifying the problem and developing questions

---

IDENTIFIED PROBLEM

GENERATED QUESTIONS

QUESTIONS OF INTEREST

RESEARCH QUESTION(S) – this must be a question / series of questions answerable by research

GENERAL NATURE OF LITERATURE TO BE CONSULTED

SPECIFIC EXAMPLES OF LITERATURE CONSULTED OF POTENTIAL USE

WORKING TITLE

IDEAS FOR RESEARCH II: refining research ideas and formulating the research design

By now you should have a fair idea about what the problem you wish to research is; and what the research questions that particularly interest you are.

RESEARCH QUESTION(S)

Think generally about: What sort of data you want.
Who you want these data from.
How you might get the data from the people you want them from.

WHAT SORT OF DATA DO YOU WANT?

WHO DO YOU WANT THE DATA FROM?

Now bring all this information together to set out the aims of the study

AIMS OF THE INTENDED RESEARCH

Finally, ask yourself how you might get the data you want from the people you want them from – start generally (e.g. ask them). Then become more specific (e.g. ask them using an interview format). Then be even more specific (e.g. ask them using an interview format adopting a partially structured approach). Other general starting points could be: watch them; ask them to keep a record; look at existing records; measure their physiological responses etc. . . .

HOW MIGHT YOU GET THE DATA YOU WANT FROM THE PEOPLE YOU WANT THEM FROM?

You should now be able to identify more formal objectives in terms of 'doing' the research.

RESEARCH OBJECTIVES

References

DoH 1990: *Taking research seriously*. London: HMSO.
DoH 1991: *Research for health: a research and development strategy for the NHS*. London: HMSO.
DoH 1993: *Report of the taskforce on the strategy for research in nursing, midwifery and health visiting*. London: HMSO.
Pacey, A. 1983: *The culture of technology*. Oxford: Blackwell.
Schon, D. 1987: *Educating the reflective practitioner*. California: Jossey Bass.

17 Closing comments

David Skidmore

Although the concept of care in the community has been with us for many years it is now taking on a new significance. In real terms it is about to become another country, largely unexplored and full of potential surprises. The new ethos of health care will mean delivering health care not only into the home, but also the workplace, the clinic, the school and residential homes. The previous chapters have offered a glimpse and some guidance regarding what we should expect. However, this is still a relatively new country and community practitioners are still in that pioneer role. The Romans used the expression *pater patriae* to designate distinguished statesmen. Literally it means: father of his country. That is the duel role of the future community practitioner: father and statesman; it is in your gift to shape, encourage and protect the country you are given responsibility for.

The role should not be confused with that of the missionary who believed that they were bringing the truth to the heathen. The countries you enter will have their own truths (or realities) and you are there merely to facilitate its prominence, not replace it with your own. The hardest skill a practitioner must develop is that of listening. You may hear what a person is saying; this is not synonymous with listening. Remember, a bore is a person who wants to talk about themselves when you want to talk about you. This is not being flippant, it is so easy to assume you understand the meaning when someone relates an experience. Buber (1970) suggests that we can only ever gain a perception of another's experience; we can never share that experience. Consequently, how can we really understand what they are saying before they have finished saying it?

In many ways this text does mankind an injustice with regard to health care. By necessity it has categorized health care and people into clear divisions. Unfortunately, life is not like that. A person can be young and old, at the same time; travel through every aspect of the community; they have physical and mental health, are carers and are cared for. All these aspects come into play when they enter any encounter. Community care takes on a different dimension – it is far more complex than hospital care. Richman (Chapter 1) referred to the *ideal type*. Parsons (1951) offered an ideal type for those entering the sick role. A sick role is legitimized by hospital admission – there are clear expectations about what the nurse–patient role is all about; no matter how we try to dress it up with named nurses and client-centered approaches. When a person enters hospital they are entitled to expect care and the practitioner expects to give it. The act of removing them from their 'community' implies that they have no control and require the attention of an expert before they can regain control. This is not the case with community care. The act of leaving a person within the community, or returning them to it, implies that they have responsibility . . . otherwise they would not be allowed to be there. There is not an ideal type for the community; community care permits individuality. The best advice that can be given to any practitioner about to intervene in the community is *ecce homo* (behold the man) and *ecce signum* (look at the proof). Yes, back to listening again. Do not base your assessment of a person's problem on your previous experience, on a diagnosis or on the observations of others. To do so may make intervention easier but it may, equally, do little to help the client.

Herrick (1987), who lived 1591–1674, offered:

Gather ye rosebuds while ye may,
Old Time it is a-flying:
And this same flower that smiles to-day,
To-morrow will be dying.

Whilst Herrick was attempting to persuade maidens to give up their virginity and enjoy the pleasures of life, one can equally translate the verse to be in agreement with Horace (1972), the Roman poet, whose Odes advise that we should seize the day. In short, it is the person's life and unlike any other. They deserve a quality of life. To transfer the verse to the practitioner one could suggest that the rosebuds are the pieces of information that a client offers; Old Time is the length of involvement, the same flower that smiles is the intervention based on diagnosis or therapeutic fashion and the last line is obvious. The knowledge you gain from books and experience is but a framework, a baseline upon which to commence intervention. If it ever becomes the truth, that is the only way to intervene, then the therapist and the therapy is lost. Just as the teacher should facilitate learning, so too should the practitioner facilitate health. The two roles are not dissimilar. Just as the poor teacher can alienate the child from learning, by virtue of the teaching style, the practitioner can alienate the client from health. In both cases, to be effective, one has to have respect for the rights of the client.

Shakespeare, in *As You Like It*, would have it that there are seven ages of man. This would be so if all men were the same. I would argue that each person has but one age, although I agree that: '. . . one man in his time plays many parts'. Our experiences make us all different and yet, inside, each person clings to that aspect which offers some security, that notion of self. Age will not wither it, inside the 80-year-old is the same person they were at 18 years. The body may be weaker and more wrinkled, but does the mirror really show this? What help then, when someone advises: you should slow down, you're old now? Being old is something that happens to other people; being chronically ill is something that happens to other people. If you listen you might gather some clues regarding how best to address a person and, ultimately, facilitate their return to health, or at least assist them to improve the quality of their life.

Enough humanism! The fact of the matter is that community nursing is on the brink of major change. It has developed against a backdrop of legislation, economics, population changes and tradition. The time has come when it must seize an identity of its own. All the preceding chapters have illustrated that it is not merely an extension of the hospital nurse's role. The community nurse is more than an agent of support for the transfer of the institution into the community. Community post-registration education and practice (PREP) can facilitate the growth of a new profession, in a new country. The principles that underpinned the UKCC's policy are noble enough:

- to ensure education for community practitioners meets contemporary health care needs;
- to ensure that the professions are prepared to meet the demands of changes in service provision; with reference to legislative change such as: the NHS and Community Act (1990), Children's Act (1989) and, of course, nurse prescribing;
- to eliminate unnecessary duplicity and fragmentation of postregistration nurse education and training.

Community PREP offers a new, unified discipline of community health care nursing that can do much to improve the quality of care delivered to clients. The advantages of such a move are:

- tailored preparation will promote clinical responsibility that will facilitate improved standards of care for clients and their families and, indeed, the service generally;
- a recordable qualification for all community nurses, on the UKCC's register, that will both protect standards and indicate skill;
- a rational and economic framework can be created which will make more effective and efficient use of resources;
- it could provide a more flexible and sensitive means of ensuring education and training are relevant and responsive to health and service needs.

There are many health care needs in the community: care of the dying, care of the physically ill, the elderly, workers, rehabilitation needs, care of schoolchildren, family health, people with learning disabilities and those with psychological dysfunction, to name but a few. Although this text has offered these areas as specialisms the practitioner should note that every community nurse should have awareness of these areas to be effective. If you cannot recognize a problem how can you direct the client to the best source of advice? I am not advocating a generic worker. To provide the best service to that community we profess to serve means that we need to preserve the specialist practitioner. However, with regard to assessment of needs each practitioner needs to have a little knowledge of every aspect;

behold the man, but do not intervene in areas in which you lack the skill. To allow any of the specialist areas to die is to betray the community if one accepts a client-centred approach.

Equally unethical is to assume that every 'community' (whatever that may be) is identical. Just as people are different, so are so-called communities. Each area has its own identity; some will have a large elderly population, others massive unemployment, cities will have a transient population and some may have a combination. Each community service should develop a community profile so that service needs can be identified. Community profiling is effectively dealt with by Hawtin *et al.* (1994) and is essential reading for all community service managers. In essence, then, an area that the community 'team' strives to serve should be dealt with in the same way that a new client is. It is rather pointless having an expert team of behavioural and cognitive therapists in an area that does not need the service. The sad fact about intervention is that it is fickle. Practitioners respond to fashion, or at least they appear to. Using psychiatry again, as an example, in the early 1970s behavioural therapy was in vogue. Indeed, it seemed that anyone and everyone with any psychiatric problem, however remote, received behavioural psychotherapy. Psycho-social intervention is now in danger of becoming equally ubiquitous. I am not saying that psychiatric community nurses should not have this skill, I am warning them that they could lose sight of the many problems beyond schizophrenia. Even the great and the good of psychiatric nursing are implying that all educational focus should be in this area. Bowers (Chapter 14) does offer a balanced view. The problem with intervention fashion seems to arise from professionals who think that they know what a society needs without really getting to know that society. This, in turn, may have its genesis in professionals creating their own problems. The 1970s was the decade when community psychiatric care really took off. Initially, the growth area was intervening in behavioural problems. The knock-on effect was that people with long-term psychiatric problems tended to be ignored. It was not a very big step to assume that this group would benefit from community care. After all, it is cheaper if you do not transfer the necessary resources. Consequently, in the 1990s, we find problems with the management of such a group in the community. Resorting to supervision registers and the 'civilized' version of house arrest is merely papering over the cracks. We are now having to cope with the consequences of bad planning.

The psychiatric experience should have taught us that health care delivery cannot be planned on a purely economic basis. In the introduction to this text it was argued that the demographic change facing the UK will make increasing demands on health care delivery. Putting a direct cost on illness is not the answer. Effective use of resources is. Each service, then, must get to know the area it serves so that it can effectively assess needs. Once the health care needs are recognized an effective team can be developed. Each member of that team must then effectively assess each client so that appropriate intervention can be planned. This may seem obvious but, even so, is not put into practice enough. Ford Prefect in *The Hitch-hikers Guide to the Galaxy* (Adams, 1978) declared: '. . . it's the simplest ideas that are the best . . .'. Indeed, but often the most difficult to operationalize when confronted with economy. Giving GPs a budget may seem a noble concept but in reality it is very restrictive. It demands that the health care they deliver is costed. Consequently, certain conditions become expensive. Evidence is now emerging that people are being removed from GPs' lists because they are too expensive to treat (Kilroy, 1995); people removed from the list have no right of appeal. Unless we start to use our resources effectively we are in danger of creating a new underclass, those with chronic medical and psychological conditions. What then? . . . open a modern workhouse to contain them? People say that history repeats itself . . . let's hope not with regard to health care.

Effective assessment, then, at both service and individual level is a vital tool if we are to offer effective community care. Each practitioner, in order to develop such skills, has to develop critical thinking. This has been alluded to throughout this book. To find out more the reader is directed to Zechmeister and Johnson (1992). Every practitioner has a duty to be critical about their intervention, it is part of being an autonomous and accountable practitioner. By and large each community nurse is autonomous and, as such, accountable. Intervening in the lives of others is not just doing a job . . . it is about having a positive regard and a deep respect for the lives of those we encounter. It is what being professional is all about.

This text has sought to introduce the reader to the various specialisms that occur in the community. There are, no doubt, omissions and any real depth has been avoided; there are several excellent texts that explore each specialism in depth. We have sought to introduce you to the arena of community nursing, to give you a good overview. Hopefully, the text has stimulated you to read some of the other texts mentioned herein. More important, we hope it has stimulated thought.

If you are about to embark on a career in community nursing, we wish you every success. Our ramblings have not been offered as truths, merely suggestions and overviews. This last chapter has advised you to behold the man, be effective in your needs assessment and above all . . . watch out for all that road rage.

References

Adams, D. 1978: *The hitch hiker's guide to the galaxy*. BBC Radio, First broadcast: 29.3.78, London.
Buber, M. 1970: *I and thou*. Edinburgh: T & T Clark,
Hawtin, M., Hughes, G. and Percy-Smith, J. 1994: *Community profiling: auditing social needs*. Buckingham: Open University Press.
Herrick, R. 1987: To the virgins, to make much of time. In Wain, J. (ed.), *The Oxford Library of English Poetry*. London, Guild, 234.
Horace 1972: *The odes*. Harmondsworth: Penguin Classics.
Kilroy, R. 1995: *Kilroy*. 19.10.95. London: BBC Television.

Parsons, T. 1951: *The social system*. Chicago: Free Press.
Shakespeare, W. 1974: *As you like it*. Harmondsworth: Penguin.
Zechmeister, E.B. and Johnson, J.E. 1992: *Critical thinking: a functional approach*. Pacific Grove, CA: Brooks/Cole.

Index

Accident Target 121
Acheson Report 171
Action set 20
Advocacy 5, 251
Advocate 4, 67, 125, 185
Agricola 190
Altruism 27
Altruistic 109
Amish 26
Anomic 18
Anomie 28
Antipositivism 37, 42
Antipositivists 40, 41
Antiwelfare 60
Apprenticeships 107
Aristotle 12, 15, 39
Attendance allowance 150
Awareness, self 18, 97, 218

Barclay Report 20
Baroque 24
Befriend 153
Bergsen 5
Bethnal Green 47
Bohemianism 29
British System (drug policy) 276
Bronchopulmonary dysplasia (BPD) 128
Buber 5, 25, 296
Buddist 189
Bureaucracy 12, 64
Burn-out 12

Cannery Row 285
Care package 146, 184
Carlyle 5
Categorical set 20
Category
    analytical 14
    drug use 274
    moral 14
    normative 14
    of home 43, 44
    organizing 14
Celtic 197
Charisma 19
Child-centred care 111
Class consciousness 18
Collaborative care 81–2
Communicare 250
Comtean 37
Consensus 12, 18
Consumerism 247, 249, 250
Consumerist model 250
Copernican 29

Crack 268, 273
Credit Accumulation and Transfer 124, 181
Crisis intervention 260
Cross Roads 145
Culture 11
Culture, dance 272
Cyber
    communities 31
    slaves 31
    space 188

Dance culture 272
Darwinism 27
Dawson Report 176
Delinquency 268
Democracy 12
Dependant care 96
Deskilling 54
Dirty work 54
Disempowering 122
Disraeli 12, 13
Dorward Report 195
Down's syndrome 238
Drugs classifications 270

Eboli 29
Ecce homo 297
Ecce signum 297
Egotist 17
Elderly 23
Elders 14, 25
Ely Hospital 240
Embryonic community 48, 51
Emotional depletion 127
Empower 122, 218
Empowering 1, 12, 112, 163, 167, 169, 211, 227
Empowerment 1–5, 30, 33, 67, 70, 122, 159, 160, 164, 167, 170, 172, 223
    community 64
    group 67
    self 71
Epistemological 50, 55
Ethics 4
Ethnographers 41
Extended family 48, 110

Family
    centred approach 110–14, 116, 119, 123, 125
    extended 48, 110
    nuclear 25, 28, 48
    society 15
    therapy 260, 261
    traditional 59, 169

Field-set 20
Finalistic 36
Framework of care 80–6, 88, 89, 95, 98, 99, 107
Friends 19, 20, 22, 53, 91, 110, 114, 145, 149, 241, 242, 252, 269
Friendship 15, 20, 22
Fry, Elizabeth 136
Functionalism 48–50
Functionalist 13

Gamp, Sarah 136
Gemeinschaft 15–18, 20, 25
  artificial 24
  pseudo 17
Genetic Engineering 17
Gerontologists 48
Gesellschaft 15, 18
Global 27, 69, 200, 206
  community 29
  economy 27
  highway 30
  village 29
Globalization 19, 28
Greece 12
Gutenberg configuration 29

Handsaari 199–201, 203, 206
Harm reduction 279, 280
Health Field Model 58, 59, 63, 71, 72
Health interview 163–5, 168
Health status 64, 133, 164, 171, 213
Heroin 267–74, 276, 278, 279
Hippocrates 189, 190
Hippy(ies) 24, 25, 272
Hitler 25
Home 2, 147, 150–2
  apnoea monitoring 126
  black box 47
  personal 46
  physical 46
  social 46
  ventilation 126
Homeless 76
Hospital Plan 134
Humanism 299
Hutterites 14, 26
Hypothesis 34, 35, 37–9

Iatrogenesis 29
Ideal-type 12, 15, 297
Individualism 13, 60
Individualistic approach 80
Individuality 242, 297
Individualized services 246
Industrial Revolution 190
Institutionalization 12, 241
Invalid care allowance 151

Jameson Report 209

Key person 165
Key powers 250
Key role 175

Key worker 153, 250, 262
Kibbutz 25
Kidscape 169
Kin 20
Kinship 12, 14–16, 22, 48, 49
Komitehs 27
Kurwille 16

Landladies 260
Lay 20, 50, 83, 139, 196, 238
Lead carer 82
Leviathan 16

Maintenance 275
Maudsley 13
Mawhinney 12
Me society 26
Milpa 14
Milpero 14
Models 71, 75, 89, 96, 101, 188, 199, 201, 202, 216, 217
  abstract-idealistic 115
  community 68
  conceptual 96
  consensual 62
  consumerist 250
  empowerment 67
  engineering 29
  functional 62
  Hansaari 199–201, 206
  health field 58, 59, 63, 71, 72
  health promotion (ideal) 64, 68, 160, 161
  medical 17, 90, 98, 134
  nursing 78, 79, 84, 88–91, 93, 95, 97–9, 101
  of care 3, 75, 76, 90–2, 98, 99, 107
  of participation 64
  of practice 72, 208
  of society 44
  Orems 75 (and Chapter 5)
  partnership 114, 115
  self-efficacy 91
  self-empowerment 71
  social 62
  technological 29
  tokenistic 64, 71
  wellness 91
  Worcester 216
Modernism 28
Moorhaven Hospital 258
Moral(s) 4, 5, 27, 44
  category 14
  crusade 28
  decay 26
  education 28
  entrepreneurism 70
  rearmament 28
Mythical community 109

Napoleon 37–9
Natural
  authority 16
  will 16, 17

Neighbourhood 15, 204
  profile 100
Neuroses 260
New Labour 25, 27
New Left 29
New Right 29, 251
New science 25
Nietzsche 4
Normalization 237, 239, 242–5, 251–3, 255
Nuclear family 25, 28, 48
Nurse prescribing 133, 175, 230
Nursing process 78, 80, 84, 86, 87, 91, 216

Oedipus complex 25
Orem 75–92
Owenite movement 19

Paedophile 5
Paracelsus 190
Parenting deficit 26
Participation 63–7, 70, 71, 253
Pater patriae 297
Paternal authority 16
Paternalism 250, 253
Paternalistic 253
Patients' Charter 134, 144
Peanut Pete 279
Phoenix House 277
Plato 12, 22
Platt Report 108
Polis 12
Poor Law 136
Positivism 33, 36, 37, 42
Positivist 28, 38
Post-industrial 15, 28–30
Post-modernism 15, 28, 30
Postnatal depression 221, 222
Powerlessness 67
Practical syllogism 39, 40
Prescientific 37
Pressure-cook family 23
Psephology 12
Pseudo-gemeinschaft 17
Psycho-social 107, 126, 128, 262, 264, 299
Puritanism 26

Quakers 19, 136
Qualitative 171
Quantitative 171, 209

Ramazzini 190, 207
Rathbone, William 136
Rational will 16
Rave scene 272
Red Cross 145
Reflexivity 22
Reganism 14
Relocation 237
Reproducible 37
Retreatist theory 269
Risk-management 262
Risk-taking 268
Rites of passage 45
Ritual 11

Ritualization 86
Role, conjugal 20
Role-set 20
Rome 12

Sainsbury 12
Scarman Report 23
Schmaltze 23
Schutzian 55
Self 45, 95, 97
  awareness 18, 97, 218
  care 95–7, 100, 101, 167
  care agency 96
  care deficit 96
  organization 96
Serfdom 26
Set
  action 20
  categorical 20
  field 20
  role 20
Shabono 22
Shaker 26
Sioux 22, 60, 90
Sisters of Charity 135
Skill mix 54, 88, 138–40, 149, 154, 177, 219, 229
  reviews 149, 154
Smack in the Eye 279
Social
  action 45
  control 23
  hierarchy 45
  isolation 252
  networks 19
  order 42
  problems 12
  relations 44–7
  role valorization 237, 242, 245, 255
  value 44
Society
  capitalistic 15
  industrial 17
  me 26
Solidarity 18, 48
Status 45, 54, 159, 239, 263
  criminal 269
  health 64, 133, 164, 171, 213
  passage 50
Steinbeck 286
Stigma 20, 261, 274, 279
Structural-functionalism 49
Structuralism 51
Structuration 45
Sui generis 46
Supracommunity 27
Suss Law 23
Syllogism 39–41
Symbol 11, 45, 248
Symbolic 44, 48, 50, 55

Tallensi 44
Talmudic 16

Target Practice 121
Task-centred 86
Technology 17, 117, 128, 129, 133, 137, 206
 and child 125, 126
Teleological 36
Thatcherism 14
Therapeutic community 19
Therapeutic pessimism 278
Thessalonians 188
Tiw 22
Tokenistic model 64, 71
Tolerance 268
Transinstitutionalization 13
Trobriand Islands 41

Underclass 28, 300
Urban wilderness 22
User-led 251

Utilitarianism 136

Vandalism 12

Warlingham Park Hospital 258
West-room 45
Wigwam communities 25
Will
 good 17
 natural 16, 17
 rational 16, 17
Workaholics 268
Workhouse 136, 300

X-tabai spirit 14

Yanomamo 22

Zug 25